# Binocular Rivalry

# Binocular Rivalry

edited by
David Alais
and
Randolph Blake

A Bradford Book
The MIT Press
Cambridge, Massachusetts
London, England

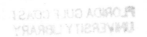

MIT Press books may be purchased at special quantity discounts for business or sales promotional use. For information, please email special_sales@mitpress.mit.edu or write to Special Sales Department, The MIT Press, 5 Cambridge Center, Cambridge, MA 02142.

This book was set in Palatino by Interactive Composition Corporation in QuarkXpress, and was printed and bound in the United States of America.

Library of Congress Cataloging-in-Publication Data

Binocular rivalry / edited by David Alais and Randolph Blake.
    p. cm.
   "A Bradford book."
   Includes bibliographical references and index.
   ISBN 0-262-01212-X (alk. paper)
    1. Binocular rivalry.  I. Alais, David.  II. Blake, Randolph.

QP487.5.B567 2005
152.14—dc22

2004042615

10  9  8  7  6  5  4  3  2  1

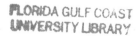

# Contents

Foreword by Robert Fox     vii

Preface     xvii

1   **Landmarks in the History of Binocular Rivalry**     1
*Randolph Blake*

2   **Ambiguities and Rivalries in the History of Binocular Vision**     29
*Nicholas J. Wade*

3   **The Nature and Depth of Binocular Rivalry Suppression**     47
*Alan W. Freeman, Vincent A. Nguyen, and David Alais*

4   **Investigations of the Neural Basis of Binocular Rivalry**     63
*Frank Tong*

5   **Parallel Pathways and Temporal Dynamics in Binocular Rivalry**     81
*Sheng He, Thomas Carlson, and Xiangchuan Chen*

6   **Human Development of Binocular Rivalry**     101
*Ilona Kovács and Michal Eisenberg*

7   **Surface Representation and Attention Modulation Mechanisms in Binocular Rivalry**     117
*Teng Leng Ooi and Zijiang J. He*

8   **Dynamics of Perceptual Bistability: Plaids and Binocular Rivalry Compared**     137
*Nava Rubin and Jean-Michel Hupé*

9   Interocular Grouping in Binocular Rivalry: Basic Attributes
    and Combinations                                              155
    *Thomas V. Papathomas, Ilona Kovács, and Tiffany Conway*

10  Binocular Rivalry and the Perception of Depth                 169
    *Ian P. Howard*

11  From Contour to Object-Face Rivalry: Multiple Neural
    Mechanisms Resolve Perceptual Ambiguity                       187
    *Timothy J. Andrews, Frank Sengpiel, and Colin Blakemore*

12  Responses of Single Neurons in the Human Brain During
    Flash Suppression                                             213
    *Gabriel Kreiman, Itzhak Fried, and Christof Koch*

13  Binocular Rivalry and the Illusion of Monocular Vision        231
    *David A. Leopold, Alexander Maier, Melanie Wilke,
    and Nikos K. Logothetis*

14  The Functional Role of Oscillatory Neuronal Synchronization
    for Perceptual Organization and Selection                     259
    *Pascal Fries, Miguel Castelo-Branco, Andreas K. Engel,
    and Wolf Singer*

15  Perceptual Rivalry as an Ultradian Oscillation                283
    *J. D. Pettigrew and O. L. Carter*

16  Binocular Rivalry in the Divided Brain                        301
    *Robert P. O'Shea and Paul M. Corballis*

17  Rivalry and Perceptual Oscillations: A Dynamical Synthesis    317
    *Hugh R. Wilson*

18  A Neural Network Model of Top-Down Rivalry                    337
    *D. P. Crewther, R. Jones, J. Munro, T. Price, S. Pulis,
    and S. Crewther*

    Contributors                                                  357
    Name Index                                                    361
    Subject Index                                                 369

# Foreword

I accepted with enthusiasm the invitation to provide some commentary on the work presented at the meeting organized by the editors of this volume. One reason is that publication of the proceedings denotes a significant milestone in the extended history of research on binocular rivalry. My interest intensified given the suggestion that I provide some historical context that would frame these contributions and complement the more comprehensive treatment by Blake given in chapter 1. Accordingly, I begin with a brief account of the conceptual themes and extant knowledge operative in the 1960s as I saw them. Then I note some extensions of those themes reflected in the current work. I close with some suggestions about the directions future inquiry may take.

As a dramatic phenomenon easy to demonstrate, the suppression of vision during rivalry invariably sparks intrinsic interest distinct from its intimate connection to stereopsis, fusion, and the related arcanum of binocular vision. My own interest arose not from any concern with binocular vision but, rather, from the role rivalry might play as a technique for investigating another issue in visual perception: the role of central processes within the organism in modulating the perception of incoming stimuli. The term *set* was widely employed to encompass research on such topics as attention, expectancy, and prior knowledge. Evidence that an anticipated or familiar stimulus could be processed more efficiently was abundant, yet it was not clear whether that efficiency was due directly to perceptual mechanisms or post-perceptual response systems. A special case of the set question concerned the role of stimulation that would induce affective states in the perceiver capable of modifying the perceptual process. The supporting evidence also implied that the triggering stimulus could be below the threshold of awareness, yet still influence subsequent processing. This controversial possibility—dubbed subliminal perception—was beset by methodological problems based, in part, on the definition of threshold. Moreover, it was difficult to envision a mechanism whereby a weak stimulus could, in effect, be smuggled into perceptual processing outside of awareness, yet then rise up and corrupt that processing.

Binocular rivalry, it seemed to me, could be an ideal phenomenon for evaluating the potency of subliminal perception. After all, rivalry effectively erases an otherwise easily perceived stimulus from awareness for durations on the order of seconds, thereby eliminating questions about the strength of the stimulus or its absence from awareness. Would it be possible to introduce during suppression a stimulus that induced an affective reaction—perhaps by making that stimulus the signal for a forthcoming electric shock? Even though the observer would report not seeing the stimulus, perhaps its unconscious registration would be revealed by autonomic responses. This kind of thinking led me to a survey of the literature on rivalry and to informal experiments that allowed me to observe rivalry's characteristics for myself. First, it was obvious that all kinds of stimuli engaged in rivalry, the key feature being stimulation of corresponding retinal areas by patterns incapable of being fused. Moreover, larger stimuli seemed to rival in a piecemeal random fashion, while smaller stimuli tended to be suppressed as complete units. Contrary to expectations based on some published accounts, I observed that rivalry was not invariably a clear-cut switch between dominance and suppression states analogous to the changes in reversible figures. Rather, there were mixed or transitory phases with both stimuli being visible. Like others before me, I found that increasing the intensity of the stimulus seen by one eye made that stimulus more visible over time. Similarly, motion of one eye's stimulus served to increase its total duration of visibility. Yet it was never possible for me to achieve complete suppression of a weaker stimulus, nor was I able to influence significantly the temporal course of rivalry by voluntary attention. This inability to suppress a given stimulus from awareness for an extended period of time thus put a crimp in my idea of exploiting suppression to completely erase an affectively charged stimulus from awareness.

This difficulty not withstanding, I was now convinced that rivalry represented a potentially useful tool for examining other questions in perception. For example, rivalry creates a significant dissociation between the total duration of physical stimulation and the total duration of phenomenal awareness, the two differing by 50% or even more under optimal conditions. It should be feasible, then, to identify visual phenomena whose magnitude or persistence vary with the duration of stimulation and learn whether those phenomena are comparable in strength when the duration of stimulation includes significant periods of time during which the stimulus is invisible owing to rivalry. My original formulation of this idea centered around the figural aftereffect, a key phenomenon in Kohler and Wallach's theory of visual cortical isomorphism, but it was years later before I got around to actually measuring aftereffects to suppressed inducing figures.

Another potentially useful application of rivalry was to index differences among individuals in terms of general organismic conditions. Already it was known that the rate of rivalry alternations could be modulated by drugs, with excitatory substances (e.g., amphetamines) increasing alternation rate and depressive substances (e.g., barbiturates) decreasing rate. Moreover, several published studies purported to show unique patterns of stimulus dominance dependent on specific personality types (e.g., scenes depicting violence being relatively more dominant in people psychometrically classified as more aggressive). Although I published studies on rivalry and individual differences myself, a nagging concern was the possible role of response bias especially when using large, complex rival figures prone to piecemeal dominance—a concern rendered more acute by the development of signal detection theory, which made the distinction between sensitivity and response bias explicit.

While fascinated with rivalry's potential applications, I became convinced that its utility would remain unrealized until we better understood the underlying mechanisms. Toward that end, I decided to employ a psychophysical "probe" technique to assess sensitivity during suppression phases, similar to work being pursued to measure threshold changes associated with Mach-band edges and with metacontrast masking. An attractive feature of using probe stimuli to assess sensitivity during suppression is the considerable control that could be maintained over the stimulus conditions and over the responses of the observer. Using the dominant phase as the control condition and the suppression phase as the independent variable or experimental condition meant that the peripheral conditions of stimulation remained identical. Therefore, changes in sensitivity must be attributed to a central inhibitory process linked to suppression. These kinds of considerations contributed to my decision to pursue an analysis of suppression for my dissertation and in later work.

My initial explorations of rivalry were clearly incomplete and rather naïve, being pursued in large part without the guidance and stimulation that the results of other investigators invariably provide. It is gratifying to see how our knowledge of rivalry has advanced over the years, as evidenced by the contents of the chapters in this volume. Yet at the same time, one can identify themes in this contemporary work that reflect prior conceptual developments. A significant factor in the emergence of interest in "set" was Hebb's seminal ideas about neural organization. He emphasized the importance of understanding central control processes as exemplified by the concepts of set and attention and encouraged the quest for identifying relevant physiological mechanisms. This is a theme embedded in several of the chapters in this volume, including those by Leopold and colleagues (chapter 13) and by Pettigrew and Carter (chapter 15). A similar focus on central mechanisms is seen in the appearance of models of attention. One of the most influential of these was the filter model, couched in information processing constructs developed by Broadbent. The model renewed focus on the rejection of suprathreshold nonattended stimuli and drew a useful distinction between early and later stages of processing where rejection might occur. Once again, one finds the fruits of these ideas in current theorizing about rivalry (see, for example, chapter 7 by Ooi and He and chapter 3 by Freeman and colleagues). Sharper focus on central mechanisms also came from the discovery by Julesz of global stereopsis generated by large sets of random elements. Initially, this work revived interest in binocular vision, but more generally it focused attention on the statistical information conveyed by sets of stimuli as distinct from the physical attributes of the constituent elements.

The theoretical issues and conceptual orientations that began in the 1960s have continued to develop, and their influence is reflected in the present chapters. Two shifts in orientation are most notable. One is the interdisciplinary character of the work, as demonstrated by the varied background of the investigators and the institutions with which they are affiliated. The insularity produced by discipline boundaries is no longer present. Second, the explosive increase in information about neural processes makes it possible for investigators to pursue relationships among several levels of analysis. And as many of the chapters demonstrate, they have taken full advantage of that freedom. Upon examining individual chapters, other more specific connections with prior work can be identified in terms of issues and in approaches to rivalry.

The somewhat neglected yet enduring topic of individual differences in rivalry is addressed directly in the chapter by Pettigrew and Carter (chapter 15). In contrast to prior studies on individual differences, which were largely atheoretical, these investigators start from a combination of clinical observations and neurophysical data to outline a theory that makes differences the critical variable. At the present state of development, it is not clear how well the theory can accommodate other characteristics of rivalry or the extent to which it is falsifiable. Nevertheless, one positive feature of any theory is to spark interest and inquiry.

Indeed, this effect is illustrated well by the chapter by O'Shea and Corballis (chapter 16). At the level of theory, they sought, perhaps in the spirit of strong inference, to provide a critical test of the idea that rivalry requires interaction between cortical hemispheres. The answer seems to be no, because they found normal rivalry in persons without interhemispheral connections. Apart from the theoretical implications of these results, the empirical contribution remains significant. It adds to the information about visual function from that small cadre of individuals with visual systems rendered unique by surgical separation of the callosal pathways.

Some attributes of the individual differences approach are reflected in chapter 6 by Kovács and Eisenberg, who obtained verbal reports of sequences of rivalry alternatives from children 4 to 7 years of age. They interpreted the results as suggesting developmental differences in maturation of the rivalry process; this may be the first study using this approach to rivalry in children with normal binocularity, as opposed to the extensive literature on orthoptics and visual training designed to promote binocular function. It is noteworthy in view of the substantial evidence indicating that other components of binocularity (e.g., stereopsis) and 3-D space perception (e.g., size constancy) become functional at much earlier stages of development.

The enduring interest in quantitative modeling implemented through simulations is represented in the contributions by Wilson (chapter 17) and by Crewther and colleagues (chapter 18). Wilson focuses on the network of inhibitory connections that would account for the temporal pattern of dominance and suppression, once rivalry begins, and in this formulation shows how the special form of "rivalry" based on rapid inter-eye stimulus exchange could be accommodated. In the former model, the process by which the conflict between stimuli induces rivalry is not addressed explicitly. That process, however, is incorporated into the network outlined by Crewther et al., which incorporates a stimulus classification scheme that compares the stimulus from each eye to determine whether the difference in stimuli warrants the initiations of suppression. The process itself is assigned to earlier stages in the system.

The psychophysical approach to rivalry, as described earlier, is exemplified in chapter 3 by Freeman, Nguyen, and Alais, who use probe stimuli to assess differences in threshold between dominance and suppression phases. Consistent with prior research, they found an elevation of threshold during suppression that operated nonselectively on attributes of the probe stimulus. In addition, the dominance/suppression threshold difference increased with increases in the complexity of the probe stimulus, a result the authors interpret as suggesting that suppression occurs at several successive stages of processing.

The systematic manipulation of stimulus dimensions intrinsic to psychophysical analyses was applied by Rubin and Hupé (chapter 8) to determine whether the temporal parameters of rivalry alternations would also be present in the bistable percept induced by a plaid motion stimulus. This stimulus, which can be composed of overlapping arrays of contours moving orthogonally, often produces a unified single direction. But after prolonged viewing, as the authors note, motion direction shifts to a bistable mode, alternating between unified and separate motion phases (typically referred to as "coherent" and "transparent" motion). Applying analogs of the stimulus strength manipulation used in rivalry, they found parallels in the pattern of bistable percepts, leading them to suggest that the reciprocal inhibitory models developed within rivalry might be profitably extended to account for bistable phenomena.

The connection between binocular rivalry and binocular vision in general is made explicit in chapter 2 by Wade, who outlines in his historical review some of the major issues that have defined research in the area. He notes that rivalry traditionally has been regarded as the default mode that becomes manifest when fusion and stereopsis cannot be achieved.

The relationship between rivalry and stereopsis is integral to chapter 10 by Howard, who examines the function of monocular occlusion in contributing to the formation of stable stereoscopic percepts. Although such occluding stimuli should, on a local retinal point-by-point scale, induce rivalry, they do not when embedded in the context of a normal binocular view. This underscores the point that the monocular stimulus arrays must be compared at high resolution by some binocular mechanism preparatory to commencement of the rivalry mode.

An interest in the stimulus conditions involved in both rivalry and binocular vision led Ooi and He (chapter 7) to focus on occlusion and the perception of surfaces as critical variables. They suggest that rivalry may be part of an inhibitory network whose more general function is the perception of stable binocular surfaces and objects. In this, attention may play a significant role.

The role of stimulus organization in influencing the pattern of rivalry alternations is the key issue examined in chapter 9 by Papathomas, Kovács, and Conway. They presented arrays of stimuli that could be grouped either by eye of origin or by stimulus attributes and requested observers to report on changes in dominance over time. The incidence of reports indicating attribute groupings was greater than expected by chance and was interpreted as suggesting the operation of stimulus grouping processes in rivalry.

Visual awareness is the central theme of chapter 4 by Tong, who equates the dominance and suppression phases of rivalry with the presence and absence of awareness. Because he regards cortical activation as indexed by fMRI as a measure of awareness, Tong suggests that studies showing a substantial reduction of activity in primary visual cortex during suppression imply that awareness is localized at that stage.

Motion and time are the dimensions focused upon by He, Carlson, and Chen (chapter 5), who review the literature from the perspective provided by the distinction between the M and P visual pathways. They conclude that stimuli presumed to engage the P pathway are more likely to be more active in rivalry and that this issue is closely related to the question of the variables that influence the duration or "switching time" of successive rivalry events.

Psychophysical analysis, by definition, can bear only inferentially on neural mechanisms, but in the research described by Kreiman, Fried, and Koch (chapter 17), inference is replaced by direct observation of single neuron responses in human observers making psychophysical reports of dominance and suppression produced by flash suppression. Although such suppression is a transient event, it resembles rivalry both at the phenomenal level and in terms of the magnitude of the effect of suppression on probe stimuli. The differences in neuron responses observed correlated well with phenomenal reports and, in general, are consistent with assumptions about neural coding.

Evidence from psychophysical, electrophysiological and brain imaging lines of inquiry relevant to rivalry and bistable stimuli are reviewed by Andrews, Sengpiel, and Blakemore in chapter 11. They conclude that rivalry and bistable perception must involve multiple mechanisms that will be selectively engaged as a function of specific conditions of stimulation.

Rivalry and bistable perception are also examined by Fries, Castelo-Branco, Engel, and Singer (chapter 14) within the context of their search for neural processes that can integrate and amplify perceptually relevant signals from distributed processing systems. Focusing on eye dominance in strabismic cats as indexed by multiple cortical recordings and on percepts induced by bistable plaid stimuli in humans, they marshal evidence and arguments that suggest synchronized neural activity may reflect the emergence of perceptual dominance in rivalry and bistability.

## CONCLUDING COMMENTS

Although each chapter makes its own unique contribution, together they demonstrate unequivocally that rivalry has moved into the mainstream of research on perception. No longer can it be dismissed as an artificial, optical curiosity limited to highly artificial conditions. The underlying reason is the relevance of rivalry to understanding two significant problems. One is the role of central cognitive processes in modifying perception. This, in a sense, is the older question about the effect of set. Now it arises with greater sophistication made possible by deeper knowledge of neural processes and is framed in terms of the concept of cognitive impenetrability. Here the issue is characterized as a conflict between early automatic processing of stimulus information and the modulating influences from higher-order processes linked to cognition.

Rivalry is the ideal phenomenon for investigating the issue because it has a foot in each camp. As a binocular process, the stimuli from both eyes reach awareness, hence potentially subject to all cognitive factors available for muster. Moreover, we know from stereopsis and fusion that a refined Vernier-like comparison process occurs in where differences measured in seconds of arc can be resolved. Finally, the conditions of rivalry would seem to provide the opportunity for a choice between competing stimulus representations. Yet, marshaled against these capacities are the attributes of suppression, which seem to operate in a much coarser automatic way. If one described spatial resolution of the binocular comparison level as akin to the precision of a scalpel, then meat axe would apply to suppression. More information about the way this paradox works would be of considerable interest. To that end, the time scale of rivalry (seconds) and its cyclic character facilitate the pursuit of relevant investigations. One other feature of the binocular comparison that should be noted, and which has not been emphasized in current research on rivalry, is that it can be regarded as a kind of stimulus categorization in terms of same versus different. The existence of fusion and rivalry implies the presence of a seemingly automatic process that measures stimuli in terms of their similarity. Rivalry occurs when stimuli are classed as dissimilar. Presumably, such a categorization is the product of well-established neural connections. Yet various sets of data imply the presence of considerable plasticity within the binocular system, as exemplified by phenomena such as variations in fusional amplitudes, ananomalous correspondence, and the results from visual training. It may be fruitful to examine rivalry from the perspective of current views on plasticity.

The second significant problem in perception to which rivalry has special relevance is the question of attention. Not only does everyone know what attention is, but most are aware of the concept of attention as a facilitory spotlight. For instance, in the inattentional blindness and change blindness paradigms, a stimulus is seen because it falls within the spotlight but otherwise goes unnoticed. Much less, however, is known about the fate of the unseen stimulus. It impinges on receptors with considerable energy and from the viewpoint of the stimulus there is every reason to believe that it, too, will achieve phenomenal status. At some point, or by some means, the upstream passage of the suprathreshold stimulus is thwarted, as if the spotlight has been turned off. There are parallels between the plight of the nonattended stimulus and the stimulus vanquished by suppression. Both, for example, are rendered vulnerable by their spatial location. It would seem reasonable to consider that the characteristics of suppression are not unique to rivalry. Rather, they might reveal the operation of a more general mechanism evolved to prevent nonattended stimuli from reaching awareness. On this view, suppression might be regarded as an involuntary turning off of the attentional spotlight, rather than the result of direct inhibition among competing stimulus elements.

These are some of the questions that might be examined in the future. The exciting thing is that this kind of inquiry can be pursued, because as the research described in this book makes clear, all the necessary elements, the people, the technology, and the interest are in place.

For bringing it all together, the editors merit our profound gratitude. As it stands, the book is a milestone. One hopes that it is only the first of a series that will summarize periodically the progress in the field.

—Robert Fox

# Preface

This book had its beginning several years ago in a discussion between the eventual editors concerning the recent arborescent growth in the field of binocular rivalry. Not only was the number of published papers increasing (approximately doubling each five years over the last fifteen-year period), but the range of experimental techniques was expanding. Among other things, this had led to new insights into the neurophysiological substrates of binocular rivalry, which in turn generated new theoretical speculation concerning the nature of rivalry and its relation to other forms of perceptual multistability. We concluded that the time was ripe for a book on binocular rivalry, to weave these threads together into a single reference volume with chapters authored by leading figures in the field. In considering potential contributors, we decided a more stimulating book would be produced if we could first bring the intended contributors together for a workshop, so that ideas contained in the potential chapters could be presented and discussed in an informal, lively environment.

With this goal in mind, we set about organizing such a meeting. The result was the San Miniato Workshop on Binocular Rivalry and Perceptual Ambiguity, held in Italy in June 2002 in the wonderful surrounds of a sixteenth-century former monastery. The three-day retreat into the Tuscan hills proved a fertile time. Nearly all the principal workers in binocular rivalry were present, and enthusiastic, vigorous discussion followed each presentation. Moreover, all participants then prepared written chapters built around their presentations, including amendments and new ideas that emerged during the course of the lively meeting. Those chapters were carefully edited by the two of us, the aim being to integrate common themes among chapters and to promote continuity of style. You the reader will judge the success of our endeavor.

As documented in the first two chapters, the phenomenon of binocular rivalry has been known for several centuries, and has been a part of experimental psychology for at least one hundred years. This book is by no means the first dedicated to binocular rivalry and related phenomena; however, it is the first for many years. The last two books dealing exclusively with binocular rivalry were Levelt's influential monograph published in 1968 and Leon Lack's dissertation published in book form in 1978. For most of the intervening years, binocular rivalry continued to be, as it had always been, the domain of experimental psychologists using psychophysical methods. This is no longer the case: the landscape changed dramatically with the neuroscience revolution of the 1980s. This era witnessed the emergence of new methods and techniques that offered novel ways to investigate the neural bases of rivalry and perceptual ambiguity. The neuroscience revolution ushered in a watershed period for the field of binocular rivalry, changing our knowledge base through techniques such as human brain imaging and multicell recordings in awake, behaving monkeys experiencing rivalry. This new approach had a large impact on the field, prompting a lot of good new science and a complete reevaluation of what constituted binocular rivalry. Now, a decade or so after these techniques were first used in rivalry, it is an opportune time to unite this body of knowledge in a single reference volume on binocular rivalry.

The eighteen chapters of this volume have been arranged in groups. Chapters 1 and 2 cover history, including the century of work in binocular rivalry since the pioneering monograph of Breese at the turn of the twentieth century. These chapters are well suited to the general reader and provide an ideal primer for the chapters that follow. Chapters 3 through 10 focus mainly on recent psychophysical investigations into binocular rivalry and other examples of ambiguous and bistable phenomena. Chapters 11 through 16 are all broadly concerned with the neurophysiology or neuroimaging of binocular rivalry and flash suppression, although several are complemented by psychophysical experiments. The book closes with two chapters that attempt to model the processes of binocular rivalry computationally, with one model based on nonlinear dynamics and the other a connectionist model whose dynamics arise from training.

Preceding the chapters is a foreword by Robert Fox, who was for several decades a key figure in the field of binocular rivalry beginning in the late 1960s. His foreword contains insights gleaned from his active participation in the field over the last thirty-five years and his knowledge of its evolution. The significance of his early studies in the United States is paralleled by the contemporaneous work of Willem Levelt in The Netherlands. Although Levelt left the field of binocular rivalry for a career in psycholinguistics soon after his monograph on rivalry appeared in 1968, his work continues to influence contemporary researchers. His monograph is cited in the majority of chapters in this book, and his insightful "second proposition" (see chapters 8 and 18) has remained influential long after he left the field.

Finally, a few words of thanks are due. No volume can appear on the library shelves without a lot of help. We gratefully acknowledge the generous financial contribution to the binocular rivalry workshop made by three Vanderbilt University centers: the John F. Kennedy Center for Research on Human Development, the Vanderbilt Vision Research Center, and the Vanderbilt Institute for Public Policy Studies. We are also grateful to La Cassa di Risparmio di San Miniato (Savings Bank of San Miniato) who administer the sixteenth-century monastery formerly of the Cappucino monks and offer it freely as a study center. Special thanks are also due to Corinne Mesana-Alais, whose multilingual talents enabled two Anglophone researchers to organize a conference in the hills of central Italy. Most important, we are deeply indebted to the participants of the workshop who so willingly engaged in enthusiastic debate and in doing so contributed greatly to the vitality of this book.

**REFERENCES**

Lack, L. C. (1978). *Selective Attention in the Control of Binocular Rivalry.* The Hague, The Netherlands: Mouton.

Levelt, W. J. M. (1968). *On Binocular Rivalry.* Soesterberg, The Netherlands: Institute for Perception.

# Binocular Rivalry

# 1 Landmarks in the History of Binocular Rivalry

## Randolph Blake

Why, in recent years, have so many perceptual psychologists, cognitive neuroscientists, neurophysiologists, philosophers, and the occasional Nobel laureate gotten excited about binocular rivalry? Why has the study of rivalry developed into a veritable industry occupying the time and resources of some of our best and brightest? It is true that many used to think that rivalry was fundamental to vision, occurring all of the time for all of us (Asher, 1953). But the weight of evidence now runs against this so-called suppression theory (O'Shea, 1987), at least the more radical version equating binocular single vision with wholesale monocular dominance (for a more refined version of suppression theory, see Wolfe, 1986). So, except for some individuals with eye misalignment, binocular rivalry is a laboratory artifact—the result of "optical trickery," as Gibson (1966) put it. Why, then, the upsurge of interest in the phenomenon?

These days a single answer to this question echoes throughout the vision literature: binocular rivalry provides a potentially powerful tool for learning about the neural concomitants of visual awareness or, as some have dubbed it, the "neural correlates of consciousness" (Crick and Koch, 1998). To illustrate rivalry's utility, consider the pair of dissimilar pictures shown in figure 1.1a (see also plate 1). Suppose the picture of the house is viewed by one eye and the picture of the face is viewed by the other eye. Even though these pictures are continuously imaged on the two retinas, we tend to see only one of the two at any given moment—the temporary "winner" dominates perception and the loser is vanquished, or suppressed, from conscious awareness.

Of course, victory by one image is only temporary, for sooner or later the suppressed image will achieve dominance and the previously dominant image will be erased from awareness; these alternations in perceptual dominance will continue for as long as the dissimilar images are viewed,

a

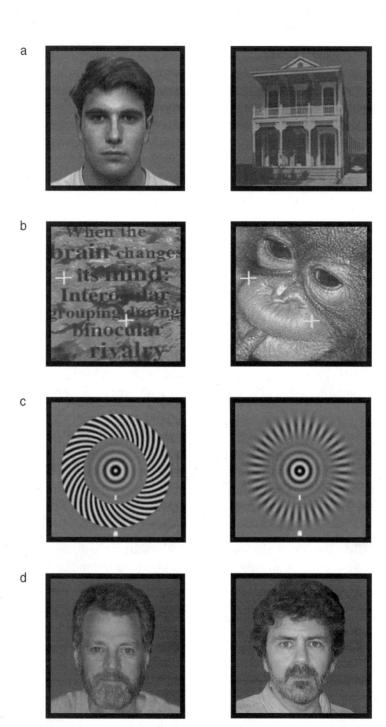

b

c

d

Randolph Blake

with the rate of alternations varying markedly among individuals (for more discussion of individual differences, see chapter 15 in this volume). Figures 1.1b–d show other examples of dichoptic half-images that produce vigorous rivalry; some of those rival figures are also shown as anaglyphs in color plate 1. Readers with access to red/green viewing glasses can experience rivalry without having to free-fuse the two rival pairs.

These fluctuations in perception during rivalry must surely result from fluctuations in neural activity associated with the two alternative perceptual outcomes. In principle, then, it should be possible to identify the nature and locus of those fluctuating neural events, thereby revealing something about the neural concomitants of visual awareness. The same line of reasoning can be applied to forms of perceptual ambiguity besides rivalry, including reversible figures such as Rubin's vase/face illusion (see chapter 11 in this volume) and bistable motion stimuli such as plaids (see chapter 8 in this volume). In these cases, too, unchanging visual stimulation triggers changing visual perception, again implicating fluctuating neural activity.

Thus this potential link between visual awareness and underlying neural events represents a chief reason for the recent, growing interest in binocular rivalry and other forms of perceptual ambiguity (Blake and Logothetis, 2002). In a related vein, there is a school of thought saying that rivalry in fact reveals a fundamental aspect of human cognition. According to this idea, human vision is routinely faced with weak, ambiguous sensory information that necessarily requires active interpretation guided by knowledge, experience, and intentions. According to this view, binocular rivalry represents a patent manifestation of this interpretative process (e.g., Leopold and Logothetis, 1999) and, for this reason, provides a promising means for isolating and studying brain areas involved in attention and selection. Chapters 7, 9, and 13 in this volume develop this notion in more detail.

◄ **Figure 1.1** Four examples of pairs of dissimilar images that, when viewed dichoptically, trigger binocular rivalry; some of these rival targets are also produced as anaglyphs in plate 1. (*a*) House/human face rival targets used by Frank Tong and colleagues to study brain activation during dominance and suppression phases of rivalry (work detailed in chapter 4). (*b*) Monkey/jungle scene targets used by Kovács et al. (1996) to examine spatial grouping in binocular rivalry (work described in chapter 9). (*c*) Concentric radial grating and spiral grating used by Wilson, Blake, and Lee (2001) to measure the spread of dominance at the time of rivalry transitions (work described in chapter 17). (*d*) Photographs of different individuals that, when viewed dichoptically, yield binocular rivalry despite similarities in global facial structure; in reality, the two individuals pictured here experience stable friendship, with their differences of view resolved harmoniously. See plate 1 for color version.

On the other hand, there is another school of thought that distinguishes between binocular rivalry and other forms of perceptual ambiguity, with rivalry attributed to reciprocal inhibition among neurons at relatively early stages of visual processing involved in stereoscopic vision (e.g., Blake, 1989). Evidence bearing on this alternative viewpoint appears in chapters 3, 4, and 16 of this volume.

This opening chapter sidesteps the controversies concerning the nature of binocular rivalry and, instead, provides an overview of the major characteristics of rivalry, characteristics that must be accommodated by any successful theoretical account of rivalry. Rather than simply catalog these characteristics of rivalry, as done elsewhere (Blake, 2001), this chapter presents them within a historical context that highlights some of the landmark discoveries about rivalry and acknowledges the individuals who made them.

## WHEATSTONE ON BINOCULAR RIVALRY

Among vision scientists, Sir Charles Wheatstone (figure 1.2a) is appropriately celebrated for his invention of the stereoscope, the optical device by which the two eyes can receive independent stimulation (technically called "dichoptic" stimulation). With the stereoscope (figure 1.2b), Wheatstone was able to show convincingly that two-dimensional, right- and left-eye views could harmoniously blend into a stable, three-dimensional impression of the visual world, and the geometry underlying this cooperative interaction formed the core of his famous paper (Wheatstone, 1838). Also that paper is the first systematic description of binocular rivalry, the vigorous, unremitting conflict in visual perception instigated when the left eye and the right eye receive radically different views. As Wade (1998) has documented, others had observed and commented on binocular rivalry before the nineteenth century.

But it is Wheatstone who deserves credit for bringing this fascinating outcome of dichoptic stimulation to the foreground of vision science. Indeed, the importance of his observations cannot be overemphasized, for without doubt they played a key role in stimulating the thinking of later giants in the field of vision, including Helmholtz (1925), William James (1891), and Sherrington (1906). Moreover, it was his invention of the stereoscope that facilitated the scientific exploration of binocular rivalry. In chapter 2 of this volume, Wade provides a colorful account of the controversy surrounding Wheatstone's simple, clever invention and the ensuing arguments over the novelty of his observations concerning stereopsis;

a

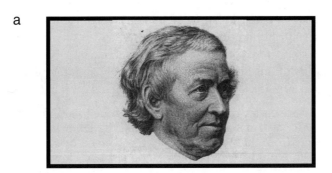

b

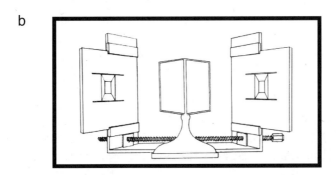

c

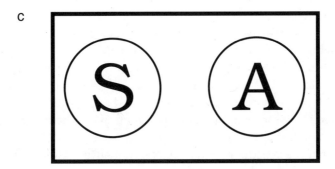

**Figure 1.2** (*a*) Drawing of Sir Charles Wheatstone, whose invention of the stereoscope brought the phenomenon of binocular rivalry to the attention of the scientific community. (*b*) Schematic of stereoscope invented by Wheatstone and used to observe rivalry. (*c*) Schematic of rival letter targets described by Wheatstone.

in the next few paragraphs of this chapter, I will concentrate on Wheatstone's seminal contributions to binocular rivalry.

In the span of two paragraphs in Wheatstone's 1838 paper, one finds succinct descriptions of three key features of binocular rivalry, made in reference to dichoptic viewing of the rival figures shown in figure 1.2c:

> If $a$ and $b$ are each presented at the same time to a different eye, the common border will remain constant, while the letter within it will change alternately from that which would be perceived by the right eye alone to that which would be perceived by the left eye alone. At the moment of change the letter which has just been seen breaks into fragments, while fragments of the letter which is about to appear mingle with them, and are immediately after replaced by the entire letter. It does not appear to be in the power of the will to determine the appearance of either of the letters, but the duration of the appearance seems to depend on causes which are under our control: thus if the two pictures be equally illuminated, the alternations appear in general of equal duration; but if one picture be more illuminated than the other, that which is less so will be perceived during a shorter time. (p. 386)

Here Wheatstone is commenting on the fragmentary appearance of rivalry during transitions in dominance as well as on the factors that can, and cannot, influence the pattern of predominance during rivalry. Concerning transitions in the rivalry state, it is typical for one small region of the suppressed figure to break through into dominance and spread wave-like throughout the rest of the region of rivalry. Ordinarily, it is impossible to anticipate exactly which portion of a previously suppressed figure will break through into dominance, but Wilson, Blake, and Lee (2001) devised unique rival targets (see figure 1.1c) along with a novel technique for triggering dominance waves at a given spatial location. This, in turn, made it possible to measure the propagation speed of the dominance waves. The results from those measurements, along with their implications, are described in chapter 17 of this volume. For our purposes it is sufficient to note that the speed and behavior of dominance waves point to a retinotopically organized visual area as the site of dominance wave propagation.

In commenting on rivalry transitions, Wheatstone noted that small patches of one figure ("fragments," as he called them) often appear intermingled with patches of the other figure—the resulting impression resembles a dynamic mosaic made up of bits and pieces of both figures. These states of mixed dominance are all the more likely when the rival figures are large in angular subtense (Meenes, 1930); other factors that influence the incidence of mixed dominance include retinal eccentricity (Blake, O'Shea, and Mueller, 1992), spatial frequency (Schor, 1977; Hollins, 1980;

Yang et al., 1992; O'Shea, Sims, and Govan, 1997), and the overall global context in which a rival target appears (e.g., Kovács et al., 1996; Alais and Blake, 1999). In chapter 6 of this volume, Kovács and Eisenberg document developmental trends in the incidence of mixed rivalry dominance and use these data to draw conclusions about changes in cortical connectivity during early childhood.

Turning to another of his seminal observations on rivalry, Wheatstone also observed an inability to use willpower to force dominance of one rival figure over the other—rivalry alternations, in other words, seem to occur spontaneously and unpredictably. Actually, opinions differ on the question of voluntary control of rivalry. Unlike Wheatstone, Helmholtz (1925) felt that he was able to hold one rival figure in dominance indefinitely:

I am able to concentrate my attention on either of the two systems [rival figures], whichever I choose, and to see it for a while exclusively, without seeing the other one at all. One way of doing it is by counting the lines in one system. (p. 498)

In keeping with his adversarial relationship with Helmholtz, Hering (1964) was skeptical of Helmholtz's claim. Hering conjectured that Helmholtz's "act of will" in fact was attributable to patterns of eye movements that favored one rival figure over the other. Evidence in favor of Hering's conjecture was subsequently reported by Breese (1899), who showed that intentional eye movements could indeed promote increased predominance of one figure over the other during rivalry. Is it possible that eye movements also play a role in triggering switches in dominance from one rival figure to the other? The answer here appears to be "no"— Peckham (1936) failed to find any correlation between fluctuations in dominance and the occurrence of eye movements, and decades later Blake, Fox, and McIntyre (1971) documented normal binocular rivalry alternations even when the rival targets were perfectly stabilized on the two retinas.

The most systematic assessment of the role of voluntary control in rivalry is provided by Lack (1978). In a series of carefully performed experiments, he convincingly showed that naïve observers could exert a degree of control over the rate of rivalry alternations, especially following relatively small amounts of practice. Moreover, Lack proved that rivalry control was not mediated by peripheral mechanisms such as changes in pupil size, accommodation, or blink rate; instead, he attributed rivalry control to a central "switching" mechanism of the sort proposed by Fox and Rasche (1969). It is noteworthy that none of Lack's observers developed an ability to completely arrest the alternations of rivalry, and on this point there seems to be consensus throughout the literature. It may well be that this inability to arrest rivalry alternations was what Wheatstone was talking about in his descriptions of willpower and binocular rivalry.

While "willpower" as exercised by Wheatstone proved ineffective in the control of rivalry, he did observe that significant control over rivalry *could* be exerted through manipulations of the relative "strengths" of the two rival figures. Specifically, a more weakly illuminated stimulus was perceived for a shorter time, according to Wheatstone. This aspect of rivalry—the relation of predominance and stimulus strength—is one of the most widely studied properties of the phenomenon. For an overview of what is known about this relation, we turn now to the seminal work by Breese (1899), a leading early figure in the study of binocular rivalry.

## B. B. BREESE

B. B. Breese (figure 1.3) completed a master's degree at Harvard under the supervision of William James and a Ph.D. at Columbia, where he was a student of James McKeen Cattell. His dissertation was on the general concept of inhibition, and this was the source of his interest in binocular rivalry. Published as a monograph in 1899, Breese's dissertation devoted many pages to discussion of what he termed "physiological" inhibition (e.g., the willful attenuation of an otherwise reflexive muscle contraction) and "psychological" inhibition (e.g., the squelching of one idea by another). With this as background, Breese turned to binocular rivalry ("inhibition of one sensation by another") as a paradigm case for studying the relation between physiological and psychological inhibition.

Using a prism stereoscope, Breese presented a red grating to one eye and a green grating to the other eye; the grating lines were oriented counterclockwise for one eye and clockwise for the other. With this basic configuration Breese was able to identify a number of conditions that influenced the dominance durations for the two rival figures. As already noted, observers could influence dominance durations simply through "willpower," but in every case Breese found that the effect of "willpower" was unwittingly accomplished by eye movements.

By having people press keys to track successive dominance periods for the two rival figures, Breese was able to quantitatively assess the effect of "strength" on rivalry predominance (defined as the percentage of total observation time that a given rival figure was dominant). Initially, he observed that, all things being equal, each rival figure was dominant

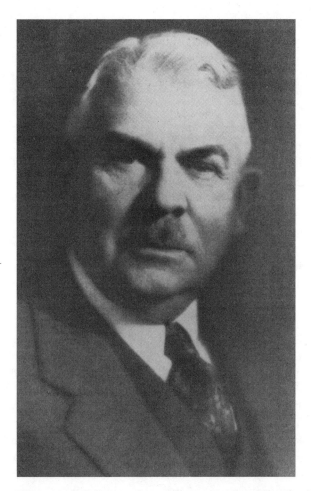

**Figure 1.3**   B. B. Breese, whose early monograph on binocular rivalry described several key features of the phenomenon. (Courtesy of Robert Frank, University of Cincinnati.)

approximately 50% of the time. He also documented that increasing the luminance intensity of both figures by an equal amount led to a four-fold increase in the rate of alternations while, at the same time, maintaining the relative parity in predominance between the two figures. In a similar vein, bilateral increases in the distinctness of the lines of the gratings increased the alternation rate without affecting relative predominance. This in itself is a remarkable set of observations, for it reveals that the process responsible for selection (i.e., predominance) is distinct from the process responsible for alternations.

When some property of one of the rival targets was varied, Breese observed changes in predominance. Specifically, unilateral fourfold decrease in luminance intensity reduced the predominance of the dimmer figure, giving its brighter competitor almost a 2:1 advantage in total dominance time. Although Breese did not comment at length on it, this decrease in predominance came about largely through an increase in the average duration of suppression of the weaker stimulus (compare tables XV and XVII in Breese, 1899).

Breese also found that the predominance of one rival figure was markedly enhanced when the contours in that figure moved. (His simple but clever method for introducing unilateral motion was to attach one stimulus card to a pendulum that swung the card back and forth behind an aperture.) Remarkably, the moving contours were visible almost continuously, with the orthogonal, stationary contours appearing and disappearing just as they did when pitted against a stationary competitor (when visible, the stationary contours appeared superimposed on the moving ones). The salience of motion during binocular rivalry has since been well documented by others (e.g., Grindley and Townsend, 1965; Blake, Yu, et al., 1998).

Breese made two other intriguing observations that warrant mention. In one experiment, he had observers tense the arm and leg on one side of the body while tracking alternations in rivalry between figures of equal strength. He found no systematic influence of muscle contraction on predominance and concluded that activation of the motor centers had no influence on activation of the visual centers. This is perhaps not so surprising, for Breese's observers relied on central fixation of the rival figures, guaranteeing that "visual centers" in both hemispheres would be engaged during rivalry.

Breese's second remarkable observation concerned the perceptual consequence of presenting the two rival figures—the red grating and the green grating—to a single eye (which was optically accomplished by using a prism). Under these conditions, Breese observed what he termed "monocular rivalry":

. . . a rivalry of the colors was perceptible. Neither disappeared entirely: but at times the red would appear very distinctly while the green would fade; then the red would fade and the green appear distinctly. The two sets of lines showed the same fluctuation, keeping pace with the changing of the intensities of the colors. Sometimes one of them would disappear altogether. This rivalry of the colors and of the lines was much slower than the rivalry in binocular vision. (p. 43)

This intriguing observation seems to have gotten lost in the mists of time for decades, but the phenomenon of monocular rivalry was rediscovered and nicely documented in the mid-1970s by Fergus Campbell and colleagues (Campbell and Howell, 1972; Campbell et al., 1973; Atkinson et al., 1973; Rauschecker, Campbell, and Atkinson, 1973); readers may be able experience monocular rivalry by viewing the overlapping red/green radial and spiral gratings in color plate 1. Whether monocular rivalry and binocular rivalry have a common neural foundation remains debatable.

Following publication of Breese's monograph, interest in binocular rivalry waned during the first half of the twentieth century. According to Lack's (1978) tally, only a handful of papers on rivalry appeared between 1909 and 1950. This lack of interest in rivalry was undoubtedly a consequence of psychology's infatuation with behaviorism and its accompanying disdain for all things mental—one sees a parallel trend in papers dealing with attention. In the case of rivalry, it was not until the middle of the twentieth century that interest in the phenomenon reemerged, although even then many publications on rivalry simply exploited the phenomenon as a tool for studying individual differences (e.g., Bagby, 1957), sex differences (Kaufer and Riess, 1960), and various kinds of "top-down" influences on perception (e.g., Bokander, 1966). However, studies aimed at learning about binocular rivalry itself did begin to appear (e.g., Wallach and Adams, 1954; Kakizaki, 1960), and some of those studies sought to place rivalry within the broader context of binocular fusion and stereopsis (Treisman, 1962; Hochberg, 1964; Ogle and Wakefield, 1967; Kaufman, 1963).

All of these studies certainly contributed to a renewed interest in the phenomenon of rivalry. In my view, however, rivalry's reappearance on the perception landscape was most forcefully promoted by work coming out of three doctoral dissertations completed within two years: one in the United States (Fox, 1963), one in England (Whittle, 1963), and one in the Netherlands (Levelt, 1965). The following sections provide an overview of the characteristics of rivalry which were illuminated by those three influential bodies of work and by the studies they spawned.

## ROBERT FOX AND THE SUPPRESSION EFFECT

During the 1940s there emerged a school of thought called "new look" psychology whose central theme was the role of motivational variables in perception. This research tradition generated experimental evidence that perception is shaped by an individual's needs, both physiological (e.g., hunger) and psychological (e.g., achievement), as well as by the individual's impulses and anxieties (Dember, 1965). Among the phenomena studied by "new look" students was perceptual defense, operationally defined as decreased perceptual awareness of words or pictures with negative connotations for the perceiver (Postman, Bruner, and McGinnies, 1948; Erdelyi, 1974). But how can one selectively avoid perception of a threatening stimulus without first perceiving what that stimulus is (Howie, 1952)? This seeming paradox was resolved by positing multiple stages of processing, with inputs reaching consciousness only after elaborate perceptual processing (Erdelyi, 1974). And given this perspective, the challenge was to develop psychophysical strategies for interrupting the processing of stimulus information at intermediate stages prior to the emergence of awareness.

It was toward that end that Robert Fox (figure 1.4) began his investigations of binocular rivalry suppression. Working at the University of Cincinnati (where, incidentally, B. B. Breese was chair of the Psychology Department for decades), Fox wanted to find a way of studying rivalry

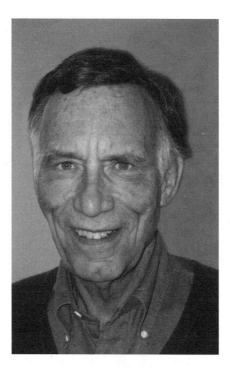

**Figure 1.4**   Recent photograph of Robert Fox, who developed and refined several important psychophysical strategies for studying binocular rivalry suppression.

that went beyond phenomenological report and its attendant susceptibility to response bias. It was in this spirit that he developed and refined the test-probe procedure, whereby visual sensitivity is assessed by briefly presenting "probe" targets to an eye during dominance and suppression phases of rivalry.

In a series of experiments beginning with his dissertation and continuing for several decades thereafter, Fox and his students documented that visual sensitivity during dominance phases is equivalent to that measured during ordinary monocular viewing, whereas visual sensitivity is depressed during suppression phases. Thus, for example, when presented during suppression phases, brief spots of light are more difficult to detect (Wales and Fox, 1970), letter forms are harder to identify (Fox and Check, 1972), and the onset of visual motion produces abnormally long reaction times (Fox and Check, 1968).

This pattern of results led Fox to characterize rivalry suppression as "nonselective," meaning that the inhibitory events underlying suppression are not specially tailored to the configuration of the rival figure; instead, those inhibitory events act more generally, or nonselectively, on all information presented within the boundaries of a suppressed stimulus. At least in Fox's mind, this property of rivalry undermined its utility as a means for introducing emotionally charged words or pictures outside of awareness—the putative inhibitory events underlying suppression were affecting all information introduced within the boundaries of the suppressed figure, making it impossible for semantic information to survive and influence perceptual judgments.[1]

In subsequent studies carried out in collaboration with Fox and others, I used a variant of the test-probe procedure to show that normally conspicuous changes in a rival figure can go undetected for several seconds when those changes are introduced during suppression. Thus, observers fail to see large changes in the spatial frequency or the orientation of a suppressed grating (Blake and Fox, 1974a); observers do not notice variations in the coherence of kinematic events (Blake, Yu, et al., 1998); and observers are "blind" to changes in the emotional expressions of human faces (Kim, Grossman, and Blake, 2002).

In fact, suppression is sufficiently broad in scope that when the dominant and suppressed stimuli are exchanged between the eyes, suppression immediately affects the previously dominant stimulus (Blake, Westendorf, and Overton, 1980). These findings, besides reaffirming the nonselectivity of suppression, were interpreted to imply a relatively "early" locus for the neural site of suppression, with "early" meaning processing stages where a wide range of visual features are compactly represented within retinotopic coordinates.

The nonselective nature of rivalry, together with evidence implying that it is an eye—not a stimulus—that is suppressed during rivalry (Blake, Westendorf, and Overton, 1980), led me to develop a neural model of rivalry based on reciprocal inhibition among orientation selective neurons varying in their ocular dominance (Blake, 1989). This model was certainly not the first to envision this kind of underlying circuitry; seeds of this idea can be identified in the writings of others (Wade, 1974; Grossberg, 1987; Sugie, 1982). The model did, however, make some rather specific predictions that stimulated subsequent work on rivalry, both psychophysical (Logothetis, Leopold, and Sheinberg, 1996) and physiological (Leopold and Logothetis, 1996; Tong and Engel, 2001). Chapters 3, 4, 9, 11, and 17 in this volume summarize some of the evidence—positive and negative— bearing on the model.

While suppression's effect is quite broad, encompassing all manner of stimulation presented within the suppressed region of an eye, suppression is at the same time quite fragile (i.e., easily perturbed). It is well known that a suppressed stimulus can be restored to dominance by abruptly increasing the contrast of that stimulus (e.g., Wilson, Blake, and Lee, 2001) or by suddenly moving the stimulus (e.g., Walker and Powell, 1979). For that matter, simply flicking a finger in front of a suppressed rival figure can trigger that figure's return to dominance (a maneuver responsible for the "Cheshire cat" illusion popularized by the San Francisco Exploratorium).

In general, suppression is highly susceptible to these kinds of transient events, and for that reason we have always been careful in our experiments to employ "ramped" contrast variations when introducing changes to a suppressed stimulus. Because of suppression's vulnerability to transients, the measured loss in visual sensitivity to briefly flashed test probes presented during suppression is only a fraction of a log-unit in magnitude. This modest loss in sensitivity could be construed to imply that the underlying inhibitory events are more subtle than one might imagine based on the wholesale invisibility of a normally salient, easily perceived stimulus (see chapter 3 in this volume).

Given suppression's nonselective breadth, does a suppressed stimulus retain any of its normal effectiveness? Scattered evidence bearing on this question existed prior to Fox's documentation of nonselective suppression. Thus, for example, Treisman (1962) reported that the positional information associated with a suppressed contour could nonetheless contribute to stereopsis. However, the most systematic work on the residual effectiveness of a suppressed stimulus was launched in Robert Fox's laboratory at Vanderbilt University. Blake and Fox (1974b) showed that several of the aftereffects associated with grating adaptation could be generated even though the adapting pattern was suppressed from vision for a substantial portion of the adapting period. Similarly, Lehmkuhle and Fox (1975) found that the translational motion aftereffect could be generated by motion signals rendered invisible by suppression.

Exploiting this approach in the study of suppression, a number of investigators have since assessed suppression's effect on the buildup of other visual aftereffects, including the tilt aftereffect (Wade and Wenderoth, 1978), the McCollough effect (White et al., 1978), the spiral motion aftereffect (Wiesenfelder and Blake, 1990), the phase-specific aftereffect (Blake and Bravo, 1985), and the plaid motion aftereffect (Van der Zwan, Wenderoth, and Alais, 1993). Summaries of the outcomes of those studies can be found elsewhere (Blake, 1995; Logothetis, 1998; Blake and Logothetis, 2002). Suffice it to say that suppression has no effect on the generation of "low-level" visual aftereffects but retards the buildup of "higher-level" aftereffects.

## PAUL WHITTLE AND GLOBAL DOMINANCE

At the same time that Fox was completing his dissertation in the United States, Paul Whittle (figure 1.5) was working at Cambridge University on an extensive series of dissertation experiments examining temporal and spatial characteristics of binocular rivalry. Some of his experiments extended Breese's earlier observations on the effect of size and blur on rivalry predominance, and other studies examined the possible role of eye movements in rivalry and the relation of rivalry alternation rate to stereoscopic acuity; some of that work was subsequently published (Whittle, 1965).

The most novel contribution of Whittle's dissertation, and the one with greatest impact, concerned his documentation of the role of figural grouping in rivalry. In these experiments, published subsequently as a journal article (Whittle, Bloor, and Pocock, 1968), Whittle sought to learn why a single, large rival target was seen in its entirety for much of the viewing period (up to 80% of the time), whereas two small, nearby rival targets seemed to rival independently of one another. Whittle reckoned that synergistic interactions among similar features forming a single "object" might promote synchronous dominance in rivalry of those features, and he set out to test this conjecture in a series of experiments.

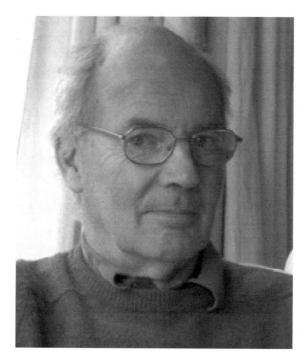

**Figure 1.5** Recent photograph of Paul Whittle, whose dissertation work highlighted the contribution of figural organization to rivalry dominance.

Whittle had observers press buttons to indicate when multifeature rival targets assumed a given state of dominance (an outcome Whittle called synchronous rivalry). He found that spatial proximity on its own was insufficient to promote synchronous rivalry of two targets—such targets were simultaneously dominant no more frequently than chance alone would dictate *when* those targets appeared to comprise separate objects. In contrast, the incidence of synchronous rivalry was greater than that expected on the basis of chance when local rival targets were arranged in a configuration suggesting the presence of an extended contour.

This, to Whittle's mind, explained why all the component parts of a large rival target could be dominant at the same time. To quote from his dissertation: "If part of a rivaling figure is visible, the rest may have a tendency to become so. This would make a patchy mixture of two figures an unstable state which would tend towards the temporary equilibrium of complete dominance of one or the other stimulus" (Whittle, 1963, p. 26). Incidentally, Whittle pointed out that these results argue against a crucial role of eye movements in rivalry, for eye movements would affect stimulus features throughout the visual field of a given eye, not just spatially adjacent, collinear features. Instead, Whittle believed that rivalry occurs within local zones throughout the visual field, with the states of these zones being independent except when local contours in adjacent zones form a single "compound object."

Thus, Whittle deserves credit for underscoring the role of figural processes in binocular rivalry.[2] In recent years, his seminal observations have been refined and extended by several research groups. In one widely cited paper, Kovács and colleagues (1996) devised "composite" rival targets consisting of bits and pieces of two complex images distributed between the two eyes in a complementary arrangement. With practice, observers can experience periods during which one image or the other is visible in its entirety (requiring interocular grouping), and these periods of complete dominance are greater than one would predict based on chance alone (see chapter 9 in this volume for further discussion of interocular grouping).

Alais and Blake (1999) showed that contour collinearity is a major factor in the production of global, figural grouping during rivalry, and Sobel and Blake (2002) discovered that global motion coherence influences dominance in the case of motion rivalry. In general, results from these and other studies (e.g., Dörrenhaus, 1975; Rogers, Rogers, and Tootle, 1977; Logothetis, 1998; Mapperson and Lovegrove, 1991) show that the pattern of global rivalry dominance depends, in part, on the structural regularity of spatially distributed rival features, even when those features are distributed between the two eyes (thereby requiring interocular grouping). This grouping propensity no doubt does play a role in promoting complete dominance of large rival figures, just as Whittle thought.

## LEVELT ON PREDOMINANCE

The last of the three landmark dissertations on rivalry was completed in 1965 by W. J. M. Levelt (figure 1.6), working at Leiden University in the Netherlands. Published in monograph form, Levelt's dissertation is still widely cited. From the outset it is worth noting that Levelt was an unabashed advocate of the view that rivalry occurs at an "early" stage in visual processing; reading his dissertation, it is clear that his thinking was influenced by the very recent physiological experiments by Hubel and Wiesel (1962) documenting the existence of cortical cells varying in their ocular dominance and demonstrating the importance of contours in evoking responses from those neurons.

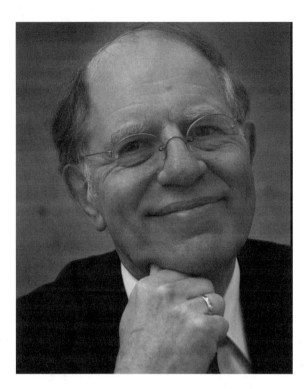

**Figure 1.6**  Recent photograph of W. J. M. Levelt, whose dissertation on binocular rivalry documented the statistical properties of rivalry alternations and the effects of stimulus "strength" on those properties. (Photograph by Erik van 't Hullenaar.)

Following several introductory chapters that provide a thorough review of extant literature on binocular rivalry is a set of chapters devoted to the determinants of binocular brightness averaging ("Fechner's paradox," as it is known) and binocular contour rivalry. For our purposes, we may focus on several significant discoveries concerning the dynamics of rivalry.

First, Levelt deserves credit for documenting the stochastic properties of successive rivalry durations. He was the first to show that individual durations of dominance phases of rivalry together comprised a gamma distribution. Noting that the best gamma fit was obtained when the parameter $\lambda$ equaled 5, Levelt interpreted this parameter as indexing the number of implicit events ("excitation spikes," as he called them) necessary for triggering a transition from suppression to dominance. He further speculated that the timing of these implicit events might be related to "flicks" in eye movements leading to a switch in dominance, but subsequent experiments showed that the optimal λ value remained 5 even when eye movements were eliminated as causal agents in rivalry alternations (Blake, Fox, and McIntyre, 1971).

Inspired by Levelt's characterization of rivalry as a stochastic process, subsequent investigations have looked in more detail at the statistical properties of dominance distributions, using various tests all of which confirm that (1) successive durations are statistically independent (Fox and Herrmann, 1967) and (2) rivalry durations do not behave as if driven by deterministic, chaotic attractors (Lehky, 1995). There are weak, second-order effects showing a trend toward longer dominance durations over the course of an extended viewing period, but these effects are probably attributable to contrast adaptation and not some property intrinsic to the alternation process itself (Lehky, 1995; Blake, Westendorf, and Fox, 1990).

The gamma distribution, first established by Levelt, has become the hallmark signature validating indirect measures of binocular rivalry in humans (Fox, Todd, and Bettinger, 1975) and in animals (e.g., Myerson, Miezin, and Allman, 1981). Moreover, there is evidence that the gamma distribution generalizes to perceptual state durations associated with bistable motion associated with viewing plaid patterns (see chapter 8 in this volume), as well as with other forms of perceptual bistability (De Marco et al., 1977; but see Strüber and Stadler, 1999).

Important as the discovery of the gamma distribution may be, Levelt's most revealing discovery concerned the lawful behavior of dominance and suppression durations with variations in the relative strengths of the rival figures. To embody these effects in a single variable, he developed the concept of "stimulus strength" and related it to "the amount of contour per area" and, for a constant amount, with the "strength of those contours" (1965, p. 74). He was able to scale stimulus strength based on measurements performed in a brightness averaging paradigm, wherein a given eye's contribution to the binocular impression of brightness was dependent on the contour density and luminance of the stimulus viewed by that eye. With "strength" gauged in this manner, Levelt was able to formulate four propositions concerning the dynamics of rivalry:

1. Increasing the stimulus strength in one eye will increase the predominance of the stimulus.

2. Increasing the stimulus strength in one eye will not affect the average duration of dominance of that eye.

3. Increasing the stimulus strength in one eye will increase the rivalry alternation rate.

4. Increasing the stimulus strength in both eyes will increase the alternation rate.

Propositions 1, 3, and 4 make intuitive sense, and at the time of Levelt's work there was ample evidence to confirm those outcomes (e.g., recall the results of Breese, 1899). But proposition 2 is counterintuitive, as Levelt himself acknowledged, for it implies that varying the strength of a stimulus has no effect on the dominance durations of that stimulus but, instead, affects the dominance durations for the contralateral stimulus. At that time, there were no data bearing on this second proposition (although tables XV and XVII in Breese, 1899, provide hints), so Levelt performed three experiments in which "strength" was manipulated unilaterally by varying blur, contrast, and average luminance.

As expected, all three manipulations produced variations in predominance, with the "stronger" stimulus being visible for a greater percentage of the overall viewing period. And, consistent with proposition 2, the average dominance durations were unaffected by changes in stimulus strength. Subsequent studies have replicated this finding (e.g., Fox and Rasche, 1969), although the independence of strength and dominance durations may break down when the disparity between monocular strength values is extreme (Mueller and Blake, 1989).

The importance of the dynamical property implied by proposition 2 cannot be overstated. For one thing, it implies that variations in predominance with stimulus strength arise from variations in the durations of suppression of a stimulus: on average, a weaker stimulus remains suppressed for a longer period of time. For that reason, varying the strength of a stimulus while it is suppressed will influence the duration of that suppression phase (Blake and Fox, 1974a), which may help us understand why transients are potent disrupters of suppression. Proposition 2 also implies that dominance and suppression are not necessarily two sides of the same coin—indeed, we now know that stimulus factors influencing suppression durations differ from those factors influencing dominance durations (Sobel and Blake, 2002).

This fact, in turn, may go some way toward reconciling seemingly conflicting views concerning the neural bases of binocular rivalry: to the extent that rivalry involves multiple processes, some governing dominance and others governing suppression, we may find that the neural events underlying those processes are distributed among visual areas within the brain (Blake and Logothetis, 2002). Finally, Levelt's proposition 2 may generalize beyond rivalry alternations, as Rubin and Hupé discuss in chapter 8 of this volume.

Levelt, along with Whittle (1963), also deserves credit for highlighting the distinction between rivalry suppression (the temporary invisibility of one monocular stimulus owing to the presence of a dissimilar stimulus imaged on the corresponding region of the other eye) and Troxler's effect (the spontaneous fading from visibility of a continuously viewed stimulus, independent of the stimulation received by the other eye). In recognition of this distinction, rivalry experiments subsequent to Levelt and Whittle's work have taken care to use stimulus conditions that preclude Troxler's effect (e.g., foveal viewing and/or flickering rival targets) or have explicitly measured the incidence of Troxler's effect and used those measures to "correct" rivalry predominance data.

## BINOCULAR RIVALRY TODAY

The historical overview provided here is by no means exhaustive—many papers on binocular rivalry not mentioned here were published during the second half of the twentieth century. To get an idea of the volume of this work, interested readers are directed to Robert O'Shea's up-to-date reference list accessible at http://psy.otago.ac.nz/r_oshea/br_bibliography.html. Moreover, much of the most revealing, provocative research on binocular rivalry has appeared since about 1990, including research on possible neurophysiological concomitants of binocular rivalry. In addition, alternative theoretical views about rivalry have been advanced recently (Logothetis, Leopold, and Sheinberg, 1996; Andrews and Purves, 1997; Lee and Blake, 1999; Pettigrew, 2001), and these theoretical accounts have sharpened the focus of recent empirical work on rivalry. Indeed, a major purpose of the following chapters is to document these exciting, recent developments, both empirical and theoretical. This chapter is intended to set the stage for what appears in the following pages and to provide the reader with a deeper appreciation of the intellectual roots of contemporary work on binocular rivalry and bistable perception.

## ACKNOWLEDGMENTS

My work on binocular rivalry is supported by a grant from the National Institutes of Health (EY13358). I am very grateful to Robert Fox for helpful discussion about some of the issues in this chapter. David Bloom provided important assistance in proofreading and coordinating references.

## NOTES

1. Experiments carried out years later confirmed that semantic information—whether linguistic or pictorial—is indeed neutralized during suppression phases of rivalry (Zimba and Blake, 1983; Blake, 1988; Cave, Blake, and McNamara, 1998).

2. The importance of perceptual grouping in rivalry, a major theme in Whittle's work, was presaged by Diaz-Caneja (1928), a little-known paper introduced to the English-speaking scientific community by Alais et al. (2000).

## REFERENCES

Alais, D., and Blake, R. (1999). Grouping visual features during binocular rivalry. *Vision Research*, 39, 4341–4353.

Alais, D., O'Shea, R. P., Mesana-Alais, C., and Wilson, I. G. (2000). On binocular alternation. *Perception*, 29, 1437–1445.

Andrews, T. J., and Purves, D. (1997). Similarities in normal and binocularly rivalrous viewing. *Proceedings of the National Academy of Sciences of the United States of America*, 94, 9905–9908.

Asher, H. (1953). Suppression theory of binocular vision. *British Journal of Ophthalmology*, 37, 37–49.

Atkinson, J., Campbell, F. W., Fiorentini, A., and Maffei, L. (1973). The dependence of monocular rivalry on spatial frequency. *Perception*, 2, 127–133.

Bagby, J. W. (1957). A cross-cultural study of perceptual predominance in binocular rivalry. *Journal of Abnormal and Social Psychology*, 54, 331–334.

Blake, R. (1988). Dichoptic reading: The role of meaning in binocular rivalry. *Perception and Psychophysics*, 44, 133–141.

Blake, R. (1989). A neural theory of binocular rivalry. *Psychological Review*, 96, 145–167.

Blake, R. (1995). Psychoanatomical strategies for studying human vision. In *Early Vision and Beyond*, T. Papathomas, C. Chubb, E. Kowler, and A. Gorea eds., 17–25. Cambridge, Mass.: MIT Press.

Blake, R. (2001). A primer on binocular rivalry, including current controversies. *Brain and Mind*, 2, 5–38.

Blake, R., and Bravo, M. (1985). Binocular rivalry suppression interferes with phase adaptation. *Perception and Psychophysics*, 38, 277–280.

Blake, R., and Fox, R. (1974a). Binocular rivalry suppression: Insensitive to spatial frequency and orientation change. *Vision Research*, 14, 687–692.

Blake, R., and Fox, R. (1974b). Adaptation to invisible gratings and the site of binocular rivalry suppression. *Nature*, 249, 488–490.

Blake, R., Fox, R., and McIntyre, C. (1971). Stochastic properties of stabilized-image binocular rivalry alternations. *Journal of Experimental Psychology*, 88, 327–332.

Blake, R., and Logothetis, N. K. (2002). Visual competition. *Nature Reviews: Neuroscience*, 3, 13–21.

Blake, R., O'Shea, R. P., and Mueller, T. J. (1992). Spatial zones of binocular rivalry in central and peripheral vision. *Visual Neuroscience*, 8, 469–478.

Blake, R., Westendorf, D., and Fox, R. (1990). Temporal perturbations of binocular rivalry? *Perception and Psychophysics*, 48, 593–602.

Blake, R., Westendorf, D. J., and Overton, R. (1980). What is suppressed during binocular rivalry? *Perception*, 9, 223–231.

Blake, R., Yu, K., Lokey, M., and Norman, H. (1998). Binocular rivalry and motion perception. *Journal of Cognitive Neuroscience*, 10, 46–60.

Bokander, I. (1966). The importance of collative-affective and intensive arousal potential in stereoscopically induced perceptual conflict. *Scandinavian Journal of Psychology, 7*, 234–238.

Breese, B. B. (1899). On inhibition. *Psychological Monographs*, 3, 1–65.

Campbell, F. W., Gilinsky, A. S., Howell, E. R., Riggs, L. A., and Atkinson, J. (1973). The dependence of monocular rivalry on orientation. *Perception*, 2, 123–125.

Campbell, F. W., and Howell, E. R. (1972). Monocular alternation: A method for the investigation of pattern vision. *Journal of Physiology*, 225, 19–21P.

Cave, C., Blake, R., and McNamara, T. (1998). Binocular rivalry disrupts visual priming. *Psychological Science*, 9, 299–302.

Crick, F., and Koch, C. (1998). Consciousness and neuroscience. *Cerebral Cortex*, 8, 97–107.

De Marco, A., Penengo, P., Trabucco, A., Borsellino, A., Carlini, F., Riani, M., and Tuccio, T. (1977). Stochastic models and fluctuations in reversal time of ambiguous figures. *Perception*, 6, 645–656.

Dember, W. N. (1965). *The Psychology of Perception*. New York: Holt, Rinehart and Winston.

Diaz-Caneja, E. (1928). Sur l'alternance binoculaire. *Annales d'Oculistique*, 165, 721–731.

Dörrenhaus, W. (1975). Musterspezifischer visueller wettstreit. *Naturwissenschaften*, 62, 578–579.

Erdelyi, M. H. (1974). A new look at the new look: Perceptual defense and vigilance. *Psychological Review*, 81, 1–25.

Fox, R. (1963). An analysis of the suppression mechanism in binocular rivalry. Ph.D. dissertation, University of Cincinnati.

Fox, R., and Check, R. (1968). Detection of motion during binocular rivalry suppression. *Journal of Experimental Psychology*, 78, 388–395.

Fox, R., and Check, R. (1972). Independence between binocular rivalry suppression duration and magnitude of suppression. *Journal of Experimental Psychology*, 93, 283–289.

Fox, R., and Herrmann, J. (1967). Stochastic properties of binocular rivalry alternations. *Perception and Psychophysics*, 2, 432–436.

Fox, R., and Rasche, F. (1969). Binocular rivalry and reciprocal inhibition. *Perception and Psychophysics,* 5, 215–217.

Fox, R., Todd, S., and Bettinger, L. A. (1975). Optokinetic nystagmus as an objective indicator of binocular rivalry. *Vision Research,* 15, 849–853.

Gibson, J. J. (1966). The problem of temporal order in stimulation and perception. *Journal of Psychology,* 62, 141–149.

Grindley, G. C., and Townsend, V. (1965). Binocular masking induced by a moving object. *Quarterly Journal of Experimental Psychology,* 17, 97–109.

Grossberg, S. (1987). Cortical dynamics of three-dimensional form, color, and brightness perception: II. Binocular theory. *Perception and Psychophysics,* 41, 117–158.

Helmholtz, H. von (1925). *Treatise on Physiological Optics,* J. P. C. Southall, ed. New York: Dover.

Hering, K. E. (1964). *Outlines of a Theory of the Light Sense,* L. M. Hurvich and D. Jameson, trans. Cambridge, Mass.: Harvard University Press.

Hochberg, J. (1964). Depth perception loss with local monocular suppression: A problem in the explanation of stereopsis. *Science,* 145, 1334–1335.

Hollins, M. (1980). The effect of contrast on the completeness of binocular rivalry suppression. *Perception and Psychophysics,* 27, 550–556.

Howie, D. (1952). Perceptual defense. *Psychological Review,* 59, 308–315.

Hubel, D. H., and Wiesel, T. N. (1962). Receptive fields, binocular interaction and functional architecture in the cat's visual cortex. *Journal of Physiology,* 160, 106–154.

James, W. (1891). *The Principles of Psychology.* London: Macmillan.

Kakizaki, S. (1960). Binocular rivalry and stimulus intensity. *Japanese Psychological Research,* 2, 94–105.

Kaufer, G., and Riess, B. F. (1960). Stereoscopic perception as a tool in psychotherapeutic research. *Perceptual and Motor Skills,* 10, 241–242.

Kaufman, L. (1963). On the spread of suppression and binocular rivalry. *Vision Research,* 3, 401–415.

Kim, C. Y., Grossman, E., and Blake, R. (2002). Biologically relevant events are undetectable during suppression phases of binocular rivalry. Society for Neuroscience, Orlando, FL.

Kovács, I., Papathomas, T. V., Yang, M., and Fehér, A. (1996). When the brain changes its mind: Interocular grouping during binocular rivalry. *Proceedings of the National Academy of Sciences of the United States of America,* 93, 15508–15511.

Lack, L. C. (1978). *Selective Attention and the Control of Binocular Rivalry.* The Hague: Mouton.

Lee, S. H., and Blake, R. (1999). Rival ideas about binocular rivalry. *Vision Research,* 39, 1447–1454.

Lehky, S. R. (1995). Binocular rivalry is not chaotic. *Proceedings of the Royal Society of London,* B259, 71–76.

Lehmkuhle, S. W., and Fox, R. (1975). Effect of binocular rivalry suppression on the motion aftereffect. *Vision Research,* 15, 855–859.

Leopold, D. A., and Logothetis, N. K. (1996). Activity changes in early visual cortex reflect monkeys' percepts during binocular rivalry. *Nature,* 379, 549–553.

Leopold, D. A., and Logothetis, N. K. (1999). Multistable phenomena: Changing views in perception. *Trends in Cognitive Sciences,* 3, 254–264.

Levelt, W. J. M. (1965). *On Binocular Rivalry.* Soesterberg, The Netherlands: Institute for Perception RVO-TNO.

Logothetis, N. (1998). Object vision and visual awareness. *Current Opinion in Neurobiology,* 8, 536–544.

Logothetis, N. K., Leopold, D. A., and Sheinberg, D. L. (1996). What is rivalling during binocular rivalry? *Nature,* 380, 621–624.

Mapperson, B., and Lovegrove, W. (1991). Orientation and spatial-frequency-specific surround effects on binocular rivalry. *Bulletin of the Psychonomic Society,* 29, 95–97.

Meenes, M. (1930). A phenomenological description of retinal rivalry. *American Journal of Psychology,* 42, 260–269.

Mueller, T. J., and Blake, R. (1989). A fresh look at the temporal dynamics of binocular rivalry. *Biological Cybernetics,* 61, 223–232.

Myerson, J., Miezin, F., and Allman, J. (1981). Binocular rivalry in macaque monkeys and humans: A comparative study in perception. *Behavior Analysis Letters,* 1, 149–159.

Ogle, K. N., and Wakefield, J. M. (1967). Stereoscopic depth and binocular rivalry. *Vision Research,* 7, 89–98.

O'Shea, R. P. (1987). Chronometric analysis supports fusion rather than suppression theory of binocular vision. *Vision Research,* 27, 781–791.

O'Shea, R. P., Sims, A. J. H., and Govan, D. G. (1997). The effect of spatial frequency and field size on the spread of exclusive visibility in binocular rivalry. *Vision Research,* 37, 175–183.

Peckham, R. H. (1936). Eye movements during "retinal rivalry." *American Journal of Psychology,* 48, 43–63.

Pettigrew, J. D. (2001). Searching for the switch: Neural bases for perceptual rivalry alternations. *Brain and Mind,* 2, 85–118.

Postman, L., Bruner, J., and McGinnies, E. (1948). Personal values as selective factors in perception. *Journal of Abnormal and Social Psychology,* 43, 142–154.

Rauschecker, J. P. J., Campbell, F. W., and Atkinson, J. (1973). Colour opponent neurones in the human visual system. *Nature,* 245, 42–43.

Rogers, R. L., Rogers, S. W., and Tootle, J. S. (1977). Stimulus complexity and rate of alternation in binocular rivalry. *Perceptual and Motor Skills,* 44, 669–670.

Schor, C. M. (1977). Visual stimuli for strabismic suppression. *Perception,* 6, 583–593.

Sherrington, C. S. (1906). *Integrative Action of the Nervous System*. New Haven, Conn.: Yale University Press.

Sobel, K. V., and Blake, R. (2002). How context influences predominance during binocular rivalry. *Perception, 31*, 813–824.

Strüber, D., and Stadler, M. (1999). Differences in top-down influences on the reversal rate of different categories of reversible figures. *Perception, 28*, 1185–1196.

Sugie, N. (1982). Neural models of brightness perception and retinal rivalry in binocular vision. *Biological Cybernetics, 43*, 13–21.

Tong, F., and Engel, S. A. (2001). Interocular rivalry revealed in the human cortical blind-spot representation. *Nature, 411*, 195–199.

Treisman, A. (1962). Binocular rivalry and stereoscopic depth perception. *Quarterly Journal of Experimental Psychology, 14*, 23–37.

Van der Zwan, R., Wenderoth, P., and Alais, D. (1993). Reduction of a pattern-induced motion aftereffect by binocular rivalry suggests the involvement of extrastriate mechanisms. *Visual Neuroscience, 10*, 703–709.

Wade, N. J. (1974). The effect of orientation in binocular contour rivalry of real images and afterimages. *Perception and Psychophysics, 15*, 227–232.

Wade, N. J. (1998). *A Natural History of Vision*. Cambridge, Mass.: MIT Press.

Wade, N. J., and Wenderoth, P. (1978). The influence of colour and contour rivalry on the magnitude of the tilt after-effect. *Vision Research, 18*, 827–836.

Wales, R., and Fox, R. (1970). Increment detection thresholds during binocular rivalry suppression. *Perception and Psychophysics, 8*, 90–94.

Walker, P., and Powell, D. J. (1979). The sensitivity of binocular rivalry to changes in the nondominant stimulus. *Vision Research, 19*, 247–249.

Wallach, H., and Adams, P. A. (1954). Binocular rivalry of achromatic colors. *American Journal of Psychology, 67*, 513–516.

Wheatstone, C. (1838). Contributions to the physiology vision—Part the first: On some remarkable, and hitherto unobserved, phenomena of binocular vision. *Philosophical Transactions of the Royal Society of London, 128*, 371–394.

White, K. D., Petry, H. M., Riggs, L. A., and Miller, J. (1978). Binocular interactions during establishment of McCollough effects. *Vision Research, 18*, 1201–1215.

Whittle, P. (1963). Binocular rivalry. Ph.D. dissertation, Cambridge University.

Whittle, P. (1965). Binocular rivalry and the contrast at contours. *Quarterly Journal of Experimental Psychology, 17*, 217–226.

Whittle, P., Bloor, D. C., and Pocock, S. (1968). Some experiments on figural effects. *Perception and Psychophysics, 4*, 183–188.

Wiesenfelder, H., and Blake, R. (1990). The neural site of binocular rivalry relative to the analysis of motion in the human visual system. *Journal of Neuroscience, 10*, 3880–3888.

Wilson, H. R., Blake, R., and Lee, S. H. (2001). Dynamics of travelling waves in visual perception. *Nature,* 412, 907–910.

Wolfe, J. (1986). Stereopsis and binocular rivalry. *Psychological Review,* 93, 269–282.

Yang, Y., Rose, D., and Blake, R. (1992). On the variety of percepts associated with dichoptic viewing of dissimilar monocular stimuli. *Perception,* 21, 47–62.

Zimba, L. D., and Blake, R. (1983). Binocular rivalry and semantic processing: Out of sight, out of mind. *Journal of Experimental Psychology—Human Perception and Performance,* 9, 807–815.

# 2 Ambiguities and Rivalries in the History of Binocular Vision

## Nicholas J. Wade

The distinction between perceptual ambiguity and binocular rivalry is a fascinating one, and it applies to present as well as past vision research. Natural vision is binocular and yields the perception of depth. Perceptual ambiguities, such as Necker's rhomboid, involve alternating depth interpretations of flat drawings. Binocular rivalry involves alternations between grossly disparate patterns in each eye. Ambiguities and rivalries reflect the failure of depth perception in either the monocular or the binocular domain. In the monocular domain, ambiguities impose apparent depth on flat pictures: the stimuli are not seen as they are— two-dimensional outlines. In the binocular domain, rivalry reflects alternating dominances of the stimuli to one eye or the other (because the differences are too large to be combined), rather than the experience of depth. Paradoxically, (alternating) depth is the monocular outcome, whereas the absence of (stereoscopic) depth is the binocular experience. Thus, both ambiguity and rivalry can be thought of as unsuccessful attempts to resolve the perception of depth, but in diametrically opposite directions.

The perception of objects in space is typically stable and veridical, whether using one eye or two. Perceptual instabilities arise as a consequence of atypical or unnatural stimulation in either the monocular or the binocular domain. Monocular instability (ambiguity) arises when particular patterns are viewed, an example of which is Necker's rhomboid (figure 2.1d). The outline is seen as a solid structure in one of two possible orientations, and alternation occurs between them. Binocular instability (rivalry) is experienced when radically different stimuli are presented to corresponding regions of each eye. This can be produced by

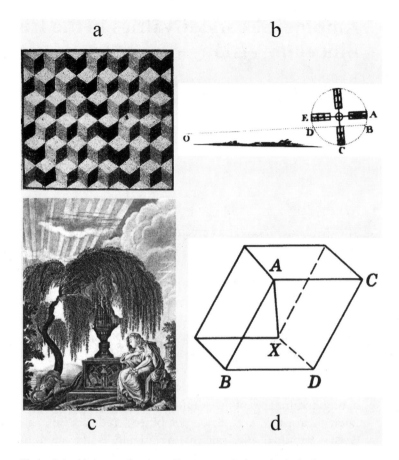

**Figure 2.1** (*a*) A second-century Roman mosaic from Antioch; the representations of cubes are spatially ambiguous. (*b*) Smith's (1738) diagram of a distant windmill where the direction of rotation appears to reverse. (*c*) The mysterious urn by Pierre Crussaire (1795); the sides of the urn represent different profiles, and faces can be seen in the foliage as well. (*d*) Necker's (1832) diagram of a reversing rhomboid.

crossing the eyes, but it is more commonly examined using a stereoscope, so that different pictures can be fixated by each eye without abnormal vergence.

I will say a little bit about the history of perceptual ambiguity before turning to binocular rivalry. The particular issue that I will discuss involves personal as well as binocular rivalries, and it highlights many of the practical problems that have been an enduring aspect of rivalry research.

Nicholas J. Wade

## AMBIGUITIES

Perceptual ambiguity refers to the alternation over time between differing interpretations of a pattern. Ambiguities often involve fluctuations in apparent depth that occur when insufficient evidence of veridical depth is available, either in pictures or when viewing distant objects. The latter is the condition under which Ptolemy (ca. A.D. 100–170) described ambiguity: distant sails of ships appeared to change between appearing concave and convex (see A. M. Smith, 1996). In contemporary vision research, ambiguities are studied almost entirely in the province of that twilight world of pictures; they feed from the flat surface. Visual ambiguities offer alternative interpretations of the depth in drawings or alternative descriptions of objects defined by equivalent contours (see figure 2.1). They occur more readily with monocular observation, and the alternatives appear successively rather than simultaneously; their perception is referred to as multistable. Ambiguities seldom arise when relatively near solid objects are viewed, and so there is the danger of basing their investigation on artificial stimuli that do not reflect the characteristics of everyday perception—viewing solid objects with two eyes.

Though we associate ambiguous stimuli with relatively recent research in perception, pictorial ambiguities have been produced in Italy for many centuries. Roman mosaics display not only the Gestalt laws of grouping but also subtle pictorial ambiguities. Geometrical mosaics, like those which have been found throughout the Roman world, often manipulate the ambiguous depth in flat designs (see Dunbabin, 1999). They abound in the borders of mosaics, like those shown in figure 2.1a.

More recent descriptions of depth fluctuations echo the conditions observed by Ptolemy. Robert Smith (1689–1768) described and illustrated the apparent reversals of direction that occur with motion of the sails of distant windmills (1738; see figure 2.1b). David Rittenhouse (1732–1796) noted that the craters of the moon, viewed through a telescope, could appear concave or convex, depending on the direction of the shadows (1786). Rittenhouse also observed similar instabilities when viewing near objects using a reduction tube; the ridges in chocolate bars could reverse. Albrecht von Haller (1708–1777) observed reversals in wax seals when they were illuminated from different directions; he also described similar effects due to the directions of shadows cast by specimens observed under the microscope (1786).

Pictorial ambiguities were made explicit by many eighteenth-century painters, including William Hogarth (1697–1764) and Pierre Crussaire

(1749–1800). For example, Crussaire illustrated a vase defined by two different profiles (figure 2.1c). This phenomenon resurfaced in the psychological domain with Rubin's vase/faces motif (Rubin, 1915). Many ambiguities are dependent on the lost dimension of pictures, depth. This loss introduces uncertainly in our vision, and this uncertainty is evidenced in the fluctuations in apparent depth that ensue. One of the commonest modern examples of perceptual reversal is that of a hollow mask, and this was described by the principal character of this chapter, David Brewster (1781–1868) in 1826 (see figure 2.2c). Brewster also observed conversions of relief with cameos and intaglios that depended on the direction of the illumination source. Louis-Albert Necker (1786–1861) corresponded with Brewster, who was an editor of *The Philosophical Magazine,* and described a perceptual alternation in a drawing of a crystal (1832; see figure 2.1d).

Charles Wheatstone (1802–1875) discussed the reversal of the Necker rhomboid in his classical memoir on the stereoscope (1838; see figure 2.2a);

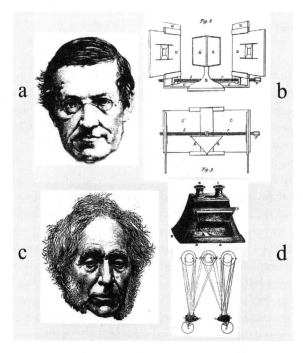

**Figure 2.2** (*a*) Charles Wheatstone (1802–1875) and (*b*) his mirror stereoscope seen from the front and from the top. (*c*) David Brewster (1781–1868) and (*d*) his lenticular stereoscope, together with the optical principles of its operation.

Nicholas J. Wade

he noted that the reversals were more frequent with monocular than with binocular vision. Indeed, the figure should be called the Wheatstone cube, and it was referred to in this way by Wallin (1905) in his detailed survey of reversing figures. Wheatstone was the first to use a skeleton 3-D cube rather than a rhomboid, and the first to note the differences in the perceived sizes of the near and far faces when reversals took place! Wheatstone is, of course, better known for his invention of the mirror stereoscope and for his subtle experiments with it. Wheatstone's important observations concerning binocular rivalry are detailed in chapter 1.

## BINOCULAR RIVALRY

In contrast to perceptual ambiguity, binocular rivalry is a natural consequence of our binocular interactions with the world; rivalry is a resolution of conditions that apply to most of what we see when using two eyes. It occurs when the differences between the images in the two eyes are too large to be combined and stereoscopic depth cannot be extracted from disparity. When we bifixate on part of an object, most of what is projected to the peripheral retina is too disparate to yield depth; since the peripheral stimuli arise from different depths, their retinal images also tend to be out of focus. We are not generally aware of this binocular rivalry because both visual resolution and attention are associated with the fixated object rather than peripheral ones. If attention shifts to a peripheral object, then the eyes generally also move to bifixate it. Binocular rivalry is rarely examined under these conditions of natural stimulation. It is typically studied with different patterns presented to corresponding foveal regions of the two eyes—as if we are bifixating two different objects. Ptolemy set up the conditions under which binocular rivalry can occur: placing a black rod and a white rod in the axis of each eye would result in rivalry (see figure 2.3a), but he did not describe the phenomenon, probably because the eyes could not remain parallel when viewing near rods (Howard and Wade, 1996). Thus, the conditions under which binocular rivalry is investigated experimentally seldom occur in normal binocular vision (but see Howard's chapter on occlusion).

Wheatstone was not the first to study binocular rivalry, but the earlier observers did not have the advantage of a stereoscope (see Wade, 1998). Ptolemy placed black and white rods in the visual axis of each eye (figure 2.3a); Giambattista della Porta (1535–1615) described rivalry between two pages of a book with a septum between them and viewed by different eyes (1593); and Jean Théophile Desaguliers (1683–1744) examined both

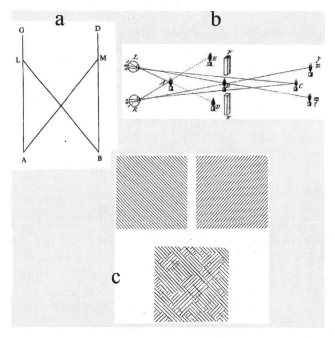

Figure 2.3  (*a*) Ptolemy's diagram for viewing different objects, such as black and white rods, at D and G, with the eyes at A and B. (*b*) Desaguliers's (1716) arrangement for viewing different objects or different colors located beyond an aperture. (*c*) Panum's (1858) orthogonal gratings and an impression of the mosaic mixture that is visible when they are viewed in a stereoscope.

color and contour rivalry, using an aperture method (1716; see figure 2.3b). However, it was Wheatstone's presentation of different letters in his stereoscope that stimulated experimental studies of binocular rivalry (see figure 1.2c in chapter 1 of this volume).

Wheatstone demonstrated that binocular vision is superior to monocular vision because it can result in stereoscopic depth perception. For the preceding 2000 years the opposite had been considered the case— monocular vision was taken to be superior to binocular. This was due to the combination of the concept of Galen's (ca. 130–200) visual spirit with the optics of Alhazen (ca. 965–1039). Galen introduced the method of separating the eyes by means of a septum, and reported that vision of a peripheral target seen by one eye when both were open was inferior to that with only one eye open. This position was repeatedly maintained until the seventeenth century, and it accorded with the Galenic theory of pneuma and the visual spirit. The source of the spirit was at the optic chiasma, and so was more concentrated when one eye was open than when both were. That is, all the visual spirit could travel to one eye rather than separating to two eyes.

In similarly placing the visual faculty at the chiasm, Roger Bacon (ca. 1220–1292) introduced the analogy of singleness of vision with a fountain: since a fountain has but one source, so is vision with two eyes single. Galen's method of separating the two eyes was applied to good effect by Porta in the context of eye dominance, and Porta also illustrated Galen's description of the apparent locations of an object seen with each eye separately and with both eyes. Porta stepped out of the Galenic mold by proposing a theory of single vision that was both parsimonious and supported by the phenomenon of binocular rivalry: we see singly with two eyes by using only one at a time. Porta's suppression theory could be contrasted with fusion theories of the type advanced by Aguilonius (1571–1650), who introduced the term *horopter* (1613).

Rivalry was easier to induce with the aid of a stereoscope, and the experimental study of it accelerated after 1838. For example, Peter Ludwig Panum (1820–1885) introduced grating stimuli to the study of rivalry (1858; see figure 2.3c), and they have proved popular ever since. Wheatstone was able to examine rivalry with the aid of the stereoscope he invented, but was his the first stereoscope and had stereoscopic pictures been produced previously?

## THE CHIMENTI CONTROVERSY

Few disputes in the history of visual science have engaged so many people from so many disciplines as that related to the Chimenti pictures (see Wade, 2003). It commenced two decades after Wheatstone's mirror stereoscope (figure 2.2b) was exposed to public gaze, and only a few years after Brewster's lenticular stereoscope had been invented (figure 2.2d).

The controversy was instigated by Brewster, and Wheatstone was ensnared by it. It concerned two drawings by Jacopo Chimenti da Empoli (ca. 1551–1640), probably executed around 1600. Chimenti was born at Empoli and spent most of his life in Florence (see Testaferrata, 1996). He painted altarpieces in Florence and Tuscany (including one in the Convent of Santa Chiara at San Miniato), and was noted for his skills as a draftsman, particularly in still-life drawings. Two drawings by Chimenti, rediscovered in the nineteenth century, stirred the world of visual science. They were exhibited in the Musée Wicar, at Lille, mounted separately and hung side by side (figure 2.4a). Their dimensions are approximately 30 × 22 cm.,

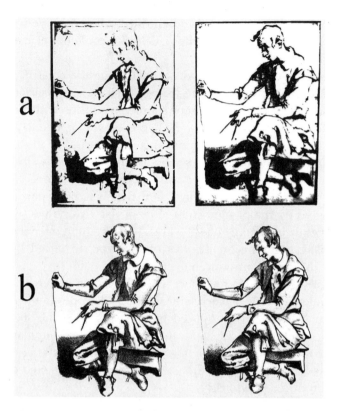

**Figure 2.4** (*a*) Photographic copies of the two Chimenti drawings from the Palais des Beaux Arts, Musée Wicar, Lille (kindly supplied by Arthur Gill). (*b*) Woodcuts of the Chimenti drawings as they were reproduced in the April 1862 issue of *The Photographic Journal*. They were transposed relative to the photographic copies so that they could be viewed with a prism or lenticular stereoscope.

and Gill (1969) stated that there was no evidence they had ever been mounted as a pair.

The drawings were seen by Alexander Crum Brown (1838–1922) on a visit to the museum in 1859. Crum Brown combined the drawings binocularly by converging his eyes to a point in front of them, and he saw the figure in depth. He considered that this union could have been achieved only if the drawings had been intended for binocular viewing. These observations were conveyed in a letter to James Forbes (1809–1868). A small diagram was included in the letter, indicating how the eyes should converge in front of the pictures in order to combine them. Forbes immediately passed Crum Brown's letter on to Brewster. Brewster, president of

Nicholas J. Wade

the Photographic Society of Scotland, read Crum Brown's letter at its monthly meeting, held in George Street Hall, Edinburgh, on March 10.

The letter was printed, with slight modifications, in the May issue of *The Photographic Journal* (Brewster, 1860a). Brewster added his own commentary on its remarkable contents, concluding:

This account of the two drawings is so distinct and evinces such knowledge of the subject, that we cannot for a moment doubt that they are binocular drawings intended by the artist to be united into relief either by the eye or by an instrument. This conclusion is the more probable as the drawings must have been executed before 1640, the year in which Chimenti died at the age of eighty-six; and it is highly probable that they were executed soon after 1593, when Baptista Porta had published the Theory of the Stereoscope, and when Chimenti was in his fortieth year. (p. 233)

Brewster had written to the director of the Musée Wicar requesting photographic copies of the drawings, but this did not prove immediately possible. Thus, Brewster's claim that the drawings were stereoscopic was made on the basis of Crum Brown's description alone; he had not seen the Chimenti pictures himself, but this did not inhibit him from including reference to the paired drawings in his entry "Stereoscope" for the eighth edition of the *Encyclopaedia Britannica*. Brewster (1860b) presented a redrawn figure from Porta (1593) purporting to illustrate the principle of the stereoscope, and also a reproduction of the diagram Crum Brown included in his letter to Forbes. Brewster even went so far as to refer to the technique of overconvergence for uniting binocular pictures as "the method of Chimenti."

## Binocular Rivalries: Brewster versus Wheatstone

One reason why Brewster was eager to press the stereoscopic case of Chimenti's drawings was to renew his claims that the basis for stereoscopic vision had been known long before Wheatstone's invention of the stereoscope (see Wade, 1983, 2002). Brewster first saw Wheatstone's mirror stereoscope at the British Association for the Advancement of Science meeting at Newcastle in August 1838. His initial response to it was positive, for he initially believed that stereoscopic phenomena could be accounted for in terms of monocular visible directions.

Prior to the invention of the stereoscope, Brewster's discussion of binocular vision had been cursory, and it had emphasized his projective concept of visible direction: "When an object, therefore, is seen single with two eyes, it is in reality double, but the two images coincide so accurately, that they appear only as one, and having twice the brightness of the image formed by either eye alone" (Brewster, 1830, p. 615). When he examined Wheatstone's reports in more detail, he realized that some of Wheatstone's stereoscopic phenomena fundamentally undermined the concept of fixed visible direction, and sought to account for them by means of rapid changes in convergence (Brewster, 1844).

Brewster first intimated the claim that the principles of binocular combination had been known for centuries in an anonymous review of several articles on binocular vision (including some of his own) in *The North British Review:*

The fundamental facts in binocular vision, on which this remarkable illusion depends, may be thus expressed:—*When we view, with both eyes, or with each eye successively, any solid object, that is, any object in relief, or in the converse of relief, any cameo or intaglio, for example, each eye sees the object differently, or, what is the same thing, dissimilar pictures of the object are painted on the two retinae.* This important fact has been long ago published by optical writers, and is well known to optical observers, though Mr. Wheatstone has claimed it "as a new fact in the theory of vision." (Anon., 1852, p. 167; italics in original)

Brewster was conflating optics and observation, that is, the geometry of optical projection with its perceptual consequences. Dissimilar projections to each eye had long been known, but the visual consequences of this were first described and demonstrated by Wheatstone (1838). Brewster's claims were extended in his book on the history of the stereoscope. He commenced: "It is, therefore, a fact well known to every person of common sagacity that *the pictures of bodies seen by both eyes are formed by the union of two dissimilar pictures formed by each.* This palpable truth was known and published by ancient mathematicians" (1856, p. 6; italics in original). They were repeated in an anonymous letter to *The Times* in October 1856. A report in the French journal *Cosmos* described a very simple arrangement of looking through two holes at two pictures. The anonymous correspondent to *The Times* pointed out that the device was not new. Wheatstone responded to the anonymous letter by pointing out that an account of his stereoscope had been published in a book by Mayo in 1833. There followed two more exchanges, penned with mounting vitriol, between Brewster and Wheatstone in October and November of that year (the correspondence is reprinted in Wade, 1983).

The battle was begun by Brewster, but the war was won by Wheatstone. Not only did Wheatstone demonstrate his mastery of literary combat, but he was also able to provide evidence that both mirror and prism stereo-scopes had been made in 1832. Brewster smarted under this public rebuke and saw the Chimenti drawings as an ideal vehicle for salvaging his reputation from the savaging it had suffered at Wheatstone's hands.

## Responses to Brewster's Speculations

Brewster's views were rapidly disseminated through photographic jour-nals. His initial description of the Chimenti drawings was read to a meet-ing of the Photographic Society of Scotland (of which he was president) in March 1860; reports of the lecture were printed in both British and Conti-nental journals, and responses were quick to appear. A brief account of Brewster's talk was printed in the April 16 issue of the *British Journal of Photography*. This journal was published fortnightly, and carried accounts of the meetings of photographic societies in Britain and France. The Chimenti pictures evoked widespread interest because they brought into question the origins of stereoscopy, and their possible stereoscopic charac-ter was determined by observation of photographs of the drawings. At a meeting of the French Photographic Society in July 1860, photographic copies were described as uniting but not providing any stereoscopic effect. This conclusion was reprinted in the August 1 issue of the *British Journal of Photography* (see Lacan, 1860). The editorial in the next issue of the *British Journal of Photography* drew attention to Lacan's report (Shadbolt, 1860).

Brewster's chagrin must have been heightened on discovering that Wheatstone had obtained photographic copies of the drawings in June 1860. Brewster's responses to these reprimands were recounted at a meet-ing of the Photographic Society of Scotland (Brewster, 1862). Crum Brown's letter was reprinted again (with other minor modifications), as was the contention that Chimenti was familiar with Porta's writings and had made the drawings for use with a stereoscope. The title of Brewster's talk and article displayed his hardening attitude regarding the prove-nance of the drawings.

The Chimenti pictures had by this time drawn the wider scientific community into the controversy, and they were discussed at meetings of photographic societies throughout Europe. For example, William Benjamin Carpenter (1813–1885) examined the pictures both with and without a stereoscope and made several critical variations in the viewing conditions (Carpenter, 1862). He was a naturalist and microscopist of note, and has been described as one of the last examples of "an almost univer-sal naturalist." Carpenter's comments were astute. He considered the dimensions of corresponding features of the two drawings, and also the possibility that their relative orientations were arbitrary. However, transposing them did not assist in any stereoscopic effect.

Brewster's second presentation to the Photographic Society of Scotland, in March 1862, had been attended by one Professor Macdonald, who obtained copies of the drawings. These were used to produce woodcuts that were printed in the April issue of *The Photographic Journal* (figure 2.4b). They were described as facsimiles, but they are more regular than the images in the photograph copied in figure 2.4a; the woodcuts also were transposed so that they could be used with a prism or lenticular stereoscope. Brewster also sent photographic copies of the pictures to Rev. Joseph Bancroft Reade (1801–1870), a pioneer of photography and a natural philosopher with wide-ranging interests. Reade (1862) commented on the effect the pictures produced; his first impression was that they were pseudoscopic (producing perception of reversed depth), but he was persuaded, in part, by Brewster's arguments that they might be stereoscopic. Reade did carry out measurements on the two drawings and remarked on the inconsistencies between them. Nonetheless, he did not consider that the issue was resolved.

Brewster did not obtain photographic copies of the drawings until 1862, by which time he was aware of the ridicule that had been heaped on his claims. Undeterred, he presented the photographs in a stereoscope to a meeting of members of the Photographic Society of Scotland, and it was noted that "The full stereoscopic relief of Chimenti's pictures was seen and acknowledged by all" (Brewster, 1862, p. 12). As is evident from the title of his article, Brewster was convinced that the drawings displayed an understanding and manipulation of disparities to yield stereoscopic depth.

Peter Guthrie Tait (1831–1901) was also a participant in this debate. He wrote a letter to Brewster, extracts of which were read before a meeting of the Photographic Society of Scotland in May 1862 and published in June (Tait, 1862). Tait's analysis of the Chimenti drawings was based on both practicalities and probabilities. Together with Brewster, he asked a student at the Edinburgh School of Design to make copies of one of the Chimenti pictures. Six of these were available for inspection at the May meeting. The issue of copies became prominent in the next episode of the drama.

### Conflict and Resolution

The Chimenti controversy spread across the Atlantic, and Edwin Emerson (1823–1908; see figure 2.5), a professor at Troy University and a keen

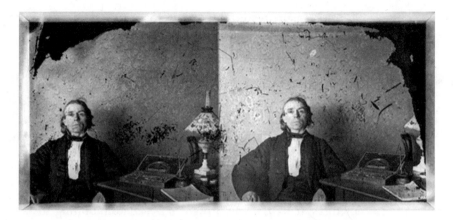

**Figure 2.5** A stereoscopic self-portrait of Edwin Emerson (1823–1908), taken around 1861, when the Chimenti controversy was raging. (Courtesy George Eastman House, Rochester, New York.)

photographer, entered into it wholeheartedly. His first report appeared in *The American Journal of Science and Arts* (Emerson, 1862). Emerson went on to describe an experiment rather like that performed by Tait: making a sketch and then trying to copy it exactly will generate differences that are both stereoscopic and pseudoscopic. Brewster's ire was raised when Emerson's article was reprinted in *The Philosophical Magazine* the next year (Emerson, 1863), and he responded in a typically robust manner (Brewster, 1864), casting aspersions on Emerson's sentience and on his science.

Brewster's riposte elicited four replies from Emerson. In the first (Emerson, 1864a) he proceeded to refute Brewster's criticisms of his earlier article. The second reply (Emerson, 1864b) highlights the improbabilities of the drawings being made to produce a stereoscopic effect. These included the dimensions of the drawings, the inappropriateness of the subject matter, and the absence of any written account about them. Emerson enlisted four impartial observers (one of whom was Ogden Rood [1831–1902], an authority on vision and art to combine the pictures); none of them described any stereoscopic effects. Rood's expertise was enlisted again for the third retort (Emerson, 1864c); he was asked to copy one of the drawings as accurately as he could, and Emerson did the same. There was a slight stereoscopic effect when they were combined. Emerson's final reply contained the most convincing evidence. He pursued the approach initially proposed by Carpenter—he measured the dimensions of the two drawings, and a colleague did so independently.

Ambiguities and Rivalries in the History of Binocular Vision

These measurements were of internal features of each drawing, such as "from the highest point of the head to the point of the left foot" (1864d, p. 203).

The outcome was clear:

As Sir David Brewster requires particulars, we enumerate:—A stereoscopic left knee, a pseudoscopic dress hanging over it, a stereoscopic left arm, but a pseudoscopic back, a pseudoscopic stool, and a pseudoscopic left foot, and a right foot still more pseudoscopic relatively to the left foot and the stool; and so we might go over the whole picture and show a *mélange* of pseudoscopic and stereoscopic lines, producing precisely the commingled and uncertain effect which a drawing and an ordinary copy of it would produce if adjusted for the stereoscope. And yet these are the pictures that Dr. Crum Brown "succeeded in uniting so as to produce *an image in relief*" and they united for him "*easily and completely!*" These are the pictures [for] which Sir David Brewster claims, gravely and persistently, a high "degree of stereoscopic effect," and on that account boldly proceeds to give the seventeenth century the high honour rightly belonging to one of the most beautiful discoveries of our own age! (1864d, p. 204)

Whether Brewster saw the error of his ways we do not know, but he did not reenter the fray. The controversy was at its height when Helmholtz was writing the third volume of his *Handbuch der physiologischen Optik*, which treated stereoscopic vision. By that stage, photographic copies of the Chimenti sketches were available, as well as the woodcuts from *The Photographic Journal*, although Helmholtz believed that the two drawings were on the same sheet of paper. He gave a sober description of the arguments, and provided another possible interpretation:

Had the artist desired to test a theory, it is more likely that he would have drawn the easy things correctly and the difficult parts, such as the man, more inaccurately. It seems more probable to me that the artist was not quite satisfied with the first figure and did it over again from another point of view, using the same sheet of paper quite by accident. (Helmholtz, 2000, p. 363)

The Chimenti controversy refuses to die. The mischief manufactured by Brewster has multiplied, and this misinformation has been mimicked many times on the Internet. Not only are the Chimenti pictures described as the first stereoscopic pictures, but it is also stated that Porta (1593) produced binocular drawings.

Nonetheless, both Wheatstone and Brewster relied on their own observations in deciding on the possible stereoscopic status of the Chimenti drawings. They did not apply the methods that were emerging in Germany to measure perception with the precision associated with physics. In the year that the Chimenti drawings were made a cause célèbre, Fechner (1860) published his account of psychophysics. However, the resolution of the controversy was a consequence of Emerson's recourse to physics rather than psychology, to measurement of the stimulus rather than the response. The history of science may look upon this controversy of observation as a triumph for optics.

This cautionary tale of the unbridled search for support of an initially untestable and ultimately untenable theory should not be considered as a historical oddity. It is a consequence of associating theories with their protagonists, and continues to be a feature of the scientific enterprise. In this regard, it is appropriate to close with a quotation from Joseph Bancroft Reade: "The eye is a treacherous guide when fortified by a little previous theory" (Reade, 1862, p. 29).

## CONCLUSION

Brewster and Wheatstone were binocular rivals in the personal and theoretical senses. Brewster's views of binocular vision were based upon analyses of visual directions that were defined in retinal terms. He referred to binocular rivalry as "ocular equivocation," and used it as evidence against Wheatstone's observations (see Brewster, 1844). Wheatstone, on the other hand, adopted a philosophically empiricist approach that was later echoed by Helmholtz. Moreover, both examined the perceptual ambiguity associated with Necker's rhomboid, and again their interpretations of it were radically different. Wheatstone (1838) dismissed Necker's suggestion that the alternations were a consequence of involuntary changes in accommodation on logical and experimental grounds. Brewster (1844) disputed Wheatstone's analysis, and argued that the alternations were due to the indistinctness of peripheral parts of the rhomboid when a central part is fixated. Thus, Brewster and Wheatstone were rivals even in the context of perceptual ambiguity.

Fortunately, the story ends on a happier note. The rivals were reconciled at the final public event that Brewster attended—the meeting of the British Association for the Advancement of Science held at Dundee in 1867. Brewster offered his hand to Wheatstone and hoped that their past disagreements were forgotten. On relating this later to a friend, Wheatstone remarked, "Do you really think he was sincere?" (Gordon, 1870, p. 389). Brewster did mellow in his final year. He even proposed that Wheatstone should be elected an honorary fellow of the Royal Society of Edinburgh.

# REFERENCES

Aguilonius [Aguilon], F. (1613). *Opticorum libri sex juxta ac mathematicis utiles.* Antwerp: Moreti.

Anon. (David Brewster). (1852). Binocular vision and the stereoscope. *The North British Review,* 17, 165–204.

Brewster, D. (1826). On the optical illusion of the conversion of cameos into intaglios, and of intaglios into cameos, with an account of other analogous phenomena. *Edinburgh Journal of Science,* 4, 99–108.

Brewster, D. (1830). Optics. In *Edinburgh Encyclopaedia,* vol. 15, 460–662. Edinburgh: Blackwoods.

Brewster, D. (1844). On the law of visible position in single and binocular vision, and on the representation of solid figures by the union of dissimilar plane pictures on the retina. *Transactions of the Royal Society of Edinburgh,* 15, 349–368.

Brewster, D. (1856). *The Stereoscope. Its History, Theory, and Construction.* London: John Murray.

Brewster, D. (1860a). Notice respecting the invention of the stereoscope in the sixteenth century, and of binocular drawings, by Jacopo Chimenti da Empoli, a Florentine artist. *The Photographic Journal,* 6, 232–233.

Brewster, D. (1860b). Stereoscope. In *Encyclopaedia Britannica,* 8th ed., vol. 20, 684–691. Edinburgh: Adam and Charles Black.

Brewster, D. (1862). On the stereoscopic pictures executed in the 16th century. *The Photographic Journal,* 8, 9–12.

Brewster, D. (1864). On the stereoscopic relief in the Chimenti pictures. *The London, Edinburgh and Dublin Philosophical Magazine and Journal of Science,* 27, 1–3.

Carpenter, W. B. (1862). Alleged stereoscopic drawings by Chimenti. *The Photographic Journal,* 8, 27–28.

Desaguliers, J. T. (1716). A plain and easy experiment to confirm Sir Isaac Newton's doctrine of the different refrangibility of the rays of light. *Philosophical Transactions of the Royal Society of London,* 29, 448–452.

Dunbabin, K. M. D. (1999). *Mosaics of the Greek and Roman World.* Cambridge: Cambridge University Press.

Emerson, E. (1862). On the perception of relief. *American Journal of Science and Arts,* 34, 312–316.

Emerson, E. (1863). On the perception of relief. *The London, Edinburgh and Dublin Philosophical Magazine and Journal of Science,* 26, 125–130.

Emerson, E. (1864a). The Chimenti pictures: A reply to Sir David Brewster. *British Journal of Photography,* 11, 111–112.

Emerson, E. (1864b). The Chimenti pictures: A reply to Sir David Brewster. *British Journal of Photography,* 11, 132–133.

Emerson, E. (1864c). The Chimenti pictures: A reply to Sir David Brewster. *British Journal of Photography*, 11, 167–169.

Emerson, E. (1864d). The Chimenti pictures: A reply to Sir David Brewster. *British Journal of Photography*, 11, 202–204.

Fechner, G. T. (1860). *Elemente der Psychophysik*. Leipzig: Breitkopf und Härtel.

Gill, A. T. (1969). Early stereoscopes. *The Photographic Journal*, 109, 641–651.

Gordon, M. M. (1870). *The Home Life of Sir David Brewster*. Edinburgh: Edmonston and Douglas.

Haller, A. von (1786). *First Lines of Physiology*, vol. 2, W. Cullen, trans. Edinburgh: Elliot.

Helmholtz, H. von (2000). *Helmholtz's Treatise on Physiological Optics*, vol. 3, J. P. C. Southall, trans. Bristol: Thoemmes.

Howard, I. P., and Wade, N. J. (1996). Ptolemy's contributions to the geometry of binocular vision. *Perception*, 25, 1189–1202.

Lacan, E. (1860). Foreign correspondence. *British Journal of Photography*, 7, 228–229.

Necker, L. A. (1832). Observations on some remarkable phenomena seen in Switzerland; and an optical phenomenon which occurs on viewing a figure of a crystal or geometrical solid. *London and Edinburgh Philosophical Magazine and Journal of Science*, 1, 329–337.

Panum, P. L. (1858). *Physiologische Untersuchungen über das Sehen mit zwei Augen*. Kiel, Germany: Schwerssche Buchhandlung.

Porta, J. della (1593). *De refractione. Optices parte. Libri novem*. Naples: Salviani.

Reade, J. B. (1862). "The Chimenti pictures." *The Photographic Journal*, 8, 29–30.

Rittenhouse, D. (1786). Explanation of an optical deception. *Transactions of the American Philosophical Society*, 2, 37–42.

Rubin, E. (1915). *Synsoplevede Figurer*. Copenhagen: Gyldendalske.

Sabra, A. I., trans. and ed. (1989). *The Optics of Ibn Al-Haytham. Books I–III. On Direct Vision*. London: The Warburg Institute.

Sakane, I. (1979). *The Expanding Visual World. A Museum of Fun*. Tokyo: Asahi Shimbun.

Shadbolt, G. (1860). Editorial. *British Journal of Photography*, 7, 231–232.

Smith, A. M. (1996). *Ptolemy's Theory of Visual Perception: An English Translation of the Optics with Introduction and Commentary*. Philadelphia: American Philosophical Society.

Smith, R. (1738). *A Compleat System of Opticks in Four Books*. Cambridge: Published by the author.

Tait, P. G. (1862). The drawings of Jacopo Chimenti. *The Photographic Journal*, 8, 69.

Testaferrata, E. (1996). Jacopo da Empoli. In *The Dictionary of Art*, J. Turner, ed., vol. 10, 187–190. London: Macmillan.

Wade, N. J. (1983). *Brewster and Wheatstone on Vision*. London: Academic Press.

Wade, N. J. (1998). *A Natural History of Vision.* Cambridge, Mass.: MIT Press.

Wade, N. J. (2002). Charles Wheatstone (1802–1875). *Perception,* 31, 265–272.

Wade, N. J. (2003). The Chimenti controversy. *Perception,* 32, 185–200.

Wallin, J. E. W. (1905). *Optical Illusions of Reversible Perspective: A Volume of Historical and Experimental Researches.* Princeton, N.J.: Published by the author.

Wheatstone, C. (1838). Contributions to the physiology of vision—Part the first. On some remarkable, and hitherto unobserved, phenomena of binocular vision. *Philosophical Transactions of the Royal Society of London,* B128, 371–394.

# 3 The Nature and Depth of Binocular Rivalry Suppression

## Alan W. Freeman, Vincent A. Nguyen, and David Alais

The binocular rivalry produced by a pair of incompatible stimuli results in alternating dominance between the two members of the pair. When one stimulus is dominant, the other is largely invisible. The latter stimulus is physically present but the associated percept is absent, implying that the neural signals evoked by that stimulus must be suppressed somewhere in the visual system. This suppression is the subject of considerable speculation, as chapters throughout this volume attest. At what stage in the visual pathway is the suppression exerted? Does the suppression occur within monocular channels or at higher levels of the pathway? How can the suppression best be measured?

In this chapter we explore the nature and locus of binocular rivalry suppression by developing and testing a model for the suppression process. The essential components of the model are as follows:

• Signals from each of the monocular stimuli travel along pathways connecting monocular cortical areas to higher areas subserving perception.

• At any moment during binocular rivalry, one of these pathways is suppressed. In particular, neurons at all stages along this pathway are suppressed.

• The depth of suppression increases along the suppressed pathway.

While the primary focus of this chapter is the suppression model, a secondary theme is the application of quantitative methods to the psychophysical study of binocular rivalry. Some of the work in binocular rivalry has relied solely on subjects' indicating which eye's stimulus is dominant at any given time. While this approach has provided invaluable insights, it requires criterion-dependent judgments on the part of the subjects. To overcome this problem, we describe new and existing psychophysical tools that provide a more quantitative approach to binocular rivalry. In so doing, we provide new data on the hitherto neglected topic of suppression depth.

## MONOCULAR SUPPRESSION

The first issue we examine is the suppression of monocular portions of the visual pathway. Logothetis, Leopold, and Sheinberg (1996) crystallized this issue by proposing two forms of suppression. Eye suppression is the nonselective loss of visual information presented to one eye without any effect on stimuli presented to the other eye. Stimulus suppression, by contrast, is selectively targeted at a stimulus feature regardless of the eye to which that feature is presented. We now describe two of our own experiments that yield evidence for eye suppression.

Figure 3.1 illustrates the protocol for the first experiment. On each trial, incompatible conditioning stimuli were presented to the two eyes of an

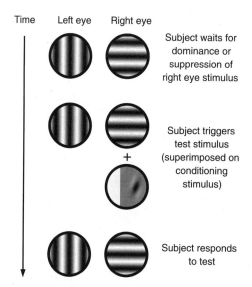

**Figure 3.1** Stimulation sequence in the first experiment. Binocularly incompatible sinusoidal gratings, 1° in diameter, were presented to the two eyes. The subject waited during the ensuing binocular rivalry until the right eye's stimulus was dominant or suppressed, depending on the type of run, and then triggered a test stimulus. The test stimulus, a Gabor patch, was superimposed on either the left or the right half of the right eye's conditioning stimulus. The subject's task was to indicate on which half it appeared.

A. W. Freeman, V. A. Nguyen, and D. Alais

adult human subject. The subject waited until the right eye's stimulus was dominant (that is, fully visible) or suppressed (invisible), and then triggered a brief test stimulus to just the right eye. The stimulus was delivered, with equal probability, to the left or right half of the right eye's view. The subject's task was to signal which alternative occurred.

Sensitivity to the test stimulus was measured over a series of trials. Test contrast was adjusted from trial to trial to find the contrast sensitivity for a fixed level (79%) of correct choice. The test stimulus was a Gabor patch with the same spatial frequency as the conditioning stimuli. Its orientation was fixed on any given run of trials, but was assigned different values from run to run. In particular, the test stimulus was aligned with the suppressed conditioning stimulus, or with the dominant stimulus, or took one of a number of intermediate orientations.

Figure 3.2A shows the results for one subject. The horizontal axis gives the orientation of the test stimulus, and the symbols under the axis provide a guide to the relative orientation of test and conditioning stimuli. The open circles show contrast sensitivity to the test stimulus when the tested eye's conditioning stimulus is dominant. In general, contrast sensitivity is lower when the test stimulus is closely aligned with the conditioning stimulus to the tested eye, presumably due to monocular masking (Phillips and Wilson, 1984). Of more immediate interest is the effect of binocular rivalry suppression. The filled circles show contrast sensitivity when the tested eye's conditioning stimulus is suppressed, and the vertical gap between open and filled circles therefore indicates the sensitivity loss due to suppression.

This loss is shown more directly in figure 3.2B, which plots the suppressed sensitivity divided by the sensitivity during dominance. Data for three subjects (including the subject represented in panel A) are shown. The dashed line indicates a lack of suppression; the gap between the plotted points and the dashed line therefore shows the depth of suppression. Sensitivity during suppression averaged 63% of that during dominance, consistent with previous measures of suppression depth (Makous and Sanders, 1978; Blake and Camisa, 1979).

What do the two hypotheses, eye suppression and stimulus suppression, predict for the dependence of suppression depth on test orientation? Eye suppression is defined to be nonselective, and therefore predicts a constant loss at all test orientations. Stimulus suppression predicts otherwise. Consider, for example, the point at the right end of the axis where the test stimulus is vertical. The open circle at this orientation in panel A

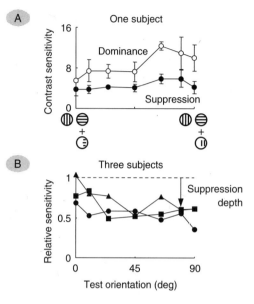

**Figure 3.2** Alignment of test and conditioning stimuli, and the effect on suppression. The horizontal axis shows the orientation of the test stimulus, and the schematic stimuli (upper panel) illustrate two representative cases. The upper part of each set of schematic stimuli illustrates the conditioning stimuli, and the lower part, the test stimulus. (*A*) The vertical axis gives contrast sensitivity during dominance (open symbols) and suppression (closed symbols) of the right eye's conditioning stimulus. Error bars give 95% confidence intervals. (*B*) These data were obtained by dividing the contrast sensitivity during suppression by that during dominance for both the subject in (*A*) and two more subjects. The gap between the dashed line and the symbols gives suppression depth. The results are more consistent with eye suppression than with stimulus suppression.

was obtained when the horizontal conditioning stimulus was dominant and the vertical was suppressed. The test stimulus has the same orientation as the suppressed conditioning stimulus and, according to the stimulus suppression hypothesis, should also be suppressed. The open circle should therefore lie below its filled counterpart (obtained when the vertical conditioning stimulus was dominant), and the suppression/dominance ratio should be greater than 1.

The ratios in panel B of the figure do not match this prediction: instead of exceeding 1 on the right, they instead appear to trend downward from left to right. A repeated-measures analysis of variance was performed on the dominance and suppression thresholds from the three subjects (using the Greenhouse–Geisser correction for intrasubject correlation). It showed no significant interaction between perceptual status and test orientation

A. W. Freeman, V. A. Nguyen, and D. Alais

$(F(2.0, 3.9) = 6.3; P = .06)$. The eye suppression hypothesis, which predicts this lack of interaction, therefore matches the data much better than does the stimulus suppression hypothesis.

This evidence for monocular suppression fits with previous psychophysical results (Blake, Westendorf, and Overton, 1980; see also chapter 1), and with several recent magnetic resonance imaging studies that are described in more detail in chapter 4. Tong and Engel (2001), for example, measured primary visual cortical activity using functional magnetic resonance imaging in human subjects presented with binocularly rivalrous stimuli. The activity, which was in the representation of the blind spot and was therefore driven by only one eye, fluctuated in synchrony with the subject's reported percepts.

## DYNAMIC SUPPRESSION

Our secondary theme in this chapter is a more quantitative approach to the measurement of binocular rivalry suppression. Variability in a binocular rivalry experiment arises from at least two sources. First, rivalry is often spatially piecemeal, meaning that one stimulus dominates at some visual field locations while the other stimulus dominates elsewhere (Blake, O'Shea, and Mueller, 1992). Second, at any given visual field location, the transition from one percept to the other is not instantaneous: there is an intermediate period where the percept cannot unambiguously be identified as one or the other (Wolfe, 1983).

We have tackled this problem with a new experimental protocol that does not require the subject to name the current percept. The protocol is illustrated in figure 3.3. One eye is presented with a static horizontal grating. The conditioning stimulus to the other eye is a sum of two gratings, one horizontal and the other vertical. The amplitude of each of these latter gratings varies sinusoidally in time but in antiphase, so that when the amplitude of one grating is maximal, the other amplitude is zero. The dynamic stimulus therefore oscillates between horizontal and vertical. When combined with the static stimulus, the conditioning stimulus varies smoothly and cyclically between binocular compatibility and incompatibility.

A test stimulus was delivered to the right eye at various times during the cycle to see how sensitivity varied with time. The test stimulus consisted of a Gabor patch tilted 30° clockwise or counterclockwise from vertical. The subject's task was to say which way it was tilted. Test contrast was varied to find the contrast yielding a fixed level of performance

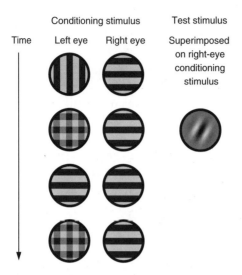

**Figure 3.3** Stimulation sequence in the second experiment. One eye was presented with a static horizontal grating. The other eye was presented with a sum of two orthogonal gratings whose amplitude varied sinusoidally in time at a frequency of 2 Hz, but in antiphase. The net effect was that the conditioning stimulus varied smoothly and cyclically between binocular compatibility and incompatibility. The figure illustrates four samples of the stimulus during one cycle. A test stimulus was superimposed briefly on the right eye's conditioning stimulus to measure contrast sensitivity at a number of times during the cycle. The diameter of the gratings was 1°.

(78% correct). Figure 3.4A shows the results. The horizontal axis gives the time at which the test stimulus was delivered, and the symbols above the axis provide a guide as to the conditioning stimulus at the time of delivery. The vertical axis gives contrast sensitivity, and data for two subjects are shown. Sensitivity is clearly modulated in synchrony with the dynamic conditioning stimulus.

Two aspects of the data indicate that this sensitivity modulation provides a dynamic analogue of the suppression measured during static binocular rivalry. First, sensitivity is least when the monocular conditioning stimuli are most incompatible, and is close to maximum when they are identical. Second, the amplitude of modulation (which averages 28% of mean sensitivity) is close to the loss of sensitivity measured during static rivalry. It seems, therefore, that the dynamic conditioning stimulus provides a way of measuring binocular rivalry suppression without the subjects having to indicate their perceptual state.

A. W. Freeman, V. A. Nguyen, and D. Alais

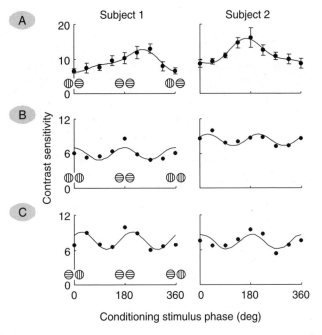

**Figure 3.4** Contrast sensitivity modulation during the dynamic conditioning stimulus cycle. The horizontal axis gives the phase of the cycle, and the schematic stimuli above the axis illustrate the relationship between left- and right-eye conditioning stimuli at selected phases. The vertical axis gives contrast sensitivity to the test stimulus, and data are shown for two subjects. (*A*) The conditioning stimuli cycle between compatibility and incompatibility, with the static stimulus presented to the tested eye. Contrast sensitivity is modulated in synchrony with the dynamic conditioning stimulus. Error bars show 95% confidence intervals, and the lines give the sum of the Fourier fundamental and second harmonic components. (*B*) The left- and right-eye conditioning stimuli are both dynamic and in phase. There can therefore be no interocular suppression. The resulting response is frequency-doubled, and is fitted with a Fourier second harmonic component. (*C*) The conditioning stimuli cycle between compatibility and incompatibility, with the dynamic stimulus presented to the tested eye. There is little or no modulation of sensitivity in synchrony with the stimulus, indicating a lack of interocular suppression. The line again gives the Fourier second harmonic.

Can this experimental protocol also tell us something about the eye suppression versus stimulus suppression issue? The answer is contained in panels B and C of figure 3.4. Panel B shows what happens when the two monocular conditioning stimuli are both dynamic and modulated in phase. The conditioning stimuli are identical in this case, so there can be no interocular suppression. Contrast sensitivity is now modulated at twice the frequency of the conditioning stimuli and is at a minimum when the stimuli are changing fastest. This modulation is presumably due to masking of the (transient) test stimulus by a rapidly changing background.

Panel C shows the result when the conditioning stimulus again varies in and out of binocular compatibility, but this time with the dynamic stimulus presented to the tested eye. Contrast sensitivity is frequency-doubled, indicative of the masking effect seen in figure 3.4B, but with almost no sign of sensitivity modulation in synchrony with the conditioning stimulus. It seems, therefore, that there is little or no interocular suppression in this last configuration.

We interpret this result to mean that the compatibility/incompatibility cycle produces interocular suppression limited to the eye presented with the static component of the conditioning stimulus. This interpretation is corroborated by the reports of our subjects, who said that they saw the dynamic conditioning stimulus but not the static one. It is also consistent with previous findings that the eye receiving the lower "stimulus strength" (in this case, lack of dynamic variation) is the one whose conditioning stimulus is more often suppressed (Levelt, 1965). These data therefore provide additional evidence for the eye suppression hypothesis.

**MODELS FOR SUPPRESSION**

The evidence for eye suppression seems to be clear. There is, however, something unexpected about the results in figure 3.2. Sensitivity during suppression averages 63% of that during dominance. Compare that sensitivity loss with the perceptual change during suppression: all trace of the suppressed stimulus disappears. How do we reconcile the minor sensitivity loss during suppression with the large perceptual loss?

Consider the hypothesis, for example, that the sensitivity and perceptual changes during suppression are mediated by the same group of neurons. The contrast–response function for these neurons is depicted in figure 3.5A, with the curve on the left representing the function during dominance. The contrast threshold during suppression is higher, and the curve during suppression has been shifted a little to the right to represent this observation. Consider now a high-contrast stimulus and its percept. The responses to this stimulus differ little between the dominance and suppression states, suggesting that the percept also will differ little. It is difficult, therefore, to see how the hypothesis of a single suppression site can account for the loss of perception during the suppression state.

We are therefore led to pursue the opposite hypothesis: that sensitivity and perceptual changes during suppression are mediated by more than

A. W. Freeman, V. A. Nguyen, and D. Alais

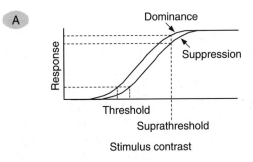

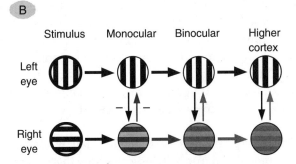

**Figure 3.5**  Models for binocular rivalry suppression. (*A*) The first model assumes that the same population of neurons is responsible for both the sensitivity loss and changes in perception during binocular rivalry. The population's contrast-response function is shown for both the dominance and the suppression phase of rivalry. The small horizontal shift between the two curves reflects the minor change in contrast sensitivity measured in the first two experiments. A consequence of the small shift is that a suprathreshold stimulus evokes similar responses in dominance and suppression. It appears, therefore, that this model cannot account for the large perceptual loss during rivalry. (*B*) The second model assumes that rivalry involves more than one neuronal population. In particular, the visual pathways are assumed to include monocular and binocular processing stages, and a feature-selective stage in higher cortex. A pathway leads from each eye, and there is mutual inhibition between these two pathways at each stage. The figure illustrates suppression of the pathway driven by the right eye; suppression of neurons along the pathway is depicted as a loss of contrast in the gratings representing the stages. Suppression is amplified as the signal progresses to higher cortex. The small changes in sensitivity during rivalry are assumed to be due to the minor suppression at the monocular stage, and perceptual losses are assumed to be due to the large suppressive effects at the feature-selective stage.

one group of neurons. There is a wealth of existing evidence supporting the idea that suppression effects are mediated over more than one area of visual cortex. Psychophysical, physiological, and imaging studies indicate reduced responses during binocular rivalry suppression at the monocular or primary cortical level (Sengpiel, Blakemore, and Harrad, 1995;

Polonsky et al., 2000; Freeman and Nguyen, 2001; Nguyen, Freeman, and Wenderoth, 2001; Tong and Engel, 2001; Lee and Blake, 2002) and also in higher visual cortex (Logothetis and Schall, 1989; Leopold and Logothetis, 1996; Sheinberg and Logothetis, 1997; Tong et al., 1998).

The model in figure 3.5B illustrates this idea. It shows two pathways for processing visual information, one leading from the left eye and the other from the right. The pathways pass through several stages, including monocular cells in primary visual cortex, binocular cells, and a feature-selective area in higher visual cortex. Suppression can occur at each stage, as indicated by the vertical arrows; these arrows indicate inhibition between groups of neurons driven by different eyes or (further along the pathway) tuned to differing visual features. Primary cortical cells presumably can mediate the location judgments made in the experiment of figure 3.2, and would therefore be responsible for the sensitivity changes illustrated in that figure. Perceptual changes due to suppression require a different group of cells, represented by the right side of the model.

Sensitivity losses during suppression are small, while perceptual losses are large. The model in figure 3.5B indicates how this difference may arise. The contrasts of the gratings at each stage of the model show the depth of suppression: low contrasts indicate large losses. A small loss in one pathway at the monocular stage results in a reduced excitatory signal to the next stage of that pathway. Consequently, inhibition at that next stage further disadvantages the suppressed pathway, and the loss there is greater than at the previous stage. Suppressive losses therefore amplify as the signal progresses along the pathway, resulting in deep suppression at the last stage.

**SUPPRESSION DEPTH**

Can increasing depth of binocular rivalry suppression be measured psychophysically? We set out to answer that question in our next experiment, illustrated in figure 3.6. As before, rivalry was induced with incompatible conditioning stimuli (shown in panel A). The stimuli were constructed from lobed circles of the type described by Wilkinson, Wilson, and Habak (1998). Briefly, the radius of the circle was varied sinusoidally around the circumference of the circle so that each cycle of the sinusoid produced one outward lobe. The conditioning stimuli consisted of a four-lobed circle presented to the left eye and an undistorted circle (0 lobes) presented to the right.

A. W. Freeman, V. A. Nguyen, and D. Alais

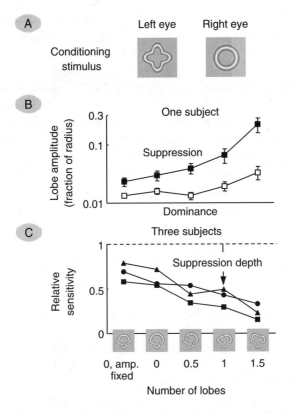

**Figure 3.6** Effect of rivalry on form discrimination. Rivalry was evoked using the conditioning stimulus shown in (*A*). The diameter of the circle and the mean diameter of the lobed circle were 1.3°. A test stimulus was briefly presented to the right eye during its dominance or suppression phase. The schematic stimuli below the horizontal axis in (*C*) illustrate the test stimuli. The subject's task was to indicate which half of the test stimulus had more lobes, and test lobe amplitude was varied to obtain a criterion response. The results for one subject are shown in (*B*). The error bars indicate 95% confidence intervals. (*C*) shows threshold during dominance divided by that during suppression, to indicate suppression depth more clearly. The subject in (*B*) and two others are represented. Suppression depth increases as the task becomes more sophisticated.

Test stimuli were presented to the right eye, and were designed to probe the visual pathway at a variety of levels; the stimuli are illustrated below the horizontal axis in panel C. Each test stimulus consisted of abutting semicircles, one containing two lobes and the other a lesser number of lobes. The two-lobed semicircle appeared with equal probability above or below the other, and the subject's task was to say where it appeared. On any given trial, lobes were randomly located around the circumference of the semicircle to prevent judgments based on single visual field locations. Lobe amplitude was adjusted from trial to trial to obtain 75% correct responses.

Consider the test stimulus (labeled *0, amp. fixed*) at the left end of the axis of panel C. This was an exceptional case in which the undistorted semicircle was not varied in amplitude. The subject's judgment in this case consisted of finding the half of the test stimulus in which there was a contrast change; this judgment presumably could be mediated by primary cortical cells. The judgments represented at the right end of the axis were considerably more sophisticated, in that they depended on the discrimination of a 1.5-lobed semicircle from a 2-lobed one. Discriminations of this type require global shape perception (Hess, Wang, and Dakin, 1999), and therefore presumably depend on activity in higher visual cortex.

Panel B shows thresholds during dominance and suppression for one subject. Panel C shows the threshold ratio for three subjects. At the left side of the graph, sensitivity during suppression averages 69% of that during dominance, a value similar to that obtained for the location judgment depicted in figure 3.2. On the right side, however, suppression is much deeper (repeated-measures $F(1.2, 2.5) = 21.3$; $P = 0.029$): as expected, a sophisticated form discrimination evokes deeper suppression than does a location judgment.

We were keen to discover whether this result applied only to the form discrimination pathway, or whether it was more general. To this end, we tried motion stimuli, as illustrated in figure 3.7. In this case the conditioning stimuli consisted of rotating spirals as represented by the symbols at the right end of the horizontal axis. The test stimulus consisted of an increment or decrement of speed in the right eye's stimulus. The subject was required to indicate whether speed increased or decreased, and the magnitude of the speed change was adjusted to find the level yielding 75% correct performance. To make the motion stimulus less sophisticated, the center of motion was shifted away from the viewing aperture. An infinite offset resulted in drifting gratings, as illustrated at the left end of the axis.

As with the form discrimination experiment, suppression deepens as the motion task becomes more sophisticated (repeated-measures $F(1.5, 4.6) = 13.5$; $P = 0.013$). Our interpretation of this result follows the same lines as before. The judgment of a speed change in a drifting grating presumably depends on activity in primary visual cortex, which contains neurons

A. W. Freeman, V. A. Nguyen, and D. Alais

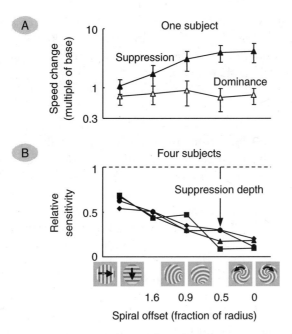

**Figure 3.7**  Effect of rivalry on motion discrimination. The schematic stimuli below the horizontal axis in (*B*) provide examples of the conditioning stimuli used. In each pair, the left and right stimuli were presented to the left and right eyes, respectively. The diameter of the circles was 1°, and arrows represent direction of motion. The test stimulus consisted of a brief speed change in the right eye's stimulus. The vertical axis in (*A*) shows the thresholds during dominance and suppression for one subject. Error bars provide 95% confidence intervals. This subject and three others are represented in (*B*), which shows the ratio of threshold during dominance and suppression. Suppression deepens as the task changes from a judgment of speed in drifting gratings to one in rotating spirals.

responsive to such stimuli. The detection of motion in rotating spirals, by contrast, requires global judgments (Cavanagh and Favreau, 1980) and therefore is presumably subserved by neurons in higher cortex (such as MST) that are specifically responsive to such stimuli (Graziano, Andersen, and Snowden, 1994).

These results dovetail nicely with recent physiological results. Logothetis and his colleagues evoked binocular rivalry in monkeys, and trained them to signal their perceptual state. Neural responses were simultaneously recorded from a variety of areas within the visual cortex. Relatively few primary cortical cells were suppressed in synchrony with the perceptual state (Leopold and Logothetis, 1996), a higher correlation was found in areas such as V4 and MT (Logothetis and Schall, 1989; Leopold and Logothetis, 1996), and in inferior temporal cortex almost all cells were found to have suppression that correlated with the percept (Sheinberg and Logothetis, 1997).

## SPECULATIONS

What do we conclude from these results? When the visual system is confronted with binocularly incompatible stimuli, it responds by suppressing one stimulus or the other. The suppression is relatively small at the monocular stages of the visual cortex. It progresses, however, to full perceptual loss of one monocular stimulus.

The end result of this progression is all-or-nothing: either a rivalrous stimulus is seen or it is not. This all-or-nothing strategy may apply to more than binocular rivalry. Recent work suggests that the same strategy applies in the case of visual attention. D. K. Lee et al. (1999) measured a variety of visual thresholds when attention was fully available for the threshold task and when attention was distracted by a concurrent task irrelevant to the threshold task. Thresholds during the near absence of attention were substantially higher than those during full attention.

Lee et al. modeled their results by calculating the effect of attention on an array of filters processing the visual image; attention sharpened the tuning functions of some filters at the expense of others. They therefore concluded that a winner-take-all strategy underlies attentive behavior. The attended stimulus evokes large responses while unattended stimuli produce negligible responses. This interpretation is supported by physiological findings that attention modulates a local competition between neurons in visual cortex (Desimone, 1998).

Thus there may be parallels between the suppressive processes in binocular rivalry and attention. It remains to be seen whether the buildup of suppression along the visual pathway, as described in this chapter, is one example of a more general mechanism within the sensory brain.

## REFERENCES

Blake, R., and Camisa, J. (1979). On the inhibitory nature of binocular rivalry suppression. *Journal of Experimental Psychology: Human Perception and Performance,* 5, 315–323.

Blake, R., O'Shea, R. P., and Mueller, T. J. (1992). Spatial zones of binocular rivalry in central and peripheral vision. *Visual Neuroscience,* 8, 469–478.

A. W. Freeman, V. A. Nguyen, and D. Alais

Blake, R., Westendorf, D. H., and Overton, R. (1980). What is suppressed during binocular rivalry? *Perception, 9*, 223–231.

Cavanagh, P., and Favreau, O. E. (1980). Motion aftereffect: A global mechanism for the perception of rotation. *Perception, 9*, 175–182.

Desimone, R. (1998). Visual attention mediated by biased competition in extrastriate visual cortex. *Philosophical Transactions of the Royal Society of London*, B353, 1245–1255.

Freeman, A. W., and Nguyen, V. A. (2001). Controlling binocular rivalry. *Vision Research, 41*, 2943–2950.

Graziano, M. S. A., Andersen, R. A., and Snowden, R. J. (1994). Tuning of MST neurons to spiral motions. *Journal of Neuroscience, 14*, 54–67.

Hess, R. F., Wang, Y.-Z., and Dakin, S. C. (1999). Are judgements of circularity local or global? *Vision Research, 39*, 4354–4360.

Lee, D. K., Itti, L., Koch, C., and Braun, J. (1999). Attention activates winner-take-all competition among visual filters. *Nature Neuroscience, 2*, 375–381.

Lee, S. H., and Blake, R. (2002). V1 activity is reduced during binocular rivalry. *Journal of Vision, 2*, 618–626.

Leopold, D. A., and Logothetis, N. K. (1996). Activity changes in early visual cortex reflect monkeys' percepts during binocular rivalry. *Nature, 379*, 549–553.

Levelt, W. J. M. (1965). *On Binocular Rivalry.* Soesterberg, The Netherlands: Institute for Perception RVO-TNO.

Logothetis, N. K., Leopold, D. A., and Sheinberg, D. L. (1996). What is rivalling during binocular rivalry? *Nature, 380*, 621–624.

Logothetis, N. K., and Schall, J. D. (1989). Neuronal correlates of subjective visual perception. *Science, 245*, 761–763.

Makous, W., and Sanders, R. K. (1978). Suppression interactions between fused patterns. In *Visual Psychophysics and Physiology*, A. C. Armington, J. Krauskopf, and B. R. Wooten, eds. New York: Academic Press.

Nguyen, V. A., Freeman, A. W., and Wenderoth, P. (2001). The depth and selectivity of suppression in binocular rivalry. *Perception and Psychophysics, 63*, 348–360.

Phillips, G. C., and Wilson, H. R. (1984). Orientation bandwidths of spatial mechanisms measured by masking. *Journal of the Optical Society of America A, 1*, 226–232.

Polonsky, A., Blake, R., Braun, J., and Heeger, D. J. (2000). Neuronal activity in human primary visual cortex correlates with perception during binocular rivalry. *Nature Neuroscience, 3*, 1153–1159.

Sengpiel, F., Blakemore, C., and Harrad, R. (1995). Interocular suppression in the primary visual cortex: A possible neural basis of binocular rivalry. *Vision Research, 35*, 179–195.

Sheinberg, D. L., and Logothetis, N. K. (1997). The role of temporal cortical areas in perceptual organization. *Proceedings of the National Academy of Sciences of the United States of America, 94*, 3408–3413.

Tong, F., and Engel, S. A. (2001). Interocular rivalry revealed in the human cortical blind-spot representation. *Nature,* 411, 195–199.

Tong, F., Nakayama, K., Vaughan, J. T., and Kanwisher, N. (1998). Binocular rivalry and visual awareness in human extrastriate cortex. *Neuron,* 21, 753–759.

Wilkinson, F., Wilson, H. R., and Habak, C. (1998). Detection and recognition of radial frequency patterns. *Vision Research,* 38, 3555–3568.

Wolfe, J. M. (1983). Influence of spatial frequency, luminance, and duration on binocular rivalry and abnormal fusion of briefly presented dichoptic stimuli. *Perception,* 12, 447–456.

# 4 Investigations of the Neural Basis of Binocular Rivalry

Frank Tong

Consciousness is selective in nature. At any moment, we are aware of only a fraction of the information that saturates our senses. Attentional capacity is one major determinant of awareness—we may fail to attend to the pressure of the socks on our toes, an object in peripheral vision, or the sound of our own breathing, but as soon as attention is directed to a particular modality, attribute, or location, we become conscious of the relevant impression. However, awareness is also determined by more basic forms of perceptual competition that can occur under conditions of sustained voluntary attention. For example, when different monocular patterns are presented to the two eyes, they rival for perceptual dominance such that only one monocular image is perceived at a time while the other is temporarily suppressed from awareness (Levelt, 1965). This phenomenon of binocular rivalry has attracted considerable scientific interest because it effectively dissociates conscious experience from the visual stimulus, and thus provides a powerful tool to investigate the neural correlates and determinants of visual awareness.

This chapter discusses investigations of the neural basis of binocular rivalry with a focus on recent human neuroimaging studies. The compelling phenomenal alternations in rivalry are believed to reflect mutual inhibitory competition between neural signals at some level of visual processing. Controversy surrounds whether rivalry results from competition between pattern-selective binocular neurons in high-level visual areas or between monocular neurons in primary visual cortex (V1) (Blake, 1989; Blake and Logothetis, 2002; Lehky, 1988; Leopold and Logothetis, 1996). Isolating the site at which binocular rivalry first occurs can therefore reveal the underlying competitive neural mechanism and, more generally, may elucidate how competing neural signals are selected for representation in awareness. The first section briefly describes early EEG studies and more recent single-unit studies of binocular rivalry. This is followed by a more detailed discussion of recent human neuroimaging studies and their contribution to our understanding of binocular rivalry.

## RIVALRY STUDIES USING ELECTROENCEPHALOGRAPHY

Electroencephalographic (EEG) recordings from the surface of the human occipital pole provided the first evidence of a neural correlate of conscious perception during binocular rivalry. Lansing (1964) found that steady-state EEG potentials to a monocular flickering light were significantly reduced when a rival static pattern was suddenly introduced to the other eye. Moreover, during steady presentation of the two rival stimuli, periodic suppression of the flickering light was accompanied by weaker steady-state EEG responses. Cobb, Morton, and Ettlinger (1967) investigated binocular rivalry between two oscillating gratings that evoked EEG modulations that were 180° out of phase. The phase of the EEG response tightly corresponded to the observer's report regarding which grating pattern appeared dominant. Moreover, in some subjects rivalry-related responses were as large as those obtained when either grating pattern was presented alone, suggesting that the physiological suppression during rivalry was essentially complete.

More recent EEG studies have measured real-time response modulations to two rival stimuli that are uniquely tagged, using different flickering frequencies (Brown and Norcia, 1997). EEG responses to the two rival gratings fluctuated in close correspondence with reported awareness and were significantly negatively correlated with one another, indicating extensive mutual inhibition. Although the precise source of EEG modulations is difficult to pinpoint, the powerful rivalry modulations found over posterior occipital sites suggest that these effects are evident in early visual areas that lie well outside the inferotemporal cortex.

Magnetoencephalography (MEG), which provides somewhat better source localization than EEG, has also revealed strong rivalry-related responses throughout occipital cortex as well as from some anterior temporal and frontal sites (Tononi et al., 1998). MEG responses during rivalry were about 50–85% of the magnitude of those evoked by physical alternations between the two monocular stimuli. Although the origin of these rivalry-related responses could not be localized precisely, their widespread nature suggested that rivalry interactions occur at an early stage of visual processing, leading to similar rivalry effects at both occipital and anterior sites.

## SINGLE-UNIT STUDIES IN AWAKE, BEHAVING MONKEYS

Unlike the powerful effects of rivalry found in occipital sites in human EEG studies, single-unit studies in alert monkeys have found weaker effects in early visual areas. Only a minority of the neurons recorded in V1, V4, and MT showed significant modulations corresponding to the monkeys' reported perception and, paradoxically, some neurons in V4 and MT were more strongly activated when their preferred stimulus was suppressed during rivalry (Leopold and Logothetis, 1996; Logothetis and Schall, 1989). Only in inferotemporal cortex did most neurons (85%) show significant modulations during rivalry, and rivalry modulations were about half as large as responses evoked by stimulus alternation (Sheinberg and Logothetis, 1997). These findings led to the proposal that rivalry results from competition among incompatible pattern representations at higher levels of the visual pathway, well after inputs from the two eyes have converged in V1.

## FUNCTIONAL MAGNETIC RESONANCE IMAGING STUDIES

### Rivalry in High-Level Extrastriate Areas

The first functional magnetic resonance imaging (fMRI) studies of binocular rivalry investigated the neural correlates of perceptual alternations in high-level visual areas. One study found that frontal–parietal attention-related areas were transiently activated during reported alternations between two rival stimuli, a face stimulus and a motion stimulus, irrespective of which of the two became dominant (Lumer, Friston, and Rees, 1998). Rivalry alternations led to stronger frontal–parietal activations than did unambiguous physical alternations. The authors suggested that frontal-parietal areas might be involved in either mediating or detecting perceptual switches during rivalry. However, behavioral studies suggest that voluntary attention has only a weak influence over binocular rivalry and does not appear to be necessary for rivalry to occur (Leopold, 1997; Meng and Tong, 2002). Moreover, other fMRI studies have found similar frontal–parietal activations when subjects report noticing a change in a challenging change-detection task (Beck et al., 2001), suggesting that these areas are involved in detecting task-relevant changes during rivalry and other attentionally demanding tasks.

My colleagues and I investigated a separate question regarding whether activity in ventral extrastriate cortex is correlated to the content of awareness

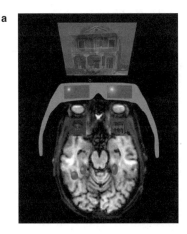

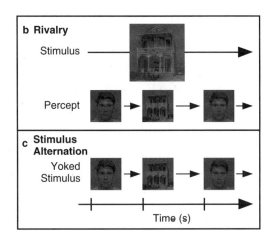

**Figure 4.1** (*a*) Schematic illustration of the binocular rivalry display and extrastriate areas of interest superimposed on a transverse MRI slice. The fusiform face area (FFA; right hemisphere) and parahippocampal place area (PPA; bilateral) are shown. During rivalry scans, a face and a house were continuously presented to different eyes (using red/green filter glasses). Observers reported alternately perceiving only the face or the house for a few seconds at a time, as illustrated in (*b*). (*c*) On stimulus alternation scans, the physical stimulus alternated between the face image and the house image, using the same temporal sequence of alternations reported in a previous rivalry scan. (Modified, with permission, from Tong et al., 1998.) See plate 2 for color version.

during rivalry (Tong et al., 1998). We monitored fMRI activity in two stimulus-selective regions of interest: the fusiform face area (FFA), which responds preferentially to face stimuli, and the parahippocampal place area (PPA), which responds preferentially to house stimuli (figure 4.1a; plate 2a). These brain areas are anterior to V4V and situated at roughly comparable levels of the visual pathway as the inferotemporal cortex in monkeys (Halgren et al., 1999).

On rivalry scans, subjects viewed a face stimulus with one eye and a house with the other eye (figure 4.1b, plate 2b). Although retinal stimulation remained constant, subjects perceived changes from house to face that were accompanied by increasing FFA activity and decreasing PPA activity; perceived changes from face to house led to the opposite pattern of responses. (figure 4.2a). Across the four subjects tested, awareness-related responses during rivalry were 91% as large as those evoked by actual alternations between the face stimulus alone and house stimulus alone, and did not reliably differ in magnitude (figure 4.2b).

The equivalence of rivalry and stimulus alternation suggested that by the time visual information reaches the FFA and PPA, binocular rivalry

**a**                              **Rivalry**

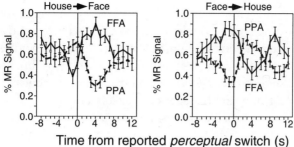

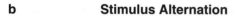

Time from reported *perceptual* switch (s)

**b**                           **Stimulus Alternation**

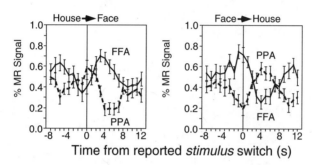

Time from reported *stimulus* switch (s)

**Figure 4.2** Average FFA (solid line) and PPA (dashed line) activity of a representative subject during reported house-to-face switches (left) and face-to-house switches (right) for rivalry (*a*) and stimulus alternation (*b*). Vertical line indicates time of the observer's perceptual report. Note that the BOLD hemodynamic signal typically exhibits a delay of 4–6 sec from initial to peak fMRI response. FFA activity is low before the house-to-face switch because the nonpreferred house was perceived beforehand. Vertical bars represent ±1 SEM. (Reproduced, with permission, from Tong et al., 1998.)

has been fully resolved such that the neural activity in these regions reflects the subject's perceptual state rather than the retinal stimulus. The magnitude of these fMRI effects was considerably larger than those found in inferotemporal neurons in the monkey, where rivalry responses were about half as large as stimulus alternation responses (Sheinberg and Logothetis, 1997). If rivalry is resolved well before these stages of processing, then these findings raise an obvious question: At what stage of the human visual pathway do rivalry competition and awareness-related activity first emerge?

## Rivalry in Primary Visual Cortex

Polonsky et al. (2000) monitored fMRI activity in human primary visual cortex during binocular rivalry between a high-contrast and a low-contrast grating (either moving or counterphasing). Previous studies have shown that fMRI responses in V1 increase monotonically as a function of stimulus contrast (Boynton et al., 1999) and appear to increase linearly as a function of neuronal firing rate (Heeger et al., 2000; Logothetis et al., 2001). If V1 activity reflects conscious perception during rivalry, then one would predict greater fMRI activity during perception of the high-contrast grating and weaker activity during perception of the low-contrast grating.

Consistent with these predictions, Polonsky et al. (2000) found highly reliable V1 response modulations during rivalry (figure 4.3a). These response modulations were about half the magnitude of those evoked by physical alternations between the high-contrast grating and low-contrast

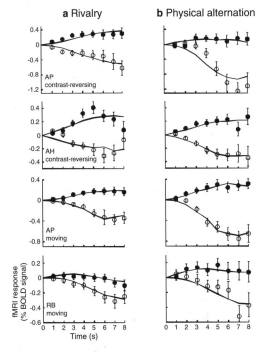

**Figure 4.3** Average fMRI activity in V1 for four subjects during reported switches to the low-contrast grating (open circles) and high-contrast grating (filled circles) for rivalry (*a*) versus physical alternation (*b*). Solid curves represent model fits. (Reproduced, with permission, from Polonsky et al., 2000.)

Frank Tong

grating (figure 4.3b). (Another fMRI study found similar magnitudes of rivalry suppression in V1 using more complex face and house stimuli [Lee and Blake, 2002].) Interestingly, the relative magnitude of fMRI responses for rivalry versus stimulus alternation remained roughly constant across visual areas (V1, 56%; V2, 42%; V3, 46%; V3A, 28%; V4V, 51%).

These findings fail to support the notion that rivalry is gradually resolved among pattern-selective neurons across multiple levels of the visual pathway (Leopold and Logothetis, 1996) and are more consistent with the notion of direct lateral competition in V1. However, Polonsky et al. (2000) were careful to conclude that their results were consistent with interocular competition theory but also amenable to pattern competition theory. Most V1 neurons are binocularly driven and far fewer are strongly monocular. Because this fMRI study could not isolate the activity of monocular V1 cells, it could not directly address whether binocular rivalry arises from competition between monocular neurons or binocular pattern-selective neurons.

### Rivalry in Monocular Visual Cortex

To test the predictions of interocular competition theory, Stephen Engel and I devised a method of measuring fMRI responses in monocular visual cortex (Tong and Engel, 2001). Inputs from the left eye and right eye form alternating bands of ocular dominance columns in human primary visual cortex that are extremely narrow (0.5–1.0 mm; Horton et al., 1990) and difficult to isolate at the resolution of conventional fMRI methods (Cheng, Waggoner, and Tanaka, 2001). However, embedded in these columns is a large monocular region corresponding to the cortical representation of the blind spot. The blind spot is a retinal region devoid of photoreceptors (size $\sim 4 \times 6°$, position $\sim 15°$ medial to fovea; see figure 4.4a, right). In human primary visual cortex, the blind spot is represented as a relatively large monocular region ($\sim 10 \times 5$ mm; J. C. Horton, personal communication) that receives direct input solely from the ipsilateral eye and not from the contralateral blind-spot eye.

To localize the V1 blind-spot representation, subjects first mapped the visual-field location of the right eye's blind spot. During fMRI localization scans, a flickering checkerboard pattern was presented to the subject's left ipsilateral eye or right blind-spot eye in the region of visual space corresponding to the blind spot and its immediate surround (figure 4.4a). Although the blind spot could not register the central portion of the checkerboard, the stimulus nonetheless appeared to be perceptually

Frank Tong

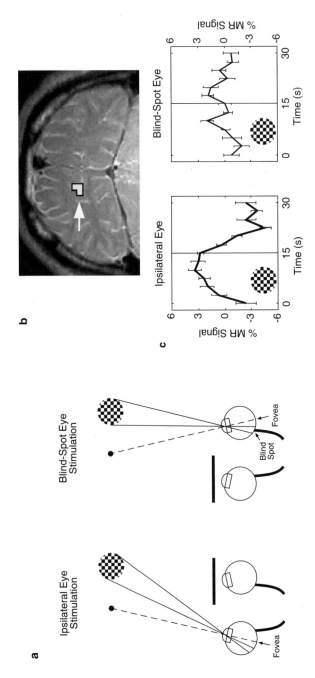

**Figure 4.4**  (*a*) Localization of the V1 blind-spot representation. Subjects maintained fixation on a reference point while viewing a flickering checkerboard pattern (stimulus size 8°, individual check sizes 1°, temporal frequency 7.5 Hz, contrast 100%) with either the left ipsilateral eye or right blind-spot eye. Note how the central portion of the checkerboard falls on the blind spot (optic nerve head, size ~4° × 6°) of the right eye but not of the left eye. (*b*) V1 representation of the right eye's blind spot appears in the left calcarine sulcus (three voxels highlighted in white, slice plane perpendicular to calcarine). (*c*) Average fMRI responses in the V1 blind-spot representation during ipsilateral eye stimulation (left) versus blind-spot eye stimulation (right). Note how this region is activated by ipsilateral stimulation only. (Reproduced, with permission, from Tong and Engel, 2001.)

filled-in due to stimulation of the region surrounding the blind spot. Figure 4.3b shows the V1 blind-spot representation of a representative subject. This region was highly monocular, responding vigorously to ipsilateral-eye stimulation (figure 4.4c, left) and negligibly to blind-spot-eye stimulation (figure 4.4c, right). Having isolated the monocular V1 blind-spot representation, we could now assess the effects of binocular rivalry in monocular visual cortex.

During rivalry scans, subjects viewed dichoptic orthogonal gratings that oscillated back and forth within a stationary circular aperture in the visual location corresponding to the blind spot and its surround (size 8°, contrast 75%, spatial frequency 0.67 cycles/°, speed 2 Hz, direction reversal every 500 msec, mean luminance 3.4 cd/m$^2$). The grating presented to the blind-spot eye was about twice the diameter of the blind spot, so the blind-spot grating appeared to be perceptually filled in. On subsequent stimulus alternation scans, the physical stimulus alternated between monocular presentations of either the ipsilateral grating alone or the blind-spot grating alone, using the same sequence of alternations reported by the subject in a previous rivalry scan.

Subjects reported normal rivalry alternations between the ipsilateral grating and the blind-spot grating with extensive periods of exclusive dominance (94%) and minimal perceptual blending (6% of total duration). The blind-spot surrounding grating effectively suppressed the entire ipsilateral grating, including its central "unpaired" region, which is consistent with the known spatial spread of rivalry interactions (Levelt, 1965). For example, a monocular point stimulus can be suppressed by a surrounding annulus even when the two stimuli do not overlap. In separate psychophysical studies we have confirmed the competitive nature of these interactions encompassing the blind spot. Increasing the contrast of either grating decreased the dominance duration of the opposing grating, as is found in foveal vision (Levelt, 1965).

Interestingly, three out of four subjects showed significantly longer dominance durations for the ipsilateral grating than for the blind-spot grating. These behavioral findings, though preliminary, are consistent with the hypothesis that rivalry dominance depends upon the ratio of monocular neurons activated by each eye (Blake, 1989).

Figure 4.5a reveals that activity in the V1 blind-spot representation was tightly linked to visual awareness during binocular rivalry for all four tested subjects. This monocular region, which receives direct input from only the ipsilateral eye, showed a sharp increase in fMRI activity soon after subjects reported that the ipsilateral grating had become perceptually

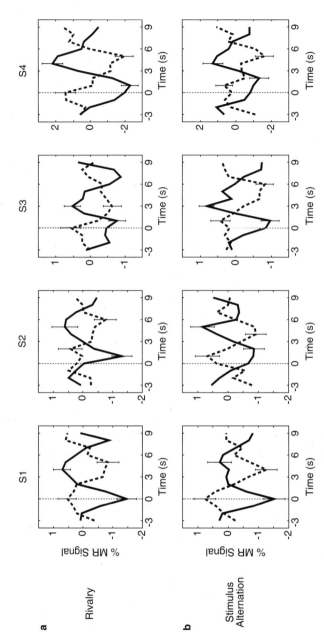

**Figure 4.5** Average fMRI activity in the V1 blind-spot representation during perceptual switches to the ipsilateral grating (solid line) and blind-spot grating (dotted line) for rivalry (a) versus stimulus alternation (b). Data of all four subjects are plotted on individually scaled y-axes. Vertical dotted lines at time 0 indicate the time of the subject's response. (a) During rivalry, fMRI activity sharply increased soon after the ipsilateral grating became dominant in awareness, and decreased when the blind-spot grating became dominant, consistent with the predictions of interocular competition. (b) Very similar fMRI responses occurred during stimulus alternations between the two monocular gratings. All fMRI responses were significant ($F > 4.0$; $p < .05$), and did not reliably differ in magnitude for rivalry versus stimulus alternation ($F < 1$). (Reproduced, with permission, from Tong and Engel, 2001.)

dominant (figure 4.4a, solid line). Conversely, fMRI activity decreased sharply when the blind-spot grating became dominant (dotted line). Thus, the signals from the ipsilateral eye to the V1 blind-spot representation were suppressed when the stimulus entering the competing eye became perceptually dominant. These findings strongly support the predictions of interocular competition theory.

fMRI responses during rivalry (figure 4.4a) were 99% as large as stimulus alternation responses (figure 4.5b) and did not reliably differ in magnitude. The fact that fMRI responses for rivalry and stimulus alternation were indistinguishable suggests that rivalry has been fully resolved among monocular neurons in the V1 blind-spot representation such that neural activity entirely reflects the subject's perceptual state. Thus, functionally equivalent neural responses are observed when the subject's conscious state alternates between the ipsilateral grating and the blind-spot grating during constant rivalry stimulation and when physical stimulus itself alternates between the ipsilateral grating alone and the blind-spot grating alone.

Our results provided the first demonstration that binocular rivalry can be fully resolved in monocular visual cortex, and thus the first physiological evidence to support interocular competition theory. Interocular competition appears to lead to the early selection of only one monocular stimulus for conscious perception and further processing by subsequent visual areas.

**GENERAL DISCUSSION**

The above studies illustrate the progression in understanding of the neural basis of binocular rivalry. Human EEG studies provided the first evidence of rivalry-related activity. Single-unit studies reported weaker effects of rivalry in early visual areas and stronger effects in inferotemporal cortex. fMRI studies found that binocular rivalry appears to be fully resolved by the time visual information reaches anterior extrastriate areas (Tong et al., 1998); that rivalry is evident in primary visual cortex, and these effects are as large as those found in higher areas such as V4 (Polonsky et al., 2000); and that rivalry modulations in monocular visual cortex are as large as those evoked by stimulus alternation, indicating that rivalry may be fully resolved by interocular competition (Tong and Engel, 2001).

These studies provide a possible answer to the question of the neural basis of binocular rivalry but also raise a number of questions. How can one account for the discrepancies between the human neuroimaging results and the single-unit data? Might top-down factors other than interocular competition account for the modulation of monocular neurons during binocular rivalry? What is the relationship between binocular rivalry and pattern rivalry? And what do these results imply about the role of V1 in conscious vision? These issues are discussed below.

## Differences Between Rivalry Studies of V1

Several factors may account for the different magnitudes of rivalry found in area V1 across studies. Although few V1 units showed significant modulations that directly corresponded to perception during rivalry (3/33 units or 9%), across the population of all recorded units, modulations in firing rate for rivalry alternations versus stimulus alternations were more comparable in magnitude for V1 and inferotemporal cortex (33% and 50%, respectively) (Leopold, 1997; Sheinberg and Logothetis, 1997; reanalyzed by Polonsky et al., 2000; Tong et al., 1998). These rivalry modulation indices (RMI) are calculated on the basis of the ratio of response magnitudes for rivalry versus stimulus alternation, where 0% indicates no rivalry modulation and 100% indicates complete rivalry modulations. Given that fMRI activity in V1 increases linearly as a function of local firing rates (Heeger et al., 2000; Logothetis et al., 2001), one would predict that fMRI data should correspond more closely to population estimates of local firing rate rather than to the percentage of individual neurons that show significant rivalry effects.

According to Polonsky et al. (2000), the remaining difference between their fMRI results and the single-unit data (RMI = 56% and 33%, respectively) may reflect any of several factors. These include genuine interspecies differences, the indirect nature of fMRI in estimating neural activity, smaller neuronal sample sizes in single-unit studies, contaminating effects of eye movements on the response of V1 units with small receptive fields, and possible confounding effects of transient responses at the time of perceptual switches. Whereas small static gratings were used in the single-unit studies of V1, large dynamic gratings were used in the human fMRI studies that would ameliorate the effects of small eye movements and any alternations induced by blinks or microsaccades. A further possibility is that the slow hemodynamic fMRI response may have facilitated detection of rivalry-related activity by blurring over the variability in the subject's response times in deciding when to report the exact moment of each rivalry alternation. The high temporal resolution of single-unit recordings might have been more adversely affected by response-time variability.

However, it remains to be explained why our fMRI results in monocular V1 (RMI = 99%) are as different from Polonsky et al.'s fMRI results (56%) as theirs is from the single-unit data (33%). In our view, the demonstration of equivalent rivalry and stimulus alternation responses likely indicates that rivalry can be fully resolved in monocular visual cortex. We have observed such complete rivalry modulations in two independent studies and in three visual areas: the fusiform face area, the parahippocampal place area (RMI for FFA/PPA = 91%), and the monocular V1 blind-spot representation (Tong and Engel, 2001; Tong et al., 1998). Such complete rivalry responses would be difficult to obtain by chance because few studies have demonstrated such equivalence between awareness-related and stimulus-driven neural activity.

By contrast, a finding of weaker rivalry responses does not necessarily indicate that rivalry interactions must continue to occur at higher levels until they are fully resolved. Many factors could dilute the strength of rivalry responses, including (a) inadequate reliability in either the accuracy or the timing of the subject's perceptual report, (b) individual differences in the strength of binocular rivalry (Halpern, Patterson, and Blake, 1987), (c) suboptimal viewing conditions that lead to frequent rivalry-blend percepts, and (d) analysis techniques that fail to exclude poor rivalry periods. Far more perceptual blending was reported by subjects in Polonsky et al.'s study (2000) than in our study (20% vs. 6%). Moreover, Polonsky et al. instructed subjects to report perceptual dominance whenever more than 75% of one stimulus was visible. This liberal criterion for rivalry dominance was chosen because the stimuli were low-contrast, large, and near central vision, factors that greatly increase the extent of piecemeal rivalry.

We used high-contrast, low-spatial-frequency moving gratings in the far periphery to maximize the exclusiveness of rivalry. Subjects were instructed to adopt a very conservative criterion to report exclusive dominance by reporting "blend" whenever they saw any amount of the second stimulus. Moreover, long blend periods (> 1 sec) and short periods of exclusive dominance (< 2 sec) were excluded from the fMRI analysis because they likely indicated short-lived or unreliable rivalry alternations. This filtering technique helped enhance the magnitude of our rivalry effects. When we selectively analyzed the poor rivalry alternations involving long blends or short periods of exclusive dominance, much weaker rivalry effects were observed (Tong et al., 1998; Tong and Engel, 2001; unpublished data). These and other factors might account for the more robust rivalry effects that we found in V1 and extrastriate cortex compared to other fMRI and single-unit studies.

**Might Interocular Rivalry Arise from Feedback Selection?**

Although competition among binocular pattern neurons alone cannot account for the rivalry effects found in monocular visual cortex, it remains possible that feedback signals from binocular neurons to monocular neurons could account for alternating monocular suppression. A recent proposal is that both V1 and extrastriate areas may contribute to grouping and segmentation processes in rivalry, although the precise site(s) of inhibitory competition remain(s) to be resolved (Blake and Logothetis, 2002).

In my view, the rivalry modulations we find in monocular visual cortex demonstrate that under ideal conditions, interocular competition can fully account for the inhibitory mechanism in binocular rivalry. Excitatory feedback projections from pattern-selective binocular neurons to monocular neurons might contribute to the spatial coherence and grouping effects found in binocular rivalry (Kovács et al., 1996). (Piecemeal rivalry remains more difficult to explain.) However, the actual site of inhibitory competition appears to strongly involve monocular neurons (see chapter 3 in this volume), and ultimately some type of mutual inhibition must account for the alternating suppression that characterizes binocular rivalry. At present there is no known mechanism by which binocular neurons might inhibit a specific monocular channel, and most extrinsic connections between visual areas appear to be excitatory rather than inhibitory (Salin and Bullier, 1995). Thus, the notion that feedback inhibition may suppress a monocular channel remains unsubstantiated. Lateral inhibition in higher extrastriate areas might contribute weakly to binocular rivalry in some circumstances but likely plays a greater role in pattern rivalry (see below). In my view, interocular competition likely accounts for most inhibitory interactions in binocular rivalry.

**Binocular Rivalry versus Pattern Rivalry: Separate or Common Mechanisms?**

Another important question is whether binocular rivalry and pattern rivalry reflect common or separate neural mechanisms. During monocular rivalry (Breese, 1899) or stimulus rivalry (Logothetis, Leopold, and Sheinberg, 1996), one can sometimes observe perceptual alternations between two different patterns despite the absence of consistent interocular competition. Although pattern rivalry typically involves weaker perceptual alternations than binocular rivalry and occurs under a more limited set of viewing conditions (e.g., low contrast) (Lee and Blake, 1999; Wade, 1975), some researchers have suggested that both types of phenomena may reflect a common neural mechanism (Andrews and Purves, 1997; Logothetis, Leopold, and Sheinberg, 1996).

However, our fMRI findings in monocular visual cortex suggest that interocular competition has an important role in binocular rivalry, whereas stimulus rivalry is unlikely to involve such an early site of competition. Single-unit recordings in area V1 of anesthetized cats provide some evidence for separate mechanisms of interocular inhibition and pattern-based (cross-orientation) inhibition (Sengpiel et al., 1998). Psychophysical studies have shown that binocular rivalry leads to a selective loss in visual sensitivity for the eye undergoing suppression (Freeman and Nguyen, 2001; Wales and Fox, 1970), whereas such monocular suppression would not occur in pattern rivalry.

I conjecture that the site of perceptual competition may determine the strength and frequency of phenomenal suppression found in various forms of rivalry. Early interocular competition in V1 may be responsible for the vigorous and often complete suppression found in binocular rivalry. By contrast, pattern-based competition in higher visual areas may be responsible for the less frequent and less complete suppression found in pattern rivalry. This proposal leads to the further suggestion that V1 may play an important role in representing the phenomenal visibility of a stimulus.

**The Role of V1 in Visual Awareness**

The powerful effects of binocular rivalry found in V1 demonstrate that neurons can reflect visual awareness at a much earlier level of the visual pathway than previously thought (Crick and Koch, 1995). These results have one of two implications. One possibility is that some aspects of conscious vision begin to emerge at the earliest stage of cortical processing among monocular V1 neurons. Alternatively, these findings may suggest a new role for V1 as the "gatekeeper" of consciousness, a primary cortical region that can select which visual signals gain access to awareness. In either case, primary visual cortex appears to have an important role in binocular rivalry, and perhaps also in conscious vision.

These findings contribute to an ongoing debate regarding the role of V1 in visual awareness (Tong, 2003). According to hierarchical models, V1 provides the necessary input to higher extrastriate areas that are crucial for awareness, but does not directly contribute to awareness per se (Crick and Koch, 1995; Rees, Kreiman, and Koch, 2002). By contrast, interactive models propose that V1 forms dynamic recurrent connections with high-level extrastriate areas, and these integrative loops are necessary for maintaining a representation in awareness (Lamme and Roelfsema, 2000; Pollen, 1999). There is evidence to support both views, although some recent studies suggest that disruption of V1 can impair awareness even when considerable extrastriate activity remains present (Goebel et al., 2001; Pascual-Leone and Walsh, 2001). The fMRI rivalry data further indicate that in the intact network, V1 activity can be tightly linked with visual awareness. Taken together, these findings raise the intriguing possibility that primary visual cortex may have an important and perhaps necessary (though not sufficient) role in conscious vision. Further investigation of V1 and its interactions with higher visual areas might provide important information on the nature of binocular rivalry, bistable perception, perceptual competition, and visual awareness.

## ACKNOWLEDGMENTS

This work was supported by the National Institutes of Health, the James S. McDonnell Foundation, and the Pew Charitable Trusts.

## REFERENCES

Andrews, T. J., and Purves, D. (1997). Similarities in normal and binocularly rivalrous viewing. *Proceedings of the National Academy of Sciences of the United States of America*, 94, 9905–9908.

Beck, D. M., Rees, G., Frith, C. D., and Lavie, N. (2001). Neural correlates of change detection and change blindness. *Nature Neuroscience*, 4, 645–650.

Blake, R. (1989). A neural theory of binocular rivalry. *Psychological Review*, 96, 145–167.

Blake, R., and Logothetis, N. K. (2002). Visual competition. *Nature Reviews: Neuroscience*, 3, 13–21.

Boynton, G. M., Demb, J. B., Glover, G. H., and Heeger, D. J. (1999). Neuronal basis of contrast discrimination. *Vision Research*, 39, 257–269.

Breese, B. B. (1899). On inhibition. *Psychological Monographs*, 3, 1–65.

Brown, R. J., and Norcia, A. M. (1997). A method for investigating binocular rivalry in real-time with the steady-state VEP. *Vision Research*, 37, 2401–2408.

Cheng, K., Waggoner, R. A., and Tanaka, K. (2001). Human ocular dominance columns as revealed by high-field functional magnetic resonance imaging. *Neuron,* 32, 359–374.

Cobb, W. A., Morton, H. B., and Ettlinger, G. (1967). Cerebral potentials evoked by pattern reversal and their suppression in visual rivalry. *Nature,* 216, 1123–1125.

Crick, F., and Koch, C. (1995). Are we aware of neural activity in primary visual cortex? *Nature,* 375, 121–123.

Freeman, A. W., and Nguyen, V. A. (2001). Controlling binocular rivalry. *Vision Research,* 41, 2943–2950.

Goebel, R., Muckli, L., Zanella, F. E., Singer, W., and Stoerig, P. (2001). Sustained extrastriate cortical activation without visual awareness revealed by fMRI studies of hemianopic patients. *Vision Research,* 41, 1459–1474.

Halgren, E., Dale, A. M., Sereno, M. I., Tootell, R. B., Marinkovic, K., and Rosen, B. R. (1999). Location of human face-selective cortex with respect to retinotopic areas. *Human Brain Mapping,* 7, 29–37.

Halpern, D. L., Patterson, R., and Blake, R. (1987). Are stereoacuity and binocular rivalry related? *American Journal of Optometry and Physiological Optics,* 64, 41–44.

Heeger, D. J., Huk, A. C., Geisler, W. S., and Albrecht, D. G. (2000). Spikes versus BOLD: What does neuroimaging tell us about neuronal activity? *Nature Neuroscience,* 3, 631–633.

Horton, J. C., Dagi, L. R., McCrane, E. P., and De Monasterio, F. M. (1990). Arrangement of ocular dominance columns in human visual cortex. *Archives of Ophthalmology,* 108, 1025–1031.

Kovács, I., Papathomas, T. V., Yang, M., and Fehér, A. (1996). When the brain changes its mind: Interocular grouping during binocular rivalry. *Proceedings of the National Academy of Sciences of the United States of America,* 93, 15508–15511.

Lamme, V. A., and Roelfsema, P. R. (2000). The distinct modes of vision offered by feedforward and recurrent processing. *Trends in Neuroscience,* 23, 571–579.

Lansing, R. W. (1964). Electroencephalographic correlates of binocular rivalry in man. *Science,* 146, 1325–1327.

Lee, S. H., and Blake, R. (1999). Rival ideas about binocular rivalry. *Vision Research,* 39, 1447–1454.

Lee, S. H., and Blake, R. (2002). V1 activity is reduced during binocular rivalry. *Journal of Vision,* 2, 618–626.

Lehky, S. R. (1988). An astable multivibrator model of binocular rivalry. *Perception,* 17, 215–228.

Leopold, D. A. (1997). Brain mechanisms of visual awareness. Ph.D. dissertation, Baylor College of Medicine.

Leopold, D. A., and Logothetis, N. K. (1996). Activity changes in early visual cortex reflect monkeys' percepts during binocular rivalry. *Nature,* 379, 549–553.

Levelt, W. J. M. (1965). *On Binocular Rivalry.* Soesterberg, The Netherlands: Institute for Perception RVO-TNO.

Logothetis, N. K., Leopold, D. A., and Sheinberg, D. L. (1996). What is rivalling during binocular rivalry? *Nature, 380,* 621–624.

Logothetis, N. K., Pauls, J., Augath, M., Trinath, T., and Oeltermann, A. (2001). Neurophysiological investigation of the basis of the fMRI signal. *Nature, 412,* 150–157.

Logothetis, N. K., and Schall, J. D. (1989). Neuronal correlates of subjective visual perception. *Science, 245,* 761–763.

Lumer, E. D., Friston, K. J., and Rees, G. (1998). Neural correlates of perceptual rivalry in the human brain. *Science, 280,* 1930–1934.

Meng, M., and Tong, F. (2002). Can attention bias bistable perception? Differences between rivalry and ambiguous figures. *Journal of Vision, 2,* 447a.

Pascual-Leone, A., and Walsh, V. (2001). Fast backprojections from the motion to the primary visual area necessary for visual awareness. *Science, 292,* 510–512.

Pollen, D. A. (1999). On the neural correlates of visual perception. *Cerebral Cortex, 9,* 4–19.

Polonsky, A., Blake, R., Braun, J., and Heeger, D. J. (2000). Neuronal activity in human primary visual cortex correlates with perception during binocular rivalry. *Nature Neuroscience, 3,* 1153–1159.

Rees, G., Kreiman, G., and Koch, C. (2002). Neural correlates of consciousness in humans. *Nature Reviews: Neuroscience, 3,* 261–270.

Salin, P. A., and Bullier, J. (1995). Corticocortical connections in the visual system: Structure and function. *Physiological Reviews, 75,* 107–154.

Sengpiel, F., Baddeley, R. J., Freeman, T. C. B., Harrad, R., and Blakemore, C. (1998). Different mechanisms underlie three inhibitory phenomena in cat area 17. *Vision Research, 38,* 2067–2080.

Sheinberg, D. L., and Logothetis, N. K. (1997). The role of temporal cortical areas in perceptual organization. *Proceedings of the National Academy of Sciences of the United States of America, 94,* 3408–3413.

Tong, F. (2003). Primary visual cortex and visual awareness. *Nature Reviews Neuroscience, 4,* 219–229.

Tong, F., and Engel, S. A. (2001). Interocular rivalry revealed in the human cortical blind-spot representation. *Nature, 411,* 195–199.

Tong, F., Nakayama, K., Vaughan, J. T., and Kanwisher, N. (1998). Binocular rivalry and visual awareness in human extrastriate cortex. *Neuron, 21,* 753–759.

Tononi, G., Srinivasan, R., Russell, D. P., and Edelman, G. M. (1998). Investigating neural correlates of conscious perception by frequency-tagged neuromagnetic responses. *Proceedings of the National Academy of Sciences of the United States of America, 95,* 3198–3203.

Wade, N. J. (1975). Monocular and binocular rivalry between contours. *Perception, 4,* 85–95.

Wales, R., and Fox, R. (1970). Increment detection thresholds during binocular rivalry suppression. *Perception and Psychophysics, 8,* 90–94.

# 5    Parallel Pathways and Temporal Dynamics in Binocular Rivalry

## Sheng He, Thomas Carlson, and Xiangchuan Chen

What we experience during binocular rivalry, alternating views of two conflicting monocular stimuli, is the final product of many steps in the visual information-processing pathway. Consequently, one of the central debates in the study of binocular rivalry is whether the neural mechanism for rivalry is located at the early or late stages of processing, often phrased as a debate between eye rivalry and stimulus rivalry (Blake and Overton, 1979; S. H. Lee and Blake, 1999; Leopold and Logothetis, 1999; Logothetis, Leopold, and Sheinberg, 1996). Over the years, many experiments have yielded important insights into the nature of rivalry, and the recent consensus seems to be that this complex phenomenon has multiple neural components (Blake and Logothetis, 2002). In the discussions of rivalry's site, however, little attention has been given to the fact that the visual system consists of parallel pathways, with the consequent possibility that the different pathways or channels may contribute differently to binocular rivalry. The most prominent parallel pathways in the early visual system are the magnocellular (M) and parvocellular (P) pathways. In the first section of this chapter we summarize the experimental data regarding the M and P pathways and their role in the binocular rivalry phenomenon. We believe that the evidence supports the view that the P pathway is more involved in binocular rivalry than the M pathway.

Turning to another important characteristic of rivalry, one of the keys to understanding binocular rivalry lies in elucidating its temporal characteristics. Although progress has been made on the behavioral description and modeling of the temporal characteristics (Blake, Westendorf, and Fox, 1990; Mueller and Blake, 1989), the neural basis of the dynamic control of rivalry is still lacking. In the second half of this chapter, we present some preliminary evidence to support the hypothesis that control of temporal dynamics during binocular rivalry is likely a local process.

# BINOCULAR RIVALRY IN PARALLEL PATHWAYS

## The M and P Pathways

The origins of the parallel pathways can be traced back to the retina. Parasol cells in the retina project to geniculate magnocellular layers that project mainly to layers $4\alpha$ and $4\beta$, and their output is projected to motion-sensitive extrastriate areas. Midget cells in the retina project to geniculate parvocellular layers of the LGN that in turn project to the V1 blob and interblob cells, which then project more dominantly to extrastriate areas that are sensitive to form and color (Dacey, 1994; DeYoe and Van Essen, 1988; B. B. Lee, 1996; Livingstone and Hubel, 1987a, 1988). Following accepted convention, this chapter terms these two the M and P pathways, respectively.

Neurons in these two pathways differ both morphologically and functionally. The parasol ganglion cells in the retina and the magnocellular cells in the LGN have large cell bodies, thick axons, and fast conductance of signal. The midget ganglion cells in the retina and the parvocellular cells in the LGN have smaller cell bodies, thinner axons, and slower conduction speed. Magnocellular cells are tuned to lower spatial frequency and higher temporal frequency signals than are the parvocellular cells. Moreover, the contrast response function for magnocellular cells shows higher gain and earlier saturation. Parvocellular cells are color opponent, and are tuned to higher spatial frequency and lower temporal frequency stimuli than are the magnocellular cells. Their contrast response is more linear.

These two neural pathways are believed to support two functionally distinct channels in vision, sometimes labeled the transient (M) and sustained (P) channels, thus emphasizing the difference in their temporal properties (Kulikowski and Tolhurst, 1973; Legge, 1978; Tolhurst, 1977). They have also been referred to as the broadband (M) and the color opponent (P) channels to emphasizes the difference in their responses to color (Derrington and Lennie, 1984; Schiller, Logothetis, and Charles, 1990b).

The segregation of the two pathways is relatively well preserved up to V1, but evidence for robust interactions between them is found in later visual areas. In the cortex, the two major anatomically distinct pathways are the dorsal action pathway and the ventral perception pathway (DeYoe and Van Essen, 1988). There is a loose link from the M pathway to the action pathway and from the P pathway to the perception pathway, but it should be noted that the selectivity of these two pathways

S. He, T. Carlson, and X. Chen

represents biases rather than exclusiveness (Maunsell, 1992). However, given the bias of these two pathways, it is reasonable to evaluate their roles in binocular rivalry.

## Evidence That Rivalry Happens Primarily in the P Pathway

While there is little mention of the parallel pathways in the binocular rivalry literature, there are a large number of studies on the influence of stimulus properties on binocular rivalry, studies that can be reinterpreted within the context of parallel pathways. Not surprisingly, the more "different" the two stimuli are, the more likely it is that they will engage in binocular rivalry. The question is whether differences along some feature dimensions are more effective than others. Generally speaking, stimuli that are high in luminance contrast, rich in contours, and small in size, and have opponent colors tend to generate strong rivalry (e.g., a high-contrast red horizontal grating presented to the left eye and high-contrast green vertical grating presented to the right eye). Conversely, stimuli that are low in contrast, have sparse contours, or differ only in temporal frequency are less likely to induce rivalry (e.g., a gray disk flickering at 2 Hz in one eye and a gray disk flickering at 10 Hz in the other eye). Mapping the properties of strong rival stimuli and weak rival stimuli back to the P and M pathways, it appears that stimuli which are processed predominantly in the M pathway are not good rivalry stimuli. Below we examine in more detail how different stimulus properties influence rivalry.

**Luminance Contrast and Rivalry**   M neurons show a nonlinear response with increased sensitivity for low-contrast stimuli (Shapley and Perry, 1986). Their responses also tend to saturate at relatively low contrast levels. P neurons show a more linear response and rarely saturate (Derrington and Lennie, 1984). Thus stimuli with low spatial frequency and low contrast presumably favor the M pathway, while stimuli with high spatial frequency and high contrast favor the P system.

The effect of luminance contrast on rivalry is consistent with a greater involvement of the P pathway in rivalry. Increasing the contrast of the two rival stimuli increases the rate of alternation (Alexander, 1951; Levelt, 1965, 1966). High-contrast images have shorter periods of suppression (Bossink, Stalmeier, and De Weert, 1993; Fox and Rasche, 1969; Levelt, 1967; Mueller and Blake, 1989; Whittle, 1965), and dominate longer (Bossink, Stalmeier, and De Weert, 1993; Mueller and Blake, 1989). It is not surprising that increasing contrast affects rivalry, because it represents an increase in the strength of the stimulus. What is important to note is that many of these studies examined contrast levels well beyond the saturation point of the M pathway and rivalry was found to be sensitive to these manipulations, supporting the P pathway's important role in binocular rivalry.

Given the M pathway's high sensitivity to low-contrast stimuli, it is of particular interest to note that rivalry is difficult to generate for low-contrast stimuli (Bossink, Stalmeier, and De Weert, 1993; Liu, Tyler, and Schor, 1992). At low contrast, when orthogonal gratings are dichoptically presented, they tend to fuse into a dichoptic plaid (Burke, Alais, and Wenderoth, 1999; Liu, Tyler, and Schor, 1992). The time necessary to engage rivalry is also substantially longer for low-contrast stimuli (Liu, Tyler, and Schor, 1992). Interocular integration at low contrast supports the hypothesis that the M pathway makes little contribution to rivalry. However, an alternative interpretation is that the mechanism which engages rivalry requires a minimal conflict threshold to induce suppression (Blake, 1977).

**Spatial Frequency and Rivalry**  The receptive field sizes of M neurons are two to three times larger than those for P neurons at a given eccentricity (Derrington and Lennie, 1984). Consequently, fine spatial details are processed predominantly in the P pathway. It was reported that high-spatial-frequency dichoptic patterns are easier to fuse between the two eyes, and this was the key evidence for Livingstone and Hubel to propose that rivalry is a property of the M pathway (Hollins, 1980; Livingstone and Hubel, 1987b). However, O'Shea and colleagues noted that the large field used in Livingstone's stimulus was not appropriate for addressing the question of spatial frequency dependence of rivalry. When smaller field sizes were tested, observers increasingly perceived rivalry (O'Shea, Sims, and Govan, 1997). They concluded that high-spatial-frequency stimuli can induce rivalry. Another possible confound in the original Livingstone and Hubel observation is the contrast levels. The effective neural contrast of the high-spatial-frequency patterns is lower than that of the low-spatial-frequency patterns.

Blake (1977) measured the rivalry contrast threshold (the minimum contrast required to induce rivalry) across spatial frequencies and found it to be in good agreement with the detection threshold for monocular gratings. Liu and colleagues further measured contrast thresholds across spatial frequencies for perceiving dichoptic plaids and for perceiving rivalry (Liu, Tyler, and Schor, 1992). They found that the fusion of dichoptic plaid was present across the spatial frequency spectrum. The thresholds for

S. He, T. Carlson, and X. Chen

perceiving dichoptic plaids were lower than the rivalry threshold, with a relatively constant offset.

These two studies seem to represent a challenge to the hypothesis that rivalry occurs primarily in the P pathway, since this hypothesis would predict that the contrast threshold for perceiving rivalry should follow the P pathway contrast sensitivity, while the threshold for perceiving dichoptic plaids should follow the M pathway contrast sensitivity function more. Resolving this issue requires the use of stimuli that more specifically target the M and P pathways, for example, with manipulation of the temporal frequencies in addition to the spatial frequencies.

**Flicker and Rivalry**   M neurons are more responsive to high-temporal-frequency information than P neurons (Derrington and Lennie, 1984), which is consistent with psychophysical measurements of flicker fusion frequency: purely chromatic flicker becomes invisible at a much lower temporal frequency than does luminance-defined flicker (DeLange, 1958). Indeed, several groups have suggested that temporal frequency can be manipulated to bias stimuli to favor either the M or the P system (Livingstone and Hubel, 1987b; Schiller and Logothetis, 1990).

Transient information seems to be immune to the rivalry process, as evidenced by the tendency of briefly presented rival figures to fuse (Anderson, Bechtoldt, and Gregory, 1978; Bower and Haley, 1964; Goldstein, 1970; Hering, 1964; Kaufman, 1963; Wade, 1973; Wolfe, 1983a, 1983b). O'Shea and Crassini (1984) found that simultaneous stimulation of the two eyes is not required to produce rivalry. If the right and left eyes' stimuli are alternated at a temporal frequency as low as 3 Hz, observers can perceive rivalry, and for temporal frequencies above 20 Hz, it is perceptually indistinguishable from normal rivalry. The implication of these observations is that the mechanism which supports rivalry has a sustained response, a characteristic of the P pathway.

Perhaps the most direct evidence of transient information's immunity to rivalry comes from a study by O'Shea and Blake (1986). They found that dramatic differences in temporal frequency of two flickers failed to generate rivalry.

**Color and Rivalry**   The P pathway is the primary pathway in color vision. Most parvocellular cells in the LGN are color opponent (Derrington, Krauskopf, and Lennie, 1984; Schiller, Logothetis, and Charles, 1990a). This is in contrast to the broadband response found for the magnocellular cells, which are essentially color-blind.

Livingstone and Hubel's suggestion that rivalry is a phenomenon of the M pathway was based, in part, on their experiments with rivalry and equiluminant color stimuli (Livingstone and Hubel, 1987b). Their conclusion was based on the observation that it was easier to fuse orthogonal red and green gratings between the two eyes at equiluminance. Unfortunately, this observation is confounded with the level of contrasts in the stimuli. Many studies have shown that interocular color differences induce strong rivalry (Kulikowski, 1992). Moreover, introducing conflicting color information to rival stimuli can extend the duration of periods of exclusive dominance and decrease the incidence of fusion between the two stimuli (Hollins and Leung, 1978; Wade, 1975). Even short-wavelength cones, with little contribution to the luminance pathway, are capable of generating rivalry (O'Shea and Williams, 1996). Rivalry suppression has also been found to have a dramatic effect on color vision (Smith et al., 1982). In fact, color sensitivity is more affected than luminance sensitivity by rivalry suppression (Ooi and Loop, 1994).

**Motion and Rivalry** The M pathway is generally considered to be crucially involved in motion processing (Livingstone and Hubel, 1988; Schiller, Logothetis, and Charles, 1990a). Yet, at the same time, it is also believed that conflicting motion between the two eyes can cause rivalry, an observation that would seem inconsistent with the hypothesis that the P pathway dominates rivalry. However, two factors need to be considered when attempting to reconcile this inconsistency: first, conflicting motion information is usually confounded with conflicting spatial information; and second, although the M pathway is dominant in motion perception, the P pathway is capable of processing slow motion (Schiller and Logothetis, 1990).

One way to avoid conflicting spatial information in a motion stimulus is through the use of motion aftereffects (MAE). Ramachandran (1991) adapted his two eyes to opposing directions of motion and then looked at a static grating. With either eye alone, he saw motion in the opposite direction of the adapting motion. When viewing the same grating with both eyes, neither motion nor rivalry was perceived. This result suggests that a conflicting motion signal in the absence of a pattern conflict is not sufficient to induce rivalry. Blake and colleagues confirmed this observation, but added that by using a dynamic test stimulus, conflicting motion signals generated by the MAE could induce binocular rivalry (Blake et al., 1998). They interpreted this result as a challenge to the view that the M pathway is spared from rivalry.

S. He, T. Carlson, and X. Chen

However, there has been extensive evidence that dynamic and static test patterns are tapping separate neural mechanisms (Culham et al., 1998). One finding of particular relevance is that dynamic test patterns can achieve perfect interocular transfer (Nishida, Ashida, and Sato, 1994), which suggests that MAEs generated with dynamic test patterns are based on a neural population after the stage of binocular integration. Static MAE test stimuli, however, show only partial transfer of the MAE. These results suggest that a conflicting motion signal originating early in the system, in the absence of pattern conflict, is not sufficient to induce binocular rivalry.

Another possible way to reduce the salience of the spatial conflict between the two motion signals is to place the two moving gratings behind identical matrix windows (figure 5.1). Locally, each element produces conflicting information in the temporal domain between the two eyes, which has been shown not to induce rivalry (O'Shea and Blake, 1986). Globally, each eye's display contains a strong motion signal. When these displays are dichoptically presented with opposing motion signals in the two eyes, observers perceive a nearly complete fusion of the two

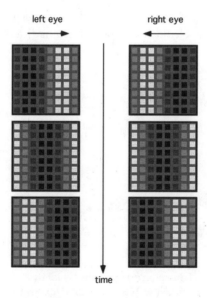

**Figure 5.1** Two moving gratings behind identical matrix windows. The identical grid patterns in the two eyes facilitate fusion between the two eyes. Although the left and right eyes' displays contain strong motion signals moving in opposite directions, they fail to induce binocular rivalry.

eyes' stimuli and not rivalry (unpublished observations). These results suggest that it is the local spatial conflict accompanying motion signals which generate rivalry, and not motion per se.

Because increasing the temporal frequency of motion signals increasingly biases the processing to the M pathway (Schiller and Logothetis, 1990), the hypothesis that rivalry is biased on the P pathway predicts that the strength of rivalry should depend on the temporal frequency of the moving stimuli. We tested this prediction by measuring the incidence of rivalry (as indexed by the proportion of time with exclusive visibility of one or the other stimulus) as a function of the temporal frequency of the motion stimuli (Carlson and He, 2000). Our results indeed show that as the temporal frequency increases, the competing motion becomes much less likely to rival (figure 5.2). However, a more recent report seemed to be inconsistent with our hypothesis (Van de Grind et al., 2001). It showed that when the conflicting motion signals are processed in the same temporal channels (e.g., slow vs. slow or fast vs. fast), observers see rivalry; but when the conflicting motion signals are processed in different temporal channels (e.g., slow vs. fast), observers see "dichoptic motion transparency."

Further studies are needed to resolve the discrepancies between our study and the one by Van de Grind et al. One important difference between

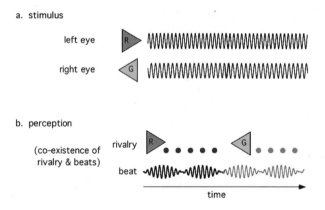

a. stimulus

left eye

right eye

b. perception

(co-existence of rivalry & beats)

rivalry

beat

time

**Figure 5.2** Schematic depiction of the co-occurrence of binocular rivalry and beats. (*a*) The left eye and the right eye were presented with two stimuli of different shapes and colors, both flickering at fast but slightly different frequencies. (*b*) Perceptual experience: shape and color differences induced strong rivalry, yet the slow beat could be seen clearly even when one of the stimuli contributing to the beat was not visible. (Adapted from Carlson and He, 2000.)

S. He, T. Carlson, and X. Chen

the two studies is the duration of stimulus presentation. In our study, observers had minutes to track their percept; in the Van de Grind study, the stimuli were presented for 1 sec in most conditions. It is also worth noting that in their study, observers were given only two response options: transparency or rivalry. It might be possible that all "nontransparent" trials were classified as rivalry, but in fact they could be nontransparent fusion of the two eyes' signals.

## Coexistence of Binocular Competition and Integration

One group of experiments deserves special attention when considering the interactions of information between the two eyes. These experiments show that some visual information is combined (integrated) between the two eyes even when the two eyes' stimuli are engaged in rivalry.

**Integration and Suppression of Motion During Rivalry**  Motion signals have been shown to integrate between the two eyes during rivalry (Andrews and Blakemore, 1999, 2002; Carney, Shadlen, and Switkes, 1987). In other words, the pattern that carries the motion may be engaged in rivalry, but the perceived direction is a result of integrating both eyes' signals (see chapter 11 in this volume).

There is sufficient evidence to suggest that components of the motion signals are preserved during suppression. Input from the suppressed eye to apparent motion is reduced, but not eliminated, for both long-range and short-range apparent motion (Wiesenfelder and Blake, 1991). Cues presented during the suppression phase of rivalry can bias ambiguous motion stimuli (Blake, Ahlstrom, and Alais, 1999). Motion adaptation studies have found that the translational MAE can survive suppression (Lehmkuhle and Fox, 1975). This finding cannot be extended to adaptation to complex motion stimuli, such as expansion, rotation, and pattern motion (Blake, 1995; Blake et al., 1998; Van der Zwan, Wenderoth, and Alais, 1993; Wiesenfelder and Blake, 1990). The results of these studies have strong implications for locus of suppression of motion signals. Simple motion signals appear to be immune to suppression. Higher-order motion signals, presumably mediated by extrastriate areas such as MT and MST, are largely suppressed.

**Stereopsis from Rival Stimuli**  For decades, the M pathway has been considered the dominant pathway in stereopsis (Hubel and Livingstone, 1987, 1990; Livingstone and Hubel, 1987a, 1987b). The idea that stereopsis is supported by the M pathway and binocular rivalry occurs primarily in the P pathway leads to the prediction of coexistence of these two phenomena. However, more recent evidence suggests that the M and P pathways both contribute to stereopsis, with the M pathway biased to the more qualitative, coarse stereo processing and the P pathway biased to the more quantitative, fine stereo matching (Kontsevich and Tyler, 2000).

Similarly, the coexistence of stereopsis matching and rivalry has been a hotly disputed subject. There are experiments and models showing that stereo perception can occur when the two images are superimposed on strongly rivalrous pairs (Julesz and Miller, 1975; Treisman, 1962; Wolfe, 1986), as well as experiments showing that stereopsis is disrupted during binocular rivalry (Amira, 1988; Blake and O'Shea, 1988; Blake, Yang, and Wilson, 1991). More recently, Harrad and colleagues found that rivalry suppression indeed initially disrupts stereopsis matching for 150–200 ms, but after that time stereopsis can overcome rivalry suppression (Harrad et al., 1994).

**Perceiving Binocular Beats During Rivalry**  Two dichoptically presented flickering stimuli with high but slightly different temporal frequencies will lead to the perception of binocular beats (Baitch and Levi, 1989; Karrer, 1967), which result from integration of luminance information from the two eyes. If rivalry were indeed occurring in the P pathway, then given that fast flicker signals are processed primarily in the M pathway, a strong prediction would be that binocular beats could be perceived even when the flickering stimuli themselves were engaged in rivalry. We tested whether binocular beats can be perceived at the same time and at the same spatial location with binocular rivalry (Carlson and He, 2000).

In this experiment, a red LED flickering at 28 Hz and a green LED flickering at 30 Hz were presented to the left and right eye, respectively. The two LEDs differed in their shape, color, and temporal frequency. The shape and color differences between the two eyes' stimuli induced strong rivalry. Interestingly, observers also perceived binocular beats, a 2 Hz modulation of luminance fluctuation, at the time when only one of the two stimuli was visible (figure 5.3). This indicates that binocular integration of luminance information can occur at the same time and within the same spatial location as binocular rivalry. Because high-frequency flicker (~30 Hz) is processed primarily in the M pathway, and color and shape information is processed mainly in the P pathway, we took this result as strong evidence supporting the hypothesis that rivalry resulted from the

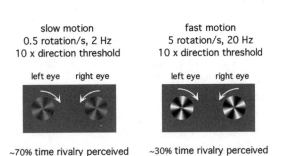

slow motion
0.5 rotation/s, 2 Hz
10 x direction threshold

fast motion
5 rotation/s, 20 Hz
10 x direction threshold

left eye    right eye          left eye    right eye

~70% time rivalry perceived     ~30% time rivalry perceived

**Figure 5.3** Two radial gratings rotating in opposite directions were presented dichoptically to observers. The grating contrasts were set to ten times the direction-discrimination threshold. At low speed (0.5 rotation per sec, 2 Hz) observers perceived the two opposite motions in rivalry about 70% of the time, whereas at high speed (five rotations per sec, 20 Hz) observers saw rivalry about 30% of the time. (Adapted from Carlson and He, 2000.)

interocular difference in visual attributes that are processed predominantly in the P pathway. Interocular differences in visual attributes that are processed predominantly in the M pathway tend to integrate.

### Some Conjectures on Why the P and M Pathways Play Different Roles in Binocular Rivalry

The experiments reviewed above imply that binocular rivalry is not an all-inclusive phenomenon spanning the full range of stimulus conditions activating the P and M pathways. When one input is inhibited during the rivalry process, not all properties associated with this stimulus are inhibited. Some of the properties are relatively immune to rivalry inhibition. Our hypothesis is that transient properties processed primarily in the M pathway are relatively immune to binocular rivalry. Rivalry is primarily a P pathway phenomenon.

At the anatomical and neurophysiological level, this differential role of the two pathways may reflect the different interocular connections in the P and M pathways. At the functional level, a more abstract idea is that properties processed in the P pathway are more critical in determining the stimulus identity, whereas properties processed in the M pathway are contributing more to the object's variable attributes and its environmental property rather than its identity. Two different identities (discrete variable) cannot be fused, but the system would benefit from some sort of averaging for the object attributes (continuous variable). It is also possible that conscious awareness is largely a property of the P pathway.

Parallel Pathways and Temporal Dynamics

# TEMPORAL CHARACTERISTICS OF BINOCULAR RIVALRY

## Rivalry Rates Are Asymmetrical across Visual Fields

The essence of binocular rivalry lies in its temporal fluctuations. Naturally, understanding binocular rivalry requires a full account of its dynamics. Many classical findings in binocular rivalry concern its dynamic properties. For example, increasing the strength of one stimulus (e.g., contrast or contour density) causes the suppression durations for that stimulus to become briefer (Levelt, 1965; see also chapters 8 and 17 in this volume). It is also well established that rivalry takes time to initiate, and briefly presented stimuli usually fuse (Wolfe, 1983b).

In this section, we examine a more specific issue in the temporal characteristics of binocular rivalry, its visual field dependence and potential asymmetries across visual fields. A number of studies have shown that rivalry rate varies tremendously at different eccentricities (Blake, O'Shea, and Mueller, 1992; Fahle, 1987). But the picture is less clear on the left–right and upper–lower asymmetry in binocular rivalry. In the early twentieth century, Breese reported his observations on rivalry in the right, left, upper, and lower visual field (Breese, 1909). Because he reported only his own observations, it is difficult to draw firm conclusions, but his data did show a somewhat faster rivalry alternation for the lower visual field than for the upper visual field, and very little difference between the right and left visual fields.

Much more recently, O'Shea and Corballis studied rivalry rate in split-brain and normal observers (see chapter 16 in this volume). The two split-brain observers had slightly higher alternation rates for stimuli presented to the left visual field compared with those to the right visual field, but this kind of asymmetry seemed to be in the opposite direction in the four normal control observers (O'Shea and Corballis, 2001).

A well-known finding in vision is the temporal–nasal hemiretina asymmetry with the nasal hemiretina usually dominant, especially for far periphery. This is true for competing colors presented for short durations (Crovitz, 1964; Crovitz and Lipscomb, 1963). Conflicting reports exist for the nasal–temporal field asymmetry for rivalry dominance. Fahle (1987) reported that the nasal hemiretina dominates over the temporal hemiretina in the far periphery, but Kaushall (1975) found that the uncrossed visual pathways (temporal hemiretinas) are dominant over the crossed pathways (nasal hemiretinas) in a binocular rivalry task.

S. He, T. Carlson, and X. Chen

In a recent study, we systematically investigated visual-field asymmetries in rivalry rate in both right-handed and left-handed observers. Our results show that for right-handed observers, the rivalry rate is higher when stimuli are presented in the right visual field, and this asymmetry is reversed for left-handed observers (Chen and He, 2003). For both groups, the rate is higher for stimuli presented in the lower visual field (see figure 5.4a). A more detailed analysis of the same data shows that the left–right asymmetry is due primarily to the long dominance times of the temporal retinas: right temporal retina for right-handed observers and left temporal retina for left-handed observers (figure 5.4b). The fact that our finding is inconsistent with the nasal hemiretina's higher ganglion cell density and higher visual sensitivity suggests that the asymmetry reported here is unlikely of retinal origin.

**The Engram of Dominant Stimulus During Rivalry Stays with the Eye**
The finding of asymmetry across the visual field suggests that rivalry is to some extent independently controlled in different parts of the visual field. This is at odds with proposals that enlist a switching mechanism outside the visual domain (Lumer, Friston, and Rees, 1998; Miller et al., 2000). What drives the alternations during rivalry? A recent finding showed that perceptual switching can be slowed or even stabilized during bistable perception (including binocular rivalry) if the stimulus is periodically removed from view (Leopold et al., 2002). The authors suggest that "recent perceptual history was the dominant factor in determining how that stimulus was interpreted on subsequent viewings" (p. 608). We tested whether this "perceptual history" is the representation of the stimulus or the representation of the dominant eye. First, we replicated the findings of Leopold et al. (2002), showing that by intermittently presenting the stimuli during binocular rivalry, perception is indeed almost stabilized. Then we made a small change in the paradigm: after the removal and upon again presenting the rival stimuli, we interchanged the two stimuli between the two eyes. Somewhat to our surprise, perception started to fluctuate again. In other words, at least for binocular rivalry, the dominant factor in determining what stimulus is perceived is not "perceptual history"; rather, it is the history of which eye was dominant. This experiment is reminiscent of a study done by Blake and colleagues (Blake, Westendorf, and Overton, 1980), which showed that when the dominant and suppressed patterns were interchanged between the eyes during a regular binocular rivalry, observers continued seeing with the dominant eye. This observation led them to conclude that "an eye, not a pattern, is

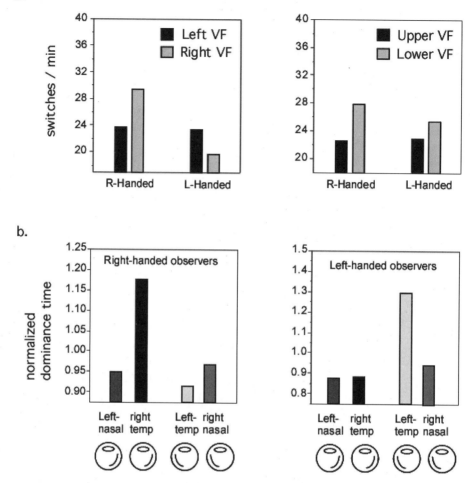

**Figure 5.4** Visual-field asymmetries of the rates of binocular rivalry. (*a*) Plot of the number of switches for stimuli presented in different parts of the visual field (VF). In right-handed observers, rivalry is faster (more switches per min) when stimuli are presented in the right visual field; the reverse is true for left-handed observers. In both groups, binocular rivalry is faster in the lower visual field than in the upper visual field. (*b*) Normalized mean dominance times for rival stimuli presented to the temporal and nasal hemiretinas. For right-handed observers, the stimuli in the right temporal hemiretina have the longest dominance duration. For left-handed observers, the stimuli in the left temporal retina have the longest dominance duration.

S. He, T. Carlson, and X. Chen

suppressed during rivalry." Of course, the suppression is not necessary for the whole eye, but rather should be interpreted as signals from a local area from one eye. Our new results show that the engram of perceptual state, and possibly the mechanism that is responsible for the rivalry alternations, is closely tied to (or "knows") the eye of origin of the competing signals.

## CONCLUDING REMARKS

The hypothesis of differential involvement of the M and P pathways in binocular rivalry is certainly a simplified one. This is especially true given that the parallel pathways are highly interconnected in the cortex—strictly independent channels do not exist in the visual system. This fact suggests that the differential involvement of these pathways in rivalry must be relative. However, the evidence reviewed in this chapter does suggest that the M and P pathways are not created equal when it comes to binocular rivalry. The visual system does not seem to be willing to tolerate interocular conflicts in the P pathway, with its significant role in processing information related to object identity, and resorts to alternating views of the two stimuli. Conflicts in the M pathway are less likely to lead to rivalry, with the visual system more willing to accept an integrated version of the inputs.

We still have a very incomplete picture in terms of understanding the temporal dynamics of the binocular rivalry process. However, the evidence reviewed here suggests that the key mechanisms responsible for rivalry switch are likely local and hemisphere specific, and have access to the originating eye of the competing signals.

## ACKNOWLEDGMENT

Our research was supported by an award from the James S. McDonnell Foundation.

## REFERENCES

Alexander, L. T. (1951). The influence of figure–ground relationships in binocular rivalry. *Journal of Experimental Psychology, 41,* 376–381.

Amira, L. (1988). When two eyes are no better than one: Depth perception is intermittently lost when binocular rivalrous suppression interacts with stereopsis. *Investigations in Ophthalmology,* (supp.) 29, 449.

Anderson, J. D., Bechtoldt, H. P., and Gregory, L. D. (1978). Binocular integration in line rivalry. *Bulletin of the Psychonomic Society*, 11, 399–402.

Andrews, T. J., and Blakemore, C. (1999). Form and motion have independent access to consciousness. *Nature Neuroscience*, 2, 405–406.

Andrews, T. J., and Blakemore, C. (2002). Integration of motion information during binocular rivalry. *Vision Research*, 42, 301–309.

Baitch, L. W., and Levi, D. M. (1989). Binocular beats: Psychophysical studies of binocular interaction in normal and stereoblind humans. *Vision Research*, 29, 27–35.

Blake, R. (1977). Threshold conditions for binocular rivalry. *Journal of Experimental Psychology: Human Perception and Performance*, 3, 251–257.

Blake, R. (1995). Psychoanatomical studies for studying human vision. In *Early Vision and Beyond*, T. Papathomas, C. Chubb, E. Kowler, and A. Gorea, eds., 17–25. Cambridge, Mass.: MIT Press.

Blake, R., Ahlstrom, U., and Alais, D. (1999). Perceptual priming by invisible motion. *Psychological Science*, 10, 145–150.

Blake, R., and Logothetis, N. K. (2002). Visual competition. *Nature Reviews: Neuroscience*, 3, 13–21.

Blake, R., and O'Shea, R. P. (1988). "Abnormal fusion" of stereopsis and binocular rivalry. *Psychological Review*, 95, 151–158.

Blake, R., O'Shea, R. P., and Mueller, T. J. (1992). Spatial zones of binocular rivalry in central and peripheral vision. *Visual Neuroscience*, 8, 469–478.

Blake, R., and Overton, R. (1979). The site of binocular rivalry suppression. *Perception*, 8, 143–152.

Blake, R., Westendorf, D. H., and Fox, R. (1990). Temporal perturbations of binocular rivalry. *Perception and Psychophysics*, 48, 593–602.

Blake, R., Westendorf, D. H., and Overton, R. (1980). What is suppressed during binocular rivalry? *Perception*, 9, 223–231.

Blake, R., Yang, Y., and Wilson, H. R. (1991). On the coexistence of stereopsis and binocular rivalry. *Vision Research*, 31, 1191–1203.

Blake, R., Yu, K., Lokey, M., and Norman, H. (1998). Binocular rivalry and motion perception. *Journal of Cognitive Neuroscience*, 10, 46–60.

Bossink, C. J., Stalmeier, P. F., and De Weert, C. M. (1993). A test of Levelt's second proposition for binocular rivalry. *Vision Research*, 33, 1413–1419.

Bower, T. G. R., and Haley, L. J. (1964). Temporal effects in binocular vision. *Psychonomic Science*, 1, 409–420.

Breese, B. (1909). Binocular rivalry. *Psychological Review*, 16, 410–415.

Burke, D., Alais, D., and Wenderoth, P. (1999). Determinants of fusion of dichoptically presented orthogonal gratings. *Perception*, 28, 73–88.

Carlson, T. A., and He, S. (2000). Visible binocular beats from invisible monocular stimuli during binocular rivalry. *Current Biology,* 10, 1055–1058.

Carney, T., Shadlen, M., and Switkes, E. (1987). Parallel processing of motion and colour information. *Nature,* 328, 647–649.

Chen, X., and He, S. (2003). Temporal characteristics of binocular rivalry: Visual field asymmetries. *Vision Research,* 43, 2207–2212.

Crovitz, H. F. (1964). Retinal locus in tachistoscopic binocular color rivalry. *Perceptual and Motor Skills,* 19, 808–810.

Crovitz, H. F., and Lipscomb, D. B. (1963). Dominance of the temporal visual fields at a short duration of stimulation. *American Journal of Psychology,* 76, 631–637.

Culham, J., Nishida, S., Ledgeway, T., Cavanagh, P., Von Grunau, M., Kwas, M., Alais, D., and Raymond, J. R. (1998). High order effects. In *Motion Aftereffect: A Modern Perspective,* George Mather, Frans Verstraten, and Stuart Anstis, eds. Cambridge, Mass.: MIT Press.

Dacey, D. M. (1994). Physiology, morphology and spatial densities of identified ganglion cell types in primate retina. *Ciba Foundation Symposium,* 184, 12–28; discussion 28–34, 63–70.

DeLange, H. (1958). Research into the dynamic nature of the human fovea -> cortex systems with intermittent and modulated light: II. Phase shift in brightness and delay in color perception. *Journal of the Optical Society of America,* 48, 784–789.

Derrington, A. M., Krauskopf, J., and Lennie, P. (1984). Chromatic mechanisms in lateral geniculate nucleus of macaque. *Journal of Physiology,* 357, 241–265.

Derrington, A. M., and Lennie, P. (1984). Spatial and temporal contrast sensitivities of neurones in lateral geniculate nucleus of macaque. *Journal of Physiology,* 357, 219–240.

DeYoe, E. A., and Van Essen, D. C. (1988). Concurrent processing streams in monkey visual cortex. *Trends in Neuroscience,* 11, 219–226.

Fahle, M. (1987). Naso-temporal asymmetry of binocular inhibition. *Investigative Ophthalmology and Visual Sciences,* 28, 1016–1017.

Fox, R., and Rasche, F. (1969). Binocular rivalry and reciprocal inhibition. *Perception and Psychophysics,* 5, 215–217.

Goldstein, A. G. (1970). Binocular fusion and contour suppression. *Perception and Psychophysics,* 7, 28–32.

Harrad, R. A., McKee, S. P., Blake, R., and Yang, Y. (1994). Binocular rivalry disrupts stereopsis. *Perception,* 23, 15–28.

Hering, K. E. (1964). *Outlines of a Theory of the Light Sense.* L. Hurvich and D. Jameson, trans. Cambridge, Mass.: Harvard University Press.

Hollins, M. (1980). The effect of contrast on the completeness of binocular rivalry suppression. *Perception and Psychophysics,* 27, 550–556.

Hollins, M., and Leung, E. H. L. (1978). The influence of color on binocular rivalry. In *Visual Psychophysics and Physiology,* J. C. Armington, J. Krauskopf, and B. R. Wooten, eds., 181–190. New York: Academic Press.

Hubel, D. H., and Livingstone, M. S. (1987). Segregation of form, color, and stereopsis in primate area 18. *Journal of Neuroscience, 7*, 3378–3415.

Hubel, D. H., and Livingstone, M. S. (1990). Color and contrast sensitivity in the lateral geniculate body and primary visual cortex of the macaque monkey. *Journal of Neuroscience*, 10, 2223–2237.

Julesz, B., and Miller, J. E. (1975). Independent spatial-frequency-tuned channels in binocular fusion and rivalry. *Perception, 4*, 125–143.

Karrer, R. (1967). Visual beat phenomena as an index to the temporal characteristics of perception. *Journal of Experimental Psychology, 75*, 372–378.

Kaufman, L. (1963). On the spread of suppression and binocular rivalry. *Vision Research, 3*, 401–415.

Kaushall, P. (1975). Functional asymmetries of the human visual system as revealed by binocular rivalry and binocular brightness matching. *American Journal of Optometry and Physiological Optics, 52*, 509–520.

Kontsevich, L. L., and Tyler, C. W. (2000). Relative contributions of sustained and transient pathways to human stereoprocessing. *Vision Research, 40*, 3245–3255.

Kulikowski, J. J. (1992). Binocular chromatic rivalry and single vision. *Ophthalmic and Physiological Optics, 12*, 168–170.

Kulikowski, J. J., and Tolhurst, D. J. (1973). Psychophysical evidence for sustained and transient detectors in human vision. *Journal of Physiology, 232*, 149–162.

Lee, B. B. (1996). Receptive field structure in the primate retina. *Vision Research, 36*, 631–644.

Lee, S. H., and Blake, R. (1999). Rival ideas about binocular rivalry. *Vision Research, 39*, 1447–1454.

Legge, G. E. (1978). Sustained and transient mechanisms in human vision: Temporal and spatial properties. *Vision Research, 18*, 69–81.

Lehmkuhle, S. W., and Fox, R. (1975). Effect of binocular rivalry suppression on the motion aftereffect. *Vision Research, 15*, 855–859.

Leopold, D. A., and Logothetis, N. K. (1999). Multistable phenomena: Changing views in perception. *Trends in Cognitive Sciences, 3*, 254–264.

Leopold, D. A., Wilke, M., Maier, A., and Logothetis, N. K. (2002). Stable perception of visually ambiguous patterns. *Nature Neuroscience, 5*, 605–609.

Levelt, W. J. M. (1965). *On Binocular Rivalry*. Soesterberg, The Netherlands: Institute for Perception.

Levelt, W. J. M. (1966). The alternation process in monocular rivalry. *British Journal of Psychology, 57*, 225–238.

Levelt, W. J. M. (1967). Note on the distribution of dominance times in binocular rivalry. *British Journal of Psychology, 58*, 143–145.

Liu, L., Tyler, C. W., and Schor, C. M. (1992). Failure of rivalry at low contrast: Evidence of a suprathreshold binocular summation process. *Vision Research, 32*, 1471–1479.

Livingstone, M. S., and Hubel, D. H. (1987a). Connections between layer 4B of area 17 and the thick cytochrome oxidase stripes of area 18 in the squirrel monkey. *Journal of Neuroscience,* 7, 3371–3377.

Livingstone, M. S., and Hubel, D. H. (1987b). Psychophysical evidence for separate channels for the perception of form, color, movement, and depth. *Journal of Neuroscience,* 7, 3416–3468.

Livingstone, M., and Hubel, D. (1988). Segregation of form, color, movement, and depth: Anatomy, physiology, and perception. *Science,* 240, 740–749.

Logothetis, N. K., Leopold, D. A., and Sheinberg, D. L. (1996). What is rivalling during binocular rivalry? *Nature,* 380, 621–624.

Lumer, E. D., Friston, K. J., and Rees, G. (1998). Neural correlates of perceptual rivalry in the human brain. *Science,* 280, 1930–1934.

Maunsell, J. H. (1992). Functional visual streams. *Current Opinions in Neurobiology,* 2, 506–510.

Miller, S. M., Liu, G. B., Ngo, T. T., Hooper, G., Riek, S., Carson, R. G., and Pettigrew, J. D. (2000). Interhemispheric switching mediates perceptual rivalry. *Current Biology,* 10, 383–392.

Mueller, T. J., and Blake, R. (1989). A fresh look at the temporal dynamics of binocular rivalry. *Biological Cybernetics,* 61, 223–232.

Nishida, S., Ashida, H., and Sato, T. (1994). Complete interocular transfer of motion after-effect with flickering test. *Vision Research,* 34, 2707–2716.

Ooi, T. L., and Loop, M. S. (1994). Visual suppression and its effect upon color and luminance sensitivity. *Vision Research,* 34, 2997–3003.

O'Shea, R. P., and Blake, R. (1986). Dichoptic temporal frequency differences do not lead to binocular rivalry. *Perception and Psychophysics,* 39, 59–63.

O'Shea, R. P., and Corballis, P. M. (2001). Binocular rivalry between complex stimuli in split-brain observers. *Brain and Mind,* 2, 151–160.

O'Shea, R. P., and Crassini, B. (1984). Binocular rivalry occurs without simultaneous presentation of rival stimuli. *Perception and Psychophysics,* 36, 266–276.

O'Shea, R. P., Sims, A. J. H., and Govan, D. G. (1997). The effect of spatial frequency and field size on the spread of exclusive visibility in binocular rivalry. *Vision Research,* 37, 175–183.

O'Shea, R. P., and Williams, D. R. (1996). Binocular rivalry with isoluminant stimuli visible only via short-wavelength-sensitive cones. *Vision Research,* 36, 1561–1571.

Ramachandran, V. S. (1991). Form, motion, and binocular rivalry. *Science,* 251, 950–951.

Schiller, P. H., and Logothetis, N. K. (1990). The color-opponent and broad-band channels of the primate visual system. *Trends in Neuroscience,* 13, 392–398.

Schiller, P. H., Logothetis, N. K., and Charles, E. R. (1990a). Functions of the colour-opponent and broad-band channels of the visual system. *Nature,* 343, 68–70.

Schiller, P. H., Logothetis, N. K., and Charles, E. R. (1990b). Role of the color-opponent and broad-band channels in vision. *Visual Neuroscience,* 5, 321–346.

Shapley, R. M., and Perry, V. H. (1986). Cat and monkey retinal ganglion cells and their visual functional roles. *Trends in Neuroscience,* 9, 229–235.

Smith, E. L., Levi, D. M., Harwerth, R. S., and White, J. M. (1982). Color vision is altered during the suppression phase of binocular rivalry. *Science, 218,* 802–804.

Tolhurst, D. J. (1977). Colour-coding properties of sustained and transient channels in human vision. *Nature, 266,* 266–268.

Treisman, A. (1962). Binocular rivalry and stereoscopic depth perception. *Quarterly Journal of Experimental Psychology, 14,* 23–37.

Van de Grind, W. A., Van Hof, P., Van der Smagt, M. J., and Verstraten, F. A. (2001). Slow and fast visual motion channels have independent binocular-rivalry stages. *Proceedings of the Royal Society of London,* B268, 437–443.

Van der Zwan, R., Wenderoth, P., and Alais, D. (1993). Reduction of a pattern-induced motion aftereffect by binocular rivalry suggests the involvement of extrastriate mechanisms. *Visual Neuroscience, 10,* 703–709.

Wade, N J (1973) Binocular rivalry and binocular fusion of after-images. *Vision Research, 13,* 999–1000.

Wade, N. J. (1975). Monocular and binocular rivalry between contours. *Perception, 4,* 85–95.

Whittle, P. (1965). Binocular rivalry and the contrast at contours. *Quarterly Journal of Experimental Psychology, 17,* 217–226.

Wiesenfelder, H., and Blake, R. (1990). The neural site of binocular rivalry relative to the analysis of motion in the human visual system. *Journal of Neuroscience, 10,* 3880–3888.

Wiesenfelder, H., and Blake, R. (1991). Apparent motion can survive binocular rivalry suppression. *Vision Research, 31,* 1589–1599.

Wolfe, J. M. (1983a). Afterimages, binocular rivalry, and the temporal properties of dominance and suppression. *Perception, 12,* 439–445.

Wolfe, J. M. (1983b). Influence of spatial frequency, luminance, and duration on binocular rivalry and abnormal fusion of briefly presented dichoptic stimuli. *Perception, 12,* 447–456.

Wolfe, J. M. (1986). Stereopsis and binocular rivalry. *Psychological Review, 93,* 269–282.

# 6   Human Development of Binocular Rivalry

## Ilona Kovács and Michal Eisenberg

A major, unresolved question regarding binocular rivalry remains the locus issue: Where in the brain is the switch that makes us perceive very different images over time despite the absence of actual physical stimulus changes? The emerging consensus is that alternations occur at distributed sites laid out along the hierarchy of cortical processing: while local stimuli will induce solutions (and alternations) at early cortical sites, more complex stimulus configurations will induce higher-level perceptual interpretations in higher cortical areas (see, e.g., chapters 1, 4, 9, and 11 in this volume). As indicated in chapters 13 and 14 of this volume, neurons related to binocular rivalry have been found at multiple sites in the brain, and the locus of the "perceptual switch" depends on the actual feature that is represented during a particular percept. Single-cell recording experiments have revealed the existence of rivalry-related neurons in the primary visual cortex, but this class of neurons is even more prevalent in higher-level temporal areas involved in object representation. Involvement of the mediotemporal lobe (see chapter 12 in this volume), and the parvo pathway (see chapter 5 in this volume) have also been implicated in rivalry.

Single-cell recordings provide one fruitful strategy for addressing the "locus" question, but we believe that another promising strategy is to examine the ontogenetic development of binocular rivalry. To what extent does this developmental trajectory correspond to the maturational course of the distributed sites participating in binocular rivalry?

A great deal of descriptive knowledge has been accumulating about visual development in the first year of human life. It is known, for example, that very young infants exhibit a preference for moving stimuli (Nelson and Horowitz, 1987), including complex patterns of motion (Kellman and Spelke, 1983), and that their sensitivity to flicker is quite good at ages as young as 2 months (Regal, 1981). Moreover, infants achieve stereoscopic vision around 4 months of age (Braddick et al., 1980), and their visual acuity increases rapidly during the first year of life (Teller et al., 1986). With respect to later development, it is known that while stereo acuity (Ciner, Schanel-Klitsch, and Herzberg, 1996) and grating acuity reach adult levels by around 2 yr, vernier acuity is not adultlike before 5 yr (Carkeet, Levi, and Manny, 1997; Zanker et al., 1992).

Beyond visual acuity, there are studies indicating that visual segmentation and form identification based on texture contrast (Atkinson and Braddick, 1992; Sireteanu and Rieth, 1992), motion contrast (Giaschi and Regan, 1997; Hollants-Gilhuijs, Ruijter, and Spekreijse, 1998a; Schrauf, Wist, and Ehrenstein, 1999), color contrast (Hollants-Gilhuijs, Ruijter, and Spekreijse, 1998b), and flicker contrast (Barnard, Crewther, and Crewther, 1998) are relatively slowly developing functions that reach maturity between 2 and 8 yr. In addition, we found significant improvement of performance in children aged between 5 and 14 yr in a contour integration task that presumably reflects the efficiency of integrating orientation information across the visual field at the level of the primary visual cortex (Kovács et al., 1999; Kovács, 2000). Considered together, a large body of evidence implies that local visual functions related to early cortical sites mature rapidly, during the first year of life, while functions related to higher cortical areas take a very long maturational course in humans, extending into the teenage years.

Assuming that binocular rivalry depends on multiple cortical sites ranging from the earliest (V1) to high-level temporal areas, and on the extended visual development found in humans, we expect to see developmental trends in binocular rivalry. Depending on the stimuli and on the age of the subject, we predict that perceptual alternations will present a pattern which differs from that seen in adults.

Developmental research in human binocular function in young infants has utilized both electrophysiological and behavioral methods. Similarity between the two eyes' images (i.e., interocular correlation) is detected by the human infant starting at 3–5 mos of age as measured by electrophysiological and preferential looking techniques (Braddick et al., 1980; Petrig et al., 1981; Braddick et al., 1983; Shimojo et al., 1986). Preferential looking techniques are used for behaviorally testing visual function in preverbal subjects. When the infant can detect binocular correlation, he or she will prefer to look at a correlated image pair as opposed to an uncorrelated one. In electrophysiological measurements, visual evoked potential (VEP) responses differ for correlated and uncorrelated image pairs after the onset of binocular vision.

With respect to the development of binocular rivalry in human infants, preferential looking studies show an early onset of rivalry, starting also at around 3–5 mos (Gwiazda, Bauer, and Held, 1989; Shimojo et al., 1986). At this age infants begin to prefer to look at fusible patterns (e.g., vertical gratings presented to each eye) compared to rivalrous patterns (e.g., vertical gratings viewed by one eye and horizontal gratings by the other). Preference for the fusible pattern is taken as evidence for sensitivity to binocular rivalry, although one could argue that it is simply sensitivity to binocular correlation.

VEP studies, in contrast, fail to demonstrate physiological rivalry before 15 mos (Brown and Norcia, 1997; Brown, Candy, and Norcia, 1999). Of course, preference studies can only indicate that infants perceive discordant binocular input, but cannot indicate whether spontaneous rivalry alternations are experienced by infants. Likewise, VEP studies are also limited in this respect because they apply temporal tagging of the left and right eye stimuli within short trial durations, where phenomenal alternations might be lost either because of the short durations or because of the possibility of piecemeal rivalry.

Taken together, the current literature on the development of binocular rivalry in human infants disagrees on the age at which rivalry emerges and, moreover, sheds no light on a most basic question: Do infants observe phenomenal alternation between percepts under rivalry conditions? For that matter, this question has not been raised in the literature with respect to older children. Therefore, the possibility of a multistep development corresponding to the distributed sites participating in rivalry has not heretofore been addressed.

In pilot studies we sought to learn what children aged 4 to 7 yr experience when they look at rivalry-inducing stimuli. Using anaglyphic techniques (red and green images and filters), we presented 36 children with various kinds of rival targets (orthogonal gratings, line drawings, photos of natural scenes) and instructed them to indicate if and when they saw changes in the stimuli during a 30-sec viewing time. Four of these 36 children did not see any alternations, 4 observed very slow alternations, 6 had fast alternations, 13 seemed to observe normal alternations, and 9 reported a patchwork of the two images. Based on these initial behavioral observations, we concluded that children in this age group do indeed observe alternations, but we suspected that this rivalry might be qualitatively and quantitatively different from the type of rivalry experienced by adults. This led us to compare the temporal characteristic of rivalry alternations in young children and adults.

## BINOCULAR RIVALRY ALTERNATIONS IN CHILDREN AND ADULTS

We tested binocular rivalry in 30 children aged 5–6 yr, and in 10 adults. Rival stimuli comprised 3 cycles/°, orthogonal sinusoidal gratings viewed anaglyphically by the two eyes (one eye viewing the horizontal and the other the vertical); both gratings subtended 2° × 2° of visual angle.

Subjects were first administered a 30-sec training session in which the horizontal and vertical gratings were shown in physical alternation (with phase durations randomly selected between 2 and 3 sec). The subjects were told that they would see a horizontal grating and a vertical grating in alternation and were instructed to press a button whenever the grating orientation changed. Each subject participated in nine successive sessions. The sessions consisted of either physically alternating gratings (control or **C**) or rivalry-inducing plaids of the orthogonal gratings (rivalry or **R**). The sequence was the following for each subject: **C** grating (with a phase duration randomly selected between 2 and 3 sec), **R** grating, **R** grating, **C** grating (phase duration between 4 and 6 sec), **R** grating, **R** grating, **C** grating (phase duration between 1 and 2 sec), **R** grating, **R** grating. This resulted in three control and six rivalry sessions. The subjects were not told about the two types of conditions, and their task remained the same throughout all sessions: press the button when the grating changes its orientation.

Our aim with the **C** gratings was twofold. First, we wanted subjects to realize the possibility that grating orientation could change irregularly over time, and we wanted them to learn to track those changes; and second, we used the **C** sessions to estimate the reliability of our subjects' reports. The three alternating speeds used in the **C** sessions were selected within the range of possible rivalry alternations. The results of the **C** sessions (figure 6.1a) show that our adult subjects were able to follow the physical alternations—the number of responses matched perfectly the number of stimulus changes. In **C** sessions with faster speed (phase durations between 1 and 2 sec and between 2 and 3 sec), children were also very reliable. However, in the slowly changing sessions (phase durations between 4 and 6 sec), 10 children tended to give 80% more responses (figure 6.1a). We called these children "overpressers," and grouped their data together.

Ilona Kovács and Michal Eisenberg

a

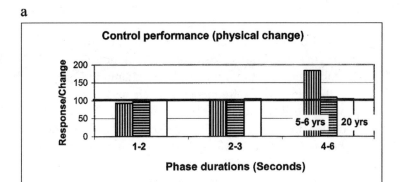

b

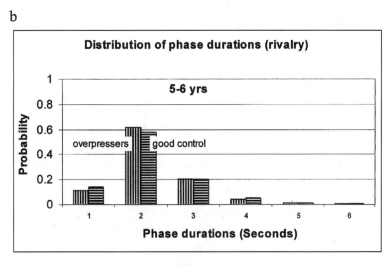

**Figure 6.1** (*a*) Control (**C**) session results, where subjects viewed physically alternating horizontal and vertical gratings. The percentage of responses with respect to the number of physical stimulus changes is shown for three different phase durations of the physically changing grating. Vertical striped bars: a group of ten children who had a tendency to press faster than the stimulus change for the largest phase duration. Horizontal striped bars: a group of 20 children who followed physical changes reliably. Empty bars: adult subjects, whose number of responses perfectly matched the number of stimulus changes. (*b*) Rivalry (**R**) session results. Normalized distribution of rivalry phase duration is shown for children who tended to overpress in the control experiment (vertical stripes), and for children providing reliable performance in the control experiment (horizontal stripes). There was no difference between the two groups in terms of their rivalry phase durations.

Then we compared the distributions of phase durations in the **R** sessions between the "overpresser" and "good control" children (figure 6.1b). The grouped data did not show any significant differences between the two groups in the **R** sessions. We conclude that the "overpresser" children were probably impatient in the very slowly changing **C** sessions, but we doubt that this affected the frequency of their responses in the **R** sessions. The peak of the **R** session distribution was at 2–3 sec, and the overpressing behavior occurred at the slower, 4–6-sec phase duration range for the **C** sessions. Therefore it was reasonable to include the overpressers in our analysis of the rivalry **R** data.

For the **R** sessions, data from all six rivalry trials were pooled. For each subject a histogram of eye-dominance durations was calculated. Figure 6.2a shows the frequency histogram of normalized phase durations under rivalry conditions in children, and figure 6.2b shows the histogram for adults. The shape of the frequency histogram of dominance durations in children resembles the adults' and can be fitted with the gamma function. The gamma function ($f(x) = [\lambda^r/(r-1)!]x^{r-1}\exp(-\lambda x)$) provides a good description of the dominance durations experienced during binocular rivalry and during viewing of other bistable perceptual figures (e.g., Logothetis, 1998; see also chapter 8 in this volume). The peak of the distribution falls at 2.1 sec for children and at 3.0 sec for adults, indicating that children experienced more rapid alternations, on average, than did adults (figure 6.2c).

## RIVALRY ALTERNATION RATE DEPENDS ON STIMULUS SIZE

The shape of the gamma distribution expresses two tendencies of multistable phenomena: (1) the tendency to change states at random with an exponential distribution ($\exp(-\lambda x)$), as shown by the decaying part of the curve; and (2) the tendency to stay at the current state due to some "inertia" ($x^{r-1}$), as shown by the ascending part of the curve. The results in figure 6.2c indicate that younger observers have less "inertia," meaning that they switch more rapidly. What might underlie this behavioral observation? We wondered whether faster switching might arise not from the lack of a neural "inertia" mechanism but, rather, from the lack of effective visual integration in children. In adult subjects, piecemeal rivalry occurs with higher probability than global alternation when rival stimuli are large (Blake, O'Shea, Mueller, 1992).

Although we kept the size of our grating stimuli within the range of global rivalry for adult observers, we cannot be sure that children also

a

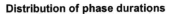

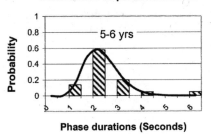

**Distribution of phase durations**

b

**Distribution of phase durations**

c

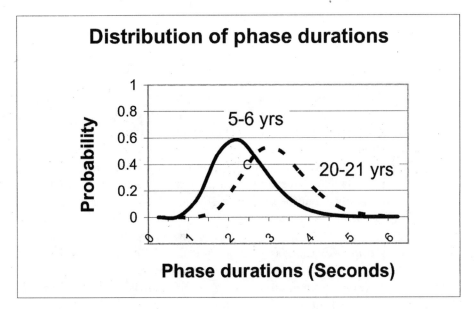

**Figure 6.2** (*a*) Distribution of normalized phase durations for children aged 5–6 yr under rivalry conditions. (*b*) Distribution of normalized phase durations for adults under rivalry conditions. (*c*) Comparison of the fitted gamma functions across children and adults. Children have shorter phase durations than adults.

observe global rivalry at this stimulus size. In the case of piecemeal alternations, one would expect the subject—who is instructed to indicate every change in stimulus orientation by pressing a single button—to increase the rate of responses. Perhaps, in other words, young children experience more piecemeal rivalry and, therefore, more "changes" during a given viewing period. To test this hypothesis, we repeated the experiment with a group of adults employing rival stimuli more likely to induce piecemeal rivalry.

Ten additional adult observers were tested with the same protocol as that used in the first experiment, with the exception of stimulus size. The size of the physically alternating and rivalry-inducing gratings was now $4° \times 4°$ of visual angle (viewing distance and stimulus spatial frequency remained the same). As figure 6.3 shows, increasing stimulus size induced faster pressing in adults. The peak of the distribution for large stimuli is at 2.4 sec, and at 3.0 sec for small stimuli—very similar to the difference between the two peaks in the child/adult comparison.

## LACK OF INTEGRATION/PIECEMEAL RIVALRY IN YOUNG CHILDREN

We observed that rivalry alternations are faster in children aged 5–6 yrs than in adults. Increasing the stimulus size can increase alternation rate in grown-up observers to the child level. Because larger stimuli induce piecemeal rivalry in adults, we may reasonably conclude that piecemeal rivalry is responsible for the similar alternation rates in children when they view the small stimulus, and in adults when they view the large stimulus. The possibility that the incidence of piecemeal rivalry is greater in children is consistent with data from contour integration studies that show the immaturity of spatial integration in children drawn from this same age group (Kovács, 2000; Kovács, et al., 1999). These studies indicate that the integration of orientation information across the visual field follows a slow developmental course, reaching maturity only after adolescence. The grating stimuli that we employed for the rivalry study also involve the integration of orientation information. When integration is immature, one would indeed expect to see more of the local-type rivalry alternations.

Having established that children differ from adults in terms of the spatiotemporal dynamimcs of rivalry, we felt it worthwhile to consider the behavior of these children on other forms of bistable perception. This seemed particularly relevant, given the evidence that alternation rates for all sorts of bistable phenomena—rivalry included—are highly correlated among adults (see chapter 15 in this volume).

a

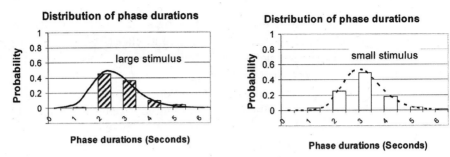

b

Distribution of phase durations

small stimulus

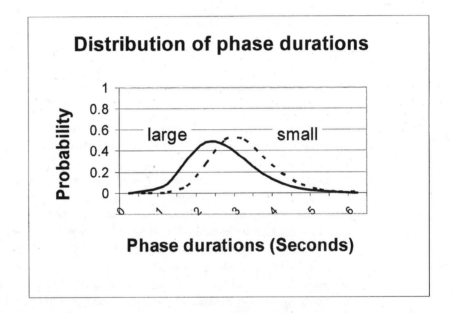

Figure 6.3   (*a*) Distribution of normalized phase durations for adults under rivalry conditions using 4° × 4° stimulus gratings. (*b*) Distribution of normalized phase durations for adults under rivalry conditions using 2° × 2° stimulus gratings. (*c*) Comparison of the fitted gamma functions across large and small stimulus conditions in adults. Large stimuli induce shorter phase durations than small stimuli.

Human Development of Binocular Rivalry

## DEVELOPMENTAL ASPECTS OF OTHER AMBIGUOUS PERCEPTS

There are only a few studies investigating the developmental aspects of bistable perception. Rock, Gopnik, and Hall (1994) looked at perceptual alternations associated with viewing images that induce figure–ground reversals in adults (e.g., Rubin's face/vase figure). Interestingly, children aged 3–4 yr report slower alternations, or none at all. Geometric optical illusions offer another class of ambiguous percepts. A few studies have indicated, although not conclusively, that there are developmental curves extending into school age (Weintraub, 1979; Hanisch, Konczak, and Dohle, 2001). Classic studies by Golin (1960) and Mooney (1957) investigated the ability of children to recognize objects in impoverished contexts. They found that the ability to integrate fragmented cues, and to use high-level cues in "solving" the images, is not fully developed until adolescence. None of these studies have dealt with the actual maturation of different brain areas related to the perceptual tasks. In the following paragraphs we briefly discuss two of our new developmental findings related to ambiguous percepts. The first is an experimental approach to the Ebbinghaus illusion, and the second is some observations with respect to two-tone ("Mooney-type") images. We will also attempt to relate them to brain maturation.

Based on our earlier results on the reduced ability of children to integrate features across the visual field (Kovács et al., 1999), we predicted that poor spatial integration might result in reduced susceptibility to visual contextual influences. The neural interactions behind integrating orientation information are also assumed to mediate context integration (see, e.g., Gilbert, 1998; Gilbert et al., 1996). Contextual modulation of the percept of a local target can be measured directly in the case of geometric illusions. We measured the magnitude of a size contrast illusion (Ebbinghaus illusion or Titchener circles) in children and in adults. Four-year-old children and adults performed 2AFC size comparisons between two target disks in the classical Ebbinghaus illusion (Kaldy and Kovács, 2003). We found that the magnitude of the illusion was significantly smaller in children than in adults: size estimations by children were closer to veridical than were the estimations of adults, indicating that these children were more immune to the effect of context.

We are led to speculate that immature cortical connectivity might be behind the reduced contextual sensitivity in children. Contextual integration might also involve higher cortical areas. Melvyn Goodale and David Milner developed a theory about the functional division of labor between

Ilona Kovács and Michal Eisenberg

higher-level cortical areas, where the dorsal (occipitoparietal) stream specializes in the visual control of action, and the ventral (occipitotemporal) stream specializes in the perception of the permanent properties of objects (Milner and Goodale, 1995).

Besides the neuroanatomical and neuropsychological evidence, Goodale and his colleagues (e.g., Haffenden and Goodale, 2000) employed psychophysical studies of the Ebbinghaus illusion. They demonstrated functional dissociation between the two streams, where the dorsal stream appeared to be less susceptible to the illusion. To date, there is not sufficient information to determine the exact contribution of V1 versus higher-level cortical areas, or the contribution of the dorsal visual stream versus the ventral one to perceptual context integration, as exemplified by size contrast (Ebbinghaus illusion) or size constancy. We are intrigued, however, by the possibility that immature cortical connectivity in V1, on the one hand, and a delayed maturation of the ventral stream, on the other hand, might be behind the more "veridical" percepts in children than in adults (Kaldy and Kovács, 2003).

In his 1957 paper, Mooney applied the now frequently used two-tone images to test the ability of children to perceive "closure," an important factor contributing to visual gestalten. The images were drawings of faces revealing only highlights and shadows in solid blacks and whites. He found that both the age and the "ability" of the subjects determined performance in a task where false and real faces were randomly presented, and each face had to be categorized according to age and gender. Subjects' performance slowly improved into the teen years. Two-tone images similar to the famous Mooney faces have also been used to demonstrate an interesting but not yet understood type of visual learning: instant or "one-shot" learning. While in most examples of visual perceptual learning, long practice periods and consolidation during sleep are required, in the case of instant learning, one presentation of a cue is sufficient to change the perceptual state of the subject.

In such a demonstration, a two-tone image is shown first (figure 6.4a), and the subject is asked what is depicted in the picture. The two-tone image is usually very difficult to recognize at first (a well-known example is the dalmatian dog that can be found in many textbooks). A better copy of the image, either a line drawing, or an original photograph (such as in figure 6.4b) is then shown for a few seconds. When the subject looks at the two-tone image again, the percept is different from that of the first presentation, although the stimulus itself (the two-tone image) has not changed at all. Due to the now unambiguous perceptual organization of the

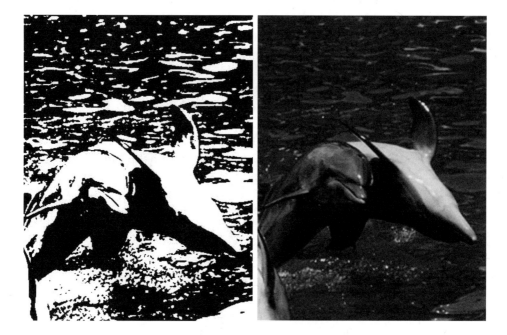

**Figure 6.4** (*a*) Two-tone image and (*b*) its gray-scale version. Most observers cannot recognize the subject of (*a*) at first. For adults, a brief, single exposure to the original, gray-scale image is sufficient for them to recognize the dolphins in subsequent viewings of the two-tone image. Such one-trial learning does not occur in children.

initially meaningless patches, recognition of the image occurs immediately and effortlessly. The effect of learning is permanent, and the subject immediately recognizes the picture without the need for the cue even years after the first cue presentation. This puzzling phenomenon shares an important property with binocular rivalry in addition to the inherent ambiguity of the stimulus: a strong reorganization of the percept occurs without any stimulus change. With this similarity in mind, we sought to study perception of two-tone images in young children.

We presented children aged 4–5 yr with two-tone images of faces, animals, and objects (see an example in figure 6.4a), then with the cue, and asked them to identify the pictures, or at least point to parts of the images (e.g., eyes, nose, mouth). Peculiarly, none of the eight children tested were able to identify the images after cue presentation, and they were not able to organize the two-tone images even when the cue was presented simultaneously. The effect is striking, since for the adult visual system the reorganization is obvious after cue presentation. Children were able to

Ilona Kovács and Michal Eisenberg

identify all original photographs, and we believe that the effect was not due to familiarity. The question is whether the inability of children aged 4–5 yr to organize two-tone images is due to their previously shown reduced low-level integration (Kovács et al., 1999) and contextual integration (Kaldy and Kovács, 2003) abilities, their difficulty in using shape from shading information (Moore and Cavanagh, 1998; Yonas, Kuskowski, and Sternfels, 1979), or their inability to use high-level cues via top-down pathways that encourages this kind of learning.

Although the first causes are present, as was shown earlier, the latter, more interesting possibility will have to be tested. According to current brain-imaging studies, this kind of perceptual learning involves the selective activation of inferotemporal regions in the adult brain, responsible for face and object identification, and a simultaneous activiation of medial and lateral parietal regions involved in attention and visual imagery (Dolan et al., 1997). Long-distance synchronization of brain activity in the gamma frequency range has also been suggested to be behind the change of perceptual state with Mooney-type images (Rodriguez et al., 1999).

## CONCLUSIONS

We conclude that since rivalry is a multilocus phenomenon, its developmental timing should follow the maturational timing of the participating areas. Children 5–6 yr of age demonstrated a local type of rivalry corresponding to activity in lower-level visual areas. Our results might also explain the failure of earlier studies to demonstrate physiological rivalry before 15 months of age (Brown and Norcia, 1997; Brown, Candy, and Norcia, 1999). Since in those studies temporal tagging was applied to follow perceptual alternations of full gratings (two different flicker frequencies were associated with the two orthogonal gratings), this VEP technique is not able to show piecemeal rivalry. It might well be that the onset of physiological piecemeal rivalry is as early as has been indicated in preferential looking techniques (Gwiazda, Bauer, and Held, 1989; Shimojo et al., 1986), that is, 3–5 mos of age.

Considering developmental observations and experiments with other ambiguous percepts (see section "Developmental Aspects of Other Ambiguous Percepts"), an intriguing conclusion arises: there are striking phenomal differences in the percepts of children and adults. We suggest that these differences can be understood in the context of imhomogeneous visual development and brain maturation.

It is also an interesting possibility that by working with subjects of different ages, one can directly investigate the different levels of binocular rivalry involving lower- or higher-level cortical sites.

## ACKNOWLEDGMENTS

We are grateful to Chetan Gandhi and Bonnie Nolan for inspiring ideas in designing the experiments, and for help in collecting data. We thank Akos Feher for software development, and Eli Eisenberg for help with the statistics.

## REFERENCES

Atkinson, J., Braddick, O., Lin, M. H., Curran, W., Guzetta, A., and Cioni, G. (1999). Form and motion coherence: Is there dorsal stream vulnerability in development? *Investigative Ophthalmology and Visual Science*, 40, S395.

Barnard, N., Crewther, S. G., and Crewther, D. P. (1998). Development of a magnocellular function in good and poor primary school-age readers. *Optometry and Vision Science*, 75, 62–68.

Blake, R., O'Shea, R. P., and Mueller, T. J. (1992). Spatial zones of binocular rivalry in central and peripheral vision. *Visual Neuroscience*, 8, 469–478.

Braddick, O., Atkinson, J., Julesz, B., Kropfl, W., Bodis-Wollner, I., and Raab, E. (1980). Cortical binocularity in infants. *Nature*, 288, 363–365.

Braddick, O., Wattam-Bell, J., Day, J., and Atkinson, J. (1983). The onset of binocular function in human infants. *Human Neurobiology*, 2, 65–69.

Brown, R. J., Candy, T. R., and Norcia, A. M. (1999). Development of rivalry and dichoptic masking in human infants. *Investigative Ophthalmology and Visual Science*, 40, 3324–3333.

Brown, R. J., and Norcia, A. M. (1997). A method for investigating binocular rivalry in real-time with the steady-state VEP. *Vision Research*, 37, 2401–2408.

Carkeet, A., Levi, D. M., and Manny, R. E. (1997). Development of vernier acuity in childhood. *Optometry and Vision Science*, 74, 741–750.

Ciner, E. B., Schanel-Klitsch, E., and Herzberg, C. (1996). Stereoacuity development: 6 months to 5 years. A new tool for testing and screening. *Optometry and Vision Science*, 73, 43–48.

Dolan, R. J., Fink, G. R., Rolls, E., Booth, M., Holmes, A., Frackowiak, R. S. J., and Friston, K. J. (1997). How the brain learns to see objects and faces in an impoverished context. *Nature*, 389, 596–599.

Giaschi, D., and Regan, D. (1997). Development of motion-defined figure–ground segregation in preschool and older children, using a letter-identification task. *Optometry and Vision Science*, 74, 61–67.

Gilbert, C. D. (1998). Adult cortical dynamics. *Physiological Reviews*, 78, 467–485.

Gilbert, C. D., Das, A., Ito, M., Kapadia, M., and Westheimer, G. (1996). Spatial integration and cortical dynamics. *Proceedings of the National Academy of Sciences of the United States of America*, 93, 615–622.

Golin, E. S. (1960). Developmental studies of visual recognition of incomplete objects. *Perceptual Motor Skills*, 11, 289–298.

Gwiazda, J., Bauer, J., and Held, R. (1989). Binocular function in human infants: Correlation of stereoptic and fusion-rivalry discriminations. *Journal of Pediatric Ophthalmology: Strabismus*, 26, 128–132.

Haffenden, A. M., and Goodale, M. A. (2000). Independent effects of pictorial displays on perception and action. *Vision Research*, 40, 1597–1607.

Hanisch, C., Konczak, J., and Dohle, C. (2001). The effect of the Ebbinghaus illusion on grasping behaviour of children. *Experimental Brain Research*, 137, 237–245.

Hollants-Gilhuijs, M. A., Ruijter, J. M., and Spekreijse, H. (1998a). Visual half-field development in children: Detection of motion-defined forms. *Vision Research*, 38, 651–657.

Hollants-Gilhuijs, M. A., Ruijter, J. M., and Spekreijse, H. (1998b). Visual half-field development in children: Detection of colour-contrast-defined forms. *Vision Research*, 38, 645–649.

Kaldy, Z., and Kovács, I. (2003). Visual context integration is not fully developed in 4-year-old children. *Perception*, 32, 657–666.

Kellman, P., and Spelke, E. (1983). Perception of partly occluded objects in infancy. *Cognitive Psychology*, 15, 483–524.

Kovács, I. (2000). Human development of perceptual organization. *Vision Research*, 40, 1301–1310.

Kovács, I., Kozma, P., Fehér, A., and Benedek, G. (1999). Late maturation of visual spatial integration in humans. *Proceedings of the National Academy of Sciences of the United States of America*, 96, 12204–12209.

Logothetis, N. K. (1998). Single units and conscious vision. *Philosophical Transactions of the Royal Society, London B*, 353, 1801–1818.

Milner, A. D., and Goodale, M. A. (1995). *The Visual Brain in Action*. Oxford: Oxford University Press.

Mooney, C. M. (1957). Age in the development of closure ability in children. *Canadian Journal of Psychology*, 1, 219–228.

Moore, C., and Cavanagh, P. (1998). Recovery of 3D volume from 2-tone images of novel objects. *Cognition*, 67, 45–71.

Nelson, C. A., and Horowitz, F. D. (1987). Visual motion perception in infancy: A review and synthesis. In *Handbook of Infant Perception*, P. Salapatek and L. Cohen, eds., vol. 2, 123–153. New York: Academic Press.

Petrig, B., Julesz, B., Kropfl, W., Baumgartner, G., and Anliker, M. (1981). Development of stereopsis and cortical binocularity in human infants: Electrophysiological evidence. *Science*, 213, 1402–1405.

Regal, D. (1981). Development of critical flicker frequency in human infants. *Vision Research*, 21, 549–555.

Rock, I., Gopnik, A., and Hall, S. (1994). Do young children reverse ambiguous figures? *Perception*, 23, 635–644.

Rodriguez, E., George, N., Lachaux, J., Martinerie, B. R., and Varela, F. J. (1999). Perception's shadow: Long-distance synchronization of human brain activity. *Nature*, 397, 430–433.

Schrauf, M., Wist, E. R., and Ehrenstein, W. H. (1999). Development of dynamic vision based on motion contrast. *Experimental Brain Research*, 124, 469–473.

Shimojo, S., Bauer, J., Jr., O'Connell, K. M., and Held, R. (1986). Pre-stereoptic binocular vision in infants. *Vision Research*, 26, 501–510.

Sireteanu, R., and Rieth, C. (1992). Texture segregation in infants and children. *Behavior Brain Research*, 49, 133–139.

Teller, D. Y., McDonald, M., Preston, K., Sebris, S. L., and Dobson, M. V. (1986). Assessment of visual acuity in infants and children: The acuity card procedure. *Developmental Medicine and Child Neurology*, 28, 779–789.

Weintraub, D. J. (1979). Ebbinghaus illusion: Context, contour, and age influence the judged size of a circle amidst circles. *Journal of Experimental Psychology: Human Perception and Performance*, 5, 353–364.

Yonas, A., Kuskowski, M., and Sternfels, S. (1979). The role of frames of reference in the development of responsiveness to shading information. *Child Development*, 50, 495–500.

Zanker, J., Mohn, G., Weber, U., Zeitler-Driess, K., and Fahle, M. (1992). The development of vernier acuity in human infants. *Vision Research*, 32, 1557–1564.

# 7 Surface Representation and Attention Modulation Mechanisms in Binocular Rivalry

Teng Leng Ooi and Zijiang J. He

This chapter focuses on two questions in binocular rivalry. The first is whether surface image properties affect rivalry dominance. This question is motivated by the notion that rivalry is mediated by an interocular inhibitory mechanism that is vital for normal binocular vision. Since representing surfaces is one major function of the binocular visual system, investigating this issue provides us with a better understanding of the interplay between surface representation constraints and the interocular inhibitory mechanism.

The second question, touched on in chapter 1, is whether attention influences rivalry perception. Can attention be used to select one rivaling image over the other? While the suggestion that it might do so dates back at least to the time of Helmholtz (1962), few studies have affirmed it (see reviews by Fox, 1991; Lack, 1978). Overall, our search for answers to these questions reveals that rivalry is mediated by a distributed intercortical network (see also chapters 11, 13, and 17 in this volume) whose computational goal is to represent binocular surfaces and objects (Ooi and He, 1999, 2003a, 2003b).

## DECIPHERING THE RULES OF BINOCULAR RIVALRY FROM BOUNDARY AND OCCLUSION CONSTRAINTS

To extract coherent 3-D surface representations from binocular images, the visual system uses an interocular inhibitory mechanism to suppress false matches between images from the two eyes (e.g., Marr and Poggio, 1979). Images (regions) can be identified and assigned as false matches by applying ecological constraints derived from the geometrical properties of surfaces in the real world (e.g., smoothness constraint) and their relationships to the two eyes (e.g., occlusion constraint). We propose that if the same interocular inhibitory mechanism is responsible for the perceptual alternation of rivalry, we should find that rivalry also respects the ecological constraints for identifying false matches.

**Binocular Corresponding Boundaries (Borders) and the Surface Occlusion Constraint**

In the natural environment, the view of one object very often partially occludes the view of another, more distant object. When the (black) occluding surface is on the left side (figure 7.1A, left), the right eye (RE) sees a fuller extent of the rear (texture) surface. The reverse is true when the occluding surface is on the right side and therefore blocks more of the RE's view (figure 7.1A, right). In both cases, binocular computation based on a point-to-point retinal correspondence is disrupted. Yet, our vision in these kinds of real-world situations is little incapacitated. Owing to the high incidence of surface occlusion in the natural environment, the visual system is able to account for the relationship between the occluding surface and the visible view from each eye by applying an occlusion constraint when representing 3-D surfaces (Gillam and Borsting, 1988; Nakayama and Shimojo, 1990).

The occlusion constraint has been generalized to binocular rivalry (Shimojo and Nakayama, 1990). Valid unpaired zones (right visual field in rear for the RE and left visual field in rear for the LE) tend to escape intermittent suppression relative to the invalid zones. In fact, the occlusion constraint also explains the lack of rivalry in the monocular zones of random-dot stereograms (Julesz, 1971). It is, however, unclear how the visual system implements the occlusion constraint and how it is applied to the typical rivalry display (e.g., figure 7.2A).

To begin, let us analyze how the 3-D occlusion constraint can be applied to rivaling scenes. Figure 7.1B shows the analysis with the assumption that the rivalry displays are images behind an occluding surface. Noticeably, besides the rivaling image, a common element in each eye's view is the boundary (indicated by the vertical arrows in the figure) that demarcates the transition between the occluding surface and the rear surface. We suggest that the visual system actively seeks binocular corresponding boundaries (Grossberg, 1987) and uses them as anchors for further processing. Once the binocular corresponding boundary is found, the visual system implements the occlusion constraint by bestowing the visual scene to the right of the corresponding boundary to the RE, and the visual scene to the left of the corresponding boundary to the LE. In this

## A          The 3D occlusion constraint

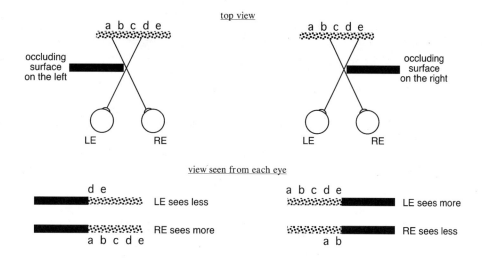

## B    Analysis of binocular rivalry using the occlusion constraint

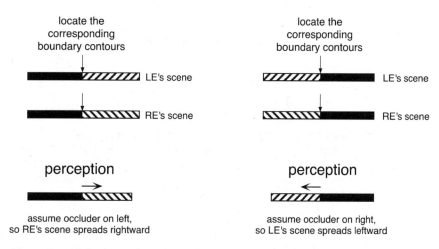

**Figure 7.1** (*A*) Surface occlusion in binocular viewing. (*B*) The corresponding boundary in each eye (indicated by the vertical arrows) is the reference upon which the monocular image spreads (view as seen from each eye). When the occluding surface is on the left, the RE sees a fuller extent of the rear surface (texture scene) than the LE. The converse is true when the occluding surface is on the right. The occlusion constraint dictates that the LE's image spreads leftward and the RE's image, rightward. Clearly, the eye-of-origin signature is required for this process.

A         A typical binocular rivalry display

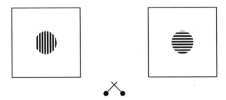

B    Applying corresponding boundary and occlusion constraint

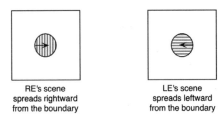

RE's scene
spreads rightward
from the boundary

LE's scene
spreads leftward
from the boundary

C         A possible 3D layout of the rivaling scenes

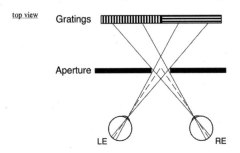

**Figure 7.2**  (*A*) A typical binocular rivalry display. (*B*) When the display in (*A*) is cross-fused, the occlusion constraint dictates that the RE's view spreads rightward from the leftmost edge of the corresponding binocular boundary, and vice versa for the LE. (*C*) A possible 3-D surface layout of the binocular rivalry display in (*A*), as seen through an aperture as the eyes fixate on the center of the aperture.

way, the respective visual scenes and eyes assume precedence in binocular surface formation.

We can apply this binocular corresponding boundary strategy to the display in figure 7.2A, which comprises a pair of same-shaped stimuli with dissimilar interior textures. It induces a robust rivalry, where waves of horizontal and vertical grating scenes compete for dominance over the rival scenes (Wilson, Blake, and Lee, 2001).

Teng Leng Ooi and Zijiang J. He

The binocular corresponding boundary contours are the circular edges of the rival stimuli (figure 7.2B). According to the occlusion constraint (when cross-fusing the display), the leftmost edge of the boundary will carry the RE's scene (vertical pattern) and the rightmost edge, the LE's scene (horizontal pattern). From their "lawful" edges, these scenes spread until they meet another boundary, or one another, as they compete for dominance. (Possibly, also at this stage, the contrast energy of the stimuli plays a role in biasing perceptual dominance.) When analyzed in this way, the rival stimuli designed in the laboratory can be reconciled with a 3-D scene where dissimilar views are seen through an aperture (figure 7.2C).

We conducted a psychophysical experiment to verify the proposal above (Ooi and He, 2003b). During the experiment (figure 7.3), the observer fixated a nonius target on a white background. Then rivalry was induced with a pair of red and green horizontal rectangles ($2.77° \times 0.57°$). This was followed 0.5 sec later by a binocular black vertical bar ($0.29° \times 1.64°$). The observer reported the perceived colors of the horizontal rectangle adjacent to the left and right edges of the black vertical bar. According to our proposal, the right edge of the black vertical bar should carry the green color (RE's view when cross-fused) and the left edge, the red color. Indeed, this was what our observers reported, indicating that the visual system can use the occlusion constraint to select the rivaling images for dominance.

**Unpaired Boundary and Dominance**

We now consider a scenario where no corresponding boundary exists within a relatively large retinal area. This is shown in figure 7.4B. Of significance, despite the dissimilarity of the patterns stimulating corresponding retinal areas (see the control display in figure 7.4A), one rarely experiences rivalry alternation. Instead, the small vertical grating patch is perceived almost continuously. We believe, from the observations in figures 7.4C–E, that an explanation of this observation rests on the unpaired boundary.

Figure 7.4C shows that simply adding a white circular outline to the corresponding retinal region (LE stimulus when cross-fused) throws the system into strong rivalry alternation. There are two possible reasons for this. The first, which we favor, is that adding the circle provides a boundary to integrate that grating area into a figure (hence making it distinct from the larger background). This makes it more similar to figure 7.4A,

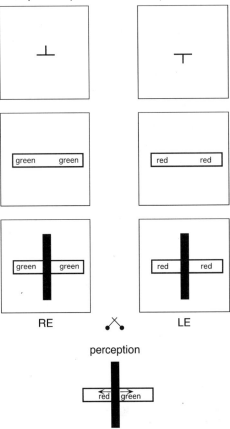

Temporal sequence of stimulus presentation

RE

LE

perception

**Figure 7.3** Temporal sequence of the stimulus display used to verify the role of the corresponding boundary and occlusion constraint in rivalry. The nonius lines ensure proper binocular fixation before the binocular rivalry stimuli are presented. This is followed 500 msec later by a black occluding bar. With cross-fusion, it is predicted that the region adjacent to the right edge of the bar is seen as green and the region adjacent to the left edge of the bar is seen as red.

where each eye receives a same-shaped circular figure with dissimilar interior patterns. The second possibility is that the added circle increases the luminance contrast energy of the LE (Levelt, 1965), leading to an increase in dominance tendency.

To choose between these possibilities, we replaced the luminance-defined circle with a circular illusory contour (figure 7.4D), on the assumption that illusory contours, unlike real contours, do not add global

Teng Leng Ooi and Zijiang J. He

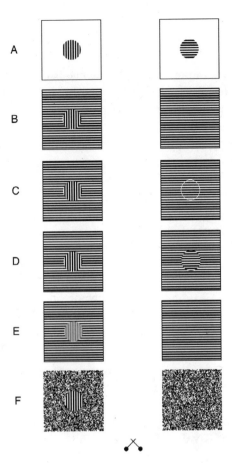

**Figure 7.4** (*A*) A robust rivalry alternation is experienced with a typical binocular rivalry display. (*B*) A relatively stable percept of the vertical grating patch is experienced even though the corresponding area in the other eye receives dissimilar pattern stimulation. Rivalry alternation resumes when a white circle (*C*) or an illusory contour (*D*) is added to the area corresponding to the boundary of the vertical grating in the other eye. (*E*) Reducing the contrast of the monocular vertical grating patch does not significantly reduce its dominance. (*F*) Rivalry alternation resumes when a random-dot background is used.

contrast energy to the LE. Yet this manipulation did not stop the robust rivalry alternations. We next modified figure 7.4B by reducing the contrast of the RE's vertical grating patch (figure 7.4E). Again, this led to little change in the rivalry dynamics, indicating that luminance contrast energy is not the primary factor for the perceptual difference between figures 7.4A and 7.4B.

Together, figures 7.4C–E underscore the importance of binocular corresponding boundaries in rivalry alternation. Having a corresponding boundary in each eye ensures that the visual scene (lawfully) attached to it is apportioned a share in perception. If one eye is deprived of a corresponding boundary (e.g., figure 7.4B), then the fellow eye with the unpaired boundary has the advantage in perception because the visual scene it carries can spread unimpeded.

We do not believe, however, that the visual system must explicitly identify the figure(s) in each eye before instigating interocular suppression. Figure 7.4F demonstrates that interocular suppression can occur at an early stage of binocular information-processing where only the boundary contours, and not the whole figure, are explicitly represented. Figure 7.4F is similar to figure 7.4B except for its background of random dots. This stimulus arrangement induces robust rivalry alternations, behaving more like figures 7.4C and 7.4D, where binocular corresponding boundaries do exist.

We attribute this to the local boundary contours (vertical components) in the random dot display (Ooi and He, 2003b). While these boundary contours do not form an explicit figure, each contour could find a correspondence with the circular boundary contour in the other eye's image (outline of the grating patch). Together, they implicitly delineate a circular boundary, and in so doing, they bestow advantage on the visual scene (random dots) it carries, leading to robust rivalry.

## A Demonstration of the Roles of the Boundary and Surface Occlusion Constraint in Binocular Rivalry

We have proposed a mechanism for interocular suppression based on corresponding binocular, or monocular unpaired, boundaries and the surface occlusion constraint. Figure 7.5 puts these ideas together. By cross-fusing the display in figure 7.5A and fixating the cross, one experiences rivalry between the gray regions and the gratings. Noticeably, the dominant percepts of the gratings originate from the black borders.

This is consistent with the analysis in figure 7.5B, where the black borders are the binocular corresponding boundaries that carry the grating scene in each eye. Thus, in rivalry, these gratings tend to dominate and spread from the respective black borders (occlusion constraint). Each eye also receives a monocular image (gray stripe), which has the unpaired boundary. Since the unpaired boundary carries the visual scene attached to it (gray stripe), it gains an advantage in rivalry and tends to dominate by spreading rightward in the RE and leftward in the LE.

A       Demonstration

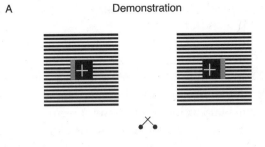

B       Analysis

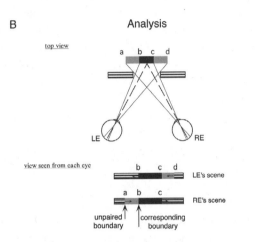

**Figure 7.5** (*A*) With cross-fusion and fixation on the cross, rivalry is experienced between the gratings and corresponding gray regions. The dominant grating percepts spread from the black borders, while the dominant gray areas extend oppositely. (*B*) Explanation for the rivalry percepts in (*A*) based upon boundary and occlusion constraint considerations. From the corresponding binocular boundaries *b* and *c*, the LE's scene spreads leftward and the RE's scene spreads rightward (occlusion constraint). The scene from the unpaired boundary *a* in the RE spreads rightward, and the scene from the unpaired boundary *d* in the LE spreads leftward.

## EVIDENCE FOR SURFACE INTEGRATION DURING BINOCULAR RIVALRY

Elements with similar image properties very likely belong to the same object or surface (similarity constraint). This constraint is exploited by the visual system for object grouping and surface integration (Marr, 1982; Nakayama, He, and Shimojo, 1995). More recently, we explored whether this constraint also affects surface integration during rivalry (Ooi and He, 2003a). We designed a rivalry display whose elements could be grouped to form transparent surfaces during rivalry (Kanizsa, 1979; Nakayama, Shimojo, and Ramachandran, 1990).

As shown in figure 7.6A (plate 3), each half-image comprises four smaller red and green square elements (57.0 × 59.1 min) adjoined to a black cross (200.2 × 28.2 min; 30.4 × 199.9 min) on a white background. To induce rivalry, each pair of corresponding small squares in the rivalry display has complementary colors (red versus green). Hypothetically, the rivalry display can produce one of sixteen possible percepts, on the supposition that each corresponding small square is treated equally and independently by the visual system.

Interestingly, when all four small squares of the same color become dominant simultaneously (all-red or all-green), a condition is created for perceiving a larger subjective square of a single color (red or green). This is because the luminance contrast polarity of the rivalry display is valid for inducing (transparent) surface integration (Metelli, 1974; Nakayama, Shimojo, and Ramachandran, 1990). Is the rivalry mechanism biased to integrate the same-color elements that are distributed between the two eyes to form a larger transparent surface? If so, the probability of perceiving all four squares with the same color as dominant will be greater than that expected on the basis of chance alone.

Of course, simultaneous dominance greater than chance could be attributed to a tendency for identically colored elements to group (as all-red or all-green squares), rather than to surface integration (Kovács et al., 1996, showed that grouping among similarly colored elements can affect rivalry perception.) To control for this, we designed a second display (figure 7.6B) that does not induce surface integration. Here, the contrast between the cross and background is reversed. All other aspects of the rivalry display remain the same. Thus, while the four small squares could be perceived simultaneously with the same color, they could no longer be integrated into a larger subjective surface.

During the experiment, the observer pressed one of three keys to indicate the perception of all-red squares, all-green squares, or a mixture of both red and green squares; rivalry perception was tracked in this way for a total of 24 min in each display. Figure 7.6C shows the averaged results, plotting the percentage of viewing time that the all-red and all-green squares were dominant. Clearly, while the observers performed above the chance level (1/8) for seeing the same-colored squares in both displays, they experienced a significantly higher predominance in the test display. This suggests that surface integration plays a role in grouping similar elements in rivalry.

Teng Leng Ooi and Zijiang J. He

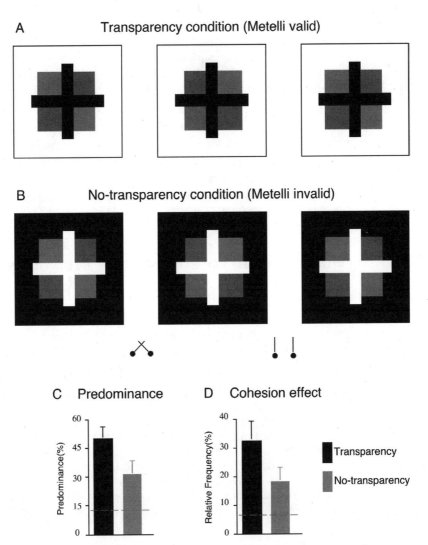

**Figure 7.6** (*A*) Transparent surface condition (Metelli valid). (*B*) No-transparency condition (Metelli invalid). For both displays, the smaller colored squares have crossed disparity with respect to the cross. Convergent fusers should free-fuse the left and middle half-images. (*C, D*). Averaged predominance and averaged cohesion indices (n = 6) for both conditions are above the chance level (12.5% and 6.25%, respectively; dashed lines). Most significantly, the predominance and cohesion indices for perceiving same-color transparent surfaces (black bars) are higher. See plate 3 for color version.

The conclusion is further emphasized in figure 7.6D, which shows that rivalry alternation is more likely to occur between the same-colored squares (e.g., all-green squares percept alternates with all-red squares percept), especially when these squares are integrated into a larger transparent surface in the test display (cohesion effect). Indeed, the tendency to switch between percepts of surfaces underscores the notion that rivalry is an integral part of the binocular visual process that seeks to disambiguate and represent surfaces. Our finding adds to the growing reports that other grouping factors (e.g., color, common motion) also affect rivalry in a way not predicted from a strictly local analysis (Alais and Blake, 1998; Alais et al., 2000; Kovács et al., 1996; Ngo et al., 2000; Papathomas et al., 1999; Sobel and Blake, 2002; Van der Zwan, Wenderoth, and Alais, 1993; see also chapter 13 in this volume).

## EVIDENCE FOR THE ROLE OF ATTENTION IN BINOCULAR RIVALRY

An early avid proponent of the role of attention in visual perception was Helmholtz (1962). Regarding rivalry, Helmholtz claimed that he could sustain a dominant percept for a longer duration by attending to it. However, prolonged concentration of attention on the dominant pattern, he noted, is not an easy task. To do so, the observer has

to have a definite purpose in mind to stimulate attention incessantly and to keep it active; such as counting the lines [of the dominant pattern] or comparing the intervals between them, etc. . . . It is natural for the attention to be distracted from one thing to another. As soon as the interest in one object has been exhausted, and there is no longer anything new in it to be perceived, it is transferred to something else, even against our will. When we wish to rivet it on an object, we must constantly seek to find something novel about it, and this is especially true when other powerful impressions of the senses are tugging at it and trying to distract it. (p. 498)

Clearly Helmholtz recognized that attention is not totally subservient to the conscious will. That which can be executed by the act of will is an "immediate" volition. The other component, which cannot be willed, is a "mediated" volition that requires intervening agencies (e.g., novel stimuli) to be summoned.

Today, we interpret Helmholtz's insightful observations to mean that there are two types of attention. Immediate volition is an endogenous attention that the observer can summon voluntarily. For instance, when commanded by, say, an arrow pointing upward, an observer can deploy his or her attention to the upper visual field (Posner, 1980). Conversely, mediated volition is an exogeneous attention that is stimulus-driven and involuntary. For example, the sudden appearance of a novel stimulus causes attention to be transiently summoned to it (Nakayama and Mackeben, 1989; Yantis, 1993). We show below that both voluntary and involuntary attention influence rivalry in distinct ways. Voluntary attention prolongs a dominant percept by preventing it from being suppressed, while involuntary attention paves the way for an image to become dominant.

### Voluntary Attention Sustains Binocular Rivalry Dominance

To show that an attended image is less likely to succumb to suppression, we combined two paradigms in our experiment (Ooi and He, 1999). The first is based on the Cheshire Cat effect, where the perceived image from one eye can be suppressed by introducing a moving stimulus over the corresponding visual field of the other eye (otherwise viewing an empty field) (Grindley and Townsend, 1965; Duensing and Miller, 1979). The second is based on Posner's (1980) spatial cuing paradigm, where a command (cue) is used to direct attention.

Figure 7.7 shows the temporal sequence of our stimulus display. A cross (48 min × 43.2 min) was used as the fixation target. Near it, a small gray square pointer (cue) was placed in the upper right quadrant to direct the observer's attention to the upper right visual field. This was followed by two monocular grating patches (3.5 cpd; 76.8 min × 75.6 min), one of which was placed at the attended location and the other placed at a diagonally opposite location. In the other eye, a pair of apparent motion (AM) tokens (81.6 min × 86.4 min; frame duration = 117 msec; ISI = 0 msec; 3 frames) was introduced to generate the perception of AM. The role of the AM was to perturb and suppress one of the two gratings in the other eye, depending on its placement.

In the cue-valid condition, the AM traverses a region of the visual field corresponding to the attended grating in the other eye. In the cue-invalid condition, the AM traverses a region corresponding to the unattended grating. We predicted that the attended grating in the cue-valid condition would be less likely to be suppressed by the perturbing AM. During the experiment, the observer reported whether the grating perturbed by the AM disappeared. For each condition, four AM gap sizes (1.26°, 1.71°, 2.16°, 2.61°) were tested, with 112 trials per gap size.

The entire experiment above was repeated with the AM generated in the eye viewing the gratings (not shown). This repetition was to demonstrate that the suppression effect (with interocular AM) stems from rivalry

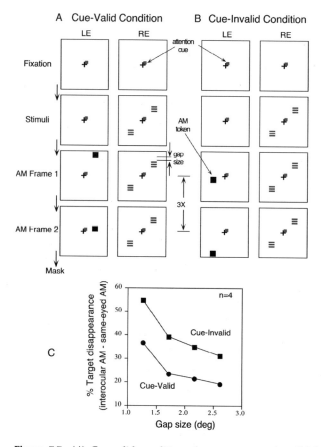

A  Cue-Valid Condition    B  Cue-Invalid Condition

**Figure 7.7**  (*A*) Cue-valid condition: the apparent motion (AM) traverses the attended grating (in visual space). (*B*) Cue-invalid condition: the AM traverses the unattended grating that is located diagonally to the attended grating (in visual space). (*C*) The average percentage difference in target disappearance plotted as a function of gap size shows fewer disappearances for the cue-valid (filled circles) than the cue-invalid (filled squares) condition.

rather than from other effects, such as Troxler's fading (see chapter 2 in this volume). Overall, we found that about 10% or fewer of such same-eyed AM trials (i.e., AM and gratings in the same eye) led to the target grating's disappearing.

Figure 7.7C plots the percent target disappearance (interocular AM – same-eye AM) as a function of the AM gap size. Clearly, fewer target disappearances occurred in the cue-valid condition than in the cue-invalid condition. This implies that voluntary attention to a particular dominant rival image counteracted the tendency of AM to induce suppression; attention effectively boosted the dominant strength of the rival target.

Teng Leng Ooi and Zijiang J. He

## Involuntary Attention Paves the Way for Binocular Rivalry Dominance

When an odd element is presented among a group of common elements, it will "pop out" and be detected quickly (Treisman and Gelade, 1980). Pop-out also acts as a cue that draws involuntary attention to its location (Nakayama and Mackeben, 1989; Joseph and Optican, 1996; Treisman and Gelade, 1980; Yantis, 1993). We reasoned that a rivalry stimulus placed in the vicinity of the odd element/cue would benefit from the attention attracted to it. Specifically, the rivalry stimulus would be more likely to be perceived (Ooi and He, 1999).

To perform the experiment (figure 7.8A), we presented six pairs of gray vertical lines in one eye and a pair of red horizontal lines in the other eye

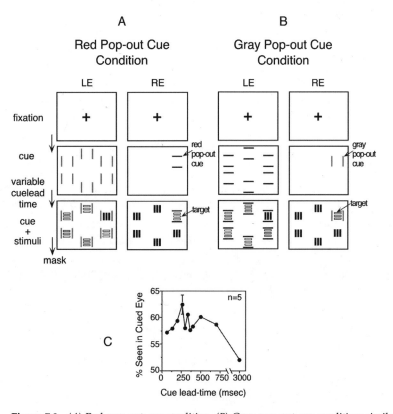

**Figure 7.8** (*A*) Red pop-out cue condition. (*B*) Gray pop-out cue condition: similar to (*A*) except that the pop-out cue is a pair of gray vertical lines and the common elements are pairs of red horizontal lines. (*C*) The combined average results from both conditions, plotted as a function of cue lead time, show performance in seeing the grating surrounded by the cue as above the chance level (50%). The vertical bar represents the average standard error of all cue lead-time intervals.

Surface Representations and Attention Modulation

(the odd element serving as the pop-out cue). After a variable cue lead time (67–3000 msec), six patches of red/green rivalry gratings were presented for 500 msec. The observer reported the color of the grating perceived in the vicinity of the pop-out cue. Eleven different cue lead-time intervals were tested, with 100 trials for each interval. In addition, another condition (figure 7.8B), where the color and orientation of the common and odd elements were switched, was tested. This was to control for the argument that the contrast energy of the odd element led to rivalry dominance.

Figure 7.8C plots the average performance in seeing the rivalry stimulus in the cued eye as a function of the cue lead time. If involuntary attention had no effect on rivalry dominance, performance would be at the 50% chance level. Our analysis shows that performance was significantly above the chance level, with a peak performance at about 250 msec, for all cue lead-time intervals except the longest one. This pattern of results suggests that involuntary attention attracted to a cued location can pave the way for a rivalry stimulus at that location to become dominant. Not coincidentally, the temporal profile of performance is consistent with the transient nature of involuntary attention (Nakayama and Mackeben, 1989).

**SUMMARY**

The studies reviewed above reveal that binocular rivalry is affected, in a predictable manner, by surface-image properties and by attentional modulation. Our psychophysical observations suggest that rivalry is not processed solely at a particular cortical level, but over several cortical levels involving both feed forward and feedback interactions (Alais and Blake, 1998; Blake, 2001; Ooi and He, 1999, 2003a, 2003b). For example, the eye-of-origin signature, which is commonly attributed to monocular neurons in the striate cortex (Blake, 1989; Blake, Westendorf, and Overton, 1980; Shimojo and Nakayama, 1990), is critical for initiating local suppression.

Meanwhile, the integration of surfaces, which occurs over several cortical levels (e.g., Bakin, Nakayama, and Gilbert, 2000; Sugita, 1999; Von der Heydt, Peterhans, and Baumgartner, 1984; Zhou, Friedman, and Von der Heydt, 2000), can also affect the outcome of rivalry.

Our psychophysical studies complement the findings of various neurophysiological studies suggesting distributed sites of binocular rivalry (Leopold and Logothetis, 1996; Logothetis, 1998; Logothetis and Schall,

1989; Lumer, Friston, and Rees, 1998; Polansky et al., 2000; Sengpiel and Blakemore, 1994; Sheinberg and Logothetis, 1997; Tong and Engel, 2001; Tong et al., 1999).

## ACKNOWLEDGMENTS

This work was supported in part by grants from the Knights Templar Eye Foundation, Inc., and the Pennsylvania College of Optometry Fund to T. L. Ooi, and a grant from the International Center of the University of Louisville to Z. J. He.

## REFERENCES

Alais, D., and Blake, R. (1998). Interactions between global motion and local binocular rivalry. *Vision Research, 38,* 637–644.

Alais, D., O'Shea, R. P., Mesana-Alais, C., and Wilson, I. G. (2000). On binocular alternation. *Perception, 29,* 1437–1445.

Bakin, J. S., Nakayama, K., and Gilbert, C. D. (2000). Visual responses in monkey areas V1 and V2 to three-dimensional surface configurations. *Journal of Neuroscience, 20,* 8188–8198.

Blake, R. (1989). A neural theory of binocular rivalry. *Psychological Review, 96,* 145–167.

Blake, R. (2001). A primer on binocular rivalry, including current controversies. *Brain and Mind, 2,* 5–38.

Blake, R., Westendorf, D. H., and Overton, R. (1980). What is suppressed during binocular rivalry? *Perception, 9,* 223–231.

Duensing, S., and Miller, B. (1979). The Cheshire Cat effect. *Perception, 8,* 269–273.

Fox, R. (1991). Binocular rivalry. In *Vision and Visual Dysfunction,* vol. 9, *Binocular Vision,* D. M. Regan, ed., 93–110. London: Macmillan.

Frisby, J. P., and Mayhew, J. E. W. (1978). The relationship between apparent depth and disparity in rivalrous texture stereograms. *Perception, 7,* 661–678.

Gillam, B., and Borsting, E. (1988). The role of monocular regions in stereoscopic displays. *Perception, 17,* 603–608.

Grindley, G. C., and Townsend, V. (1965). Binocular masking induced by a moving object. *Quarterly Journal of Experimental Psychology, 17,* 97–109.

Grossberg, S. (1997). Cortical dynamics of three-dimensional form, color, and brightness perception: II. Binocular theory. *Perception and Psychophysics, 41,* 117–158.

Helmholtz, H. von (1962). *Treatise on Physiological Optics,* trans. from 3rd German ed., J. P. C. Southall, trans. New York: Dover.

Hering, K. E. (1879). *Spatial Sense and Movement of the Eye,* C. A. Radde, trans. Baltimore: American Academy of Optometry.

Joseph, J., and Optican, L. (1996). Involuntary attentional shifts due to orientation differences. *Perception and Psychophysics,* 58, 651–665.

Julesz, B. (1971). *Foundation of Cyclopean Perception.* Chicago: University of Chicago Press.

Kanizsa, G. (1979). *Organization in Vision: Essays on Gestalt Perception.* New York: Praeger.

Kovács, I., Papathomas, T. V., Yang, M., and Fehér, A. (1996). When the brain changes its mind: Interocular grouping during binocular rivalry. *Proceedings of National Academy of Sciences of the United States of America,* 93, 15508–15511.

Lack, L. (1978). *Selective Attention and the Control of Binocular Rivalry.* The Hague: Mouton.

Leopold, D. A., and Logothetis, N. K. (1996). Activity changes in early visual cortex reflect monkeys' percepts during binocular rivalry. *Nature,* 379, 549–553.

Levelt, W. J. M. (1965). *On Binocular Rivalry.* Soesterberg, The Netherlands: Institute for Perception.

Logothetis, N. K. (1998). Single units and conscious vision. *Philosophical Transactions of the Royal Society of London,* B353, 1801–1818.

Logothetis, N. K., and Schall, J. D. (1989). Neuronal correlates of subjective visual perception. *Science,* 245, 761–763.

Lumer, E. D., Friston, K. J., and Rees, G. (1998). Neural correlates of perceptual rivalry in the human brain. *Science,* 280, 1930–1934.

Marr, D. (1982). *Vision.* San Francisco: Freeman.

Marr, D., and Poggio, T. (1979). A computational theory of human stereo vision. *Proceedings of the Royal Society of London,* B204, 301–328.

Metelli, F. (1974). The perception of transparency. *Scientific American,* 230, 90–98.

Myerson, J., Miezin, F., and Allman, J. (1981). Binocular rivalry in macaque monkeys and humans: A comparative study in perception. *Behaviour Analysis Letters,* 1, 149–159.

Nakayama, K., He, Z. J., and Shimojo, S. (1995). Visual surface representation: A critical link between lower-level and higher-level vision. In *An Invitation to Cognitive Science: Visual Cognition,* S. Kosslyn and D. O. Osherson, eds., 1–70. Cambridge, Mass.: MIT Press.

Nakayama, K., and Mackeben, M. (1989). Sustained and transient components of focal visual attention. *Vision Research,* 29, 1631–1647.

Nakayama, K., and Shimojo, S. (1990). Da Vinci stereopsis: Depth and subjective contours from unpaired image points. *Vision Research,* 30, 1811–1825.

Nakayama, K., Shimojo, S., and Ramachandran, V. S. (1990). Transparency: Relation to depth, subjective contours, luminance, and neon color spreading. *Perception,* 19, 497–513.

Ngo, T. T., Miller, S. M., Liu, G. B., and Pettigrew, J. D. (2000). Binocular rivalry and perceptual coherence. *Current Biology,* 10, R134–R136.

Ooi, T. L., and He, Z. J. (1999). Binocular rivalry and visual awareness: The role of attention. *Perception,* 28, 551–574.

Ooi, T. L., and He, Z. J. (2003a). A distributed intercortical processing of binocular rivalry: Psychophysical evidence. *Perception,* 32, 155–166.

Ooi, T. L., and He, Z. J. (2003b). On the initiation and spreading of interocular suppression from binocular vertical contours. *Journal of Vision*, 3, 452a.

Papathomas, T. V., Kovács, I., Fehér, A., and Julesz, B. (1999). Visual dilemmas: Competition between the eyes and between percepts in binocular rivalry. In *What Is Cognitive Science?*, E. LePore and Z. Pylyshyn, eds., 263–294. Malden, Mass.: Basil Blackwell.

Polonsky, A., Blake, R., Braun, J., and Heeger, D. J. (2000). Neuronal activity in human primary visual cortex correlates with perception during binocular rivalry. *Nature Neuroscience*, 3, 1153–1159.

Posner, M. I. (1980). Orienting of attention. *Quarterly Journal of Experimental Psychology*, 32, 3–25.

Sengpiel, F., and Blakemore, C. (1994). Interocular control of neuronal responsiveness in cat visual cortex. *Nature*, 368, 847–850.

Sheinberg, D. L., and Logothetis, N. K. (1997). The role of temporal cortical areas in perceptual organization. *Proceedings of National Academy of Sciences of the United States of America*, 94, 3408–3413.

Shimojo, S., and Nakayama, K. (1990). Real world occlusion constraints and binocular rivalry. *Vision Research*, 30, 69–80.

Sobel, K. V., and Blake, R. (2002). How context influences predominance during binocular rivalry. *Perception*, 31, 813–824.

Sugita, Y. (1999). Grouping of image fragments in primary visual cortex. *Nature*, 401, 269–272.

Tong, F., and Engel, S. A. (2001). Interocular rivalry revealed in the human cortical blind-spot representation. *Nature*, 411, 195–199.

Tong, F., Nakayama, K., Vaughan, J. T., and Kanwisher, N. (1998). Binocular rivalry and visual awareness in human extrastriate cortex. *Neuron*, 21, 753–759.

Treisman, A. M., and Gelade, G. (1980). A feature integration theory of attention. *Cognitive Psychology*, 12, 97–136.

Van der Zwan, R., Wenderoth, P., and Alais, D. (1993). Reduction of a pattern-induced motion aftereffect by binocular rivalry suggests the involvement of extrastriate mechanisms. *Visual Neuroscience*, 10, 703–709.

Von der Heydt, R., Peterhans, E., and Baumgartner, G. (1984). Illusory contours and cortical neuron responses. *Science*, 224, 1260–1262.

Von der Heydt, R., Zhou, H., and Friedman, H. S. (2000). Representation of stereoscopic edges in monkey visual cortex. *Vision Research*, 40, 1955–1967.

Walker, P. (1978). Binocular rivalry: Central or peripheral selective processes? *Psychological Bulletin*, 85, 376–389.

Wilson, H. R., Blake, R., and Lee, S. H. (2001). Dynamics of travelling waves in visual perception. *Nature*, 412, 907–910.

Yantis, S. (1993). Stimulus-driven attentional capture. *Current Directions in Psychological Science*, 2, 156–161.

Zhou, H., Friedman, H. S., and Von der Heydt, R. (2000). Coding of border ownership in monkey visual cortex. *Journal of Neuroscience*, 20, 6594–6611.

# 8 Dynamics of Perceptual Bistability: Plaids and Binocular Rivalry Compared

## Nava Rubin and Jean-Michel Hupé

This chapter presents a set of findings about the dynamics of bistable alternations in the perception of plaids. A plaid is a pattern composed of two superimposed gratings. When the plaid is set in motion, it becomes an ambiguous stimulus: it can be seen as one pattern moving in a single direction (coherence) or as two gratings, each moving in a different direction, with one sliding over the other (transparency). The two possibilities are illustrated in figure 8.1A. In prolonged viewing, the perception of moving plaids switches back and forth between the coherent and the transparent interpretations, a classic example of perceptual bistability. Hans Wallach, who was the first to use superimposed gratings to study motion perception, discussed their bistability at some length (Wallach, 1935, 1976; Wuerger, Shapley, and Rubin, 1996). However, in the modern literature this aspect of plaid perception has been virtually forgotten. Since Adelson and Movshon (1982) reintroduced plaids as a tool for studying motion processing, researchers have been using brief-presentation 2AFC methods, overlooking the dynamical aspect (but see Von Grunau and Dubé, 1993). We therefore decided to give the bistable alternations in plaid perception a closer look.

We had two complementary goals in this research. The first was to develop methods for studying the dynamics of perceptual alternations in plaids in order to further our understanding of global motion computation. Like all visual information, motion information is fragmented in the first stages of cortical processing, distributed over many neurons with small spatial receptive fields. Therefore, the brain must combine local motion cues into global motion percepts. Global motion computation is nontrivial because real-world scenes contain multiple, often overlapping objects that can move in different directions, leading to a complex array of local motion measurements. Thus, on the one hand, there is a need to

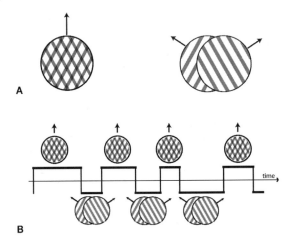

**Figure 8.1** (*A*) The two possible interpretations of a moving plaid: a coherently moving pattern (left) or two gratings sliding transparently over one another (right); the lateral offset between the gratings is for illustrative purposes, to show the impression of a slight depth difference between the gratings that accompanies the percept of transparent motion. (*B*) The dynamics of bistable alternations in the perception of moving plaids can be measured by requesting observers to continually indicate their percept (analogous to the paradigm commonly used in binocular rivalry).

integrate local motion signals that arise from the same object, while on the other hand it is necessary to segment motion cues that arise from different objects (Braddick, 1993). Plaids provide a clear illustration of those conflicting demands: in the "coherent" interpretation the integration process is dominant, while in the "transparent" interpretation the motion segmentation process is stronger (the grating components of the plaid are segmented from one another). However, most studies of plaids have used methods involving brief presentations.

By contrast, in other domains—most notably binocular rivalry—the dynamics of bistable alternations associated with prolonged viewing have revealed important insights about the underlying mechanisms. For example, the periods spent perceiving each percept vary systematically when the relative strength of the stimuli is manipulated (e.g., by changing the contrast of one or both monocular stimuli; see chapter 1 in this volume). We hypothesized that in developing dynamics-based methods (akin to those used in binocular rivalry) to measure the likelihood of the coherent and transparent percepts in plaids, we might shed new light on the mechanisms underlying motion integration and segmentation, and the interplay between them. Indeed, as we shall see below, our results indicate that

Nava Rubin and Jean-Michel Hupé

dynamics-based measures can be more sensitive than brief-presentation measures, thereby revealing effects that were not known until now.

As research toward the first goal progressed, a second, complementary goal emerged. If our first goal can be summarized as "using dynamics of bistability to learn about plaids," the second goal can be stated as "using plaids to further our understanding of bistability." At the heart of this second goal is the idea that bistability reveals general principles about brain architecture. Consider this fundamental characteristic of bistability: when a stimulus has more than one plausible interpretation, observers will alternate between perceiving one interpretation and another, but they will always experience only one percept at a time.[1] This is such a basic observation, valid in such varied domains of bistability (e.g., Necker cubes, binocular rivalry, vase/face illusion), that it is rarely questioned. But why should it be so? Why should we not be able to perceive both stimulus interpretations simultaneously?

One answer is that bistability reflects real-world constraints: a location in space cannot be occupied by two different objects simultaneously (binocular rivalry); an object cannot be convex and concave at the same time (the Necker cube); and so on. But this can be only one part of the answer—the other part has to do with brain architecture. The very fact of bistability suggests that the brain has built-in mechanisms to enforce mutual exclusivity: given a stimulus with more than one plausible interpretation, the neural representation of only one of those interpretations is allowed to dominate at each moment.[2] It is unlikely that the brain developed specialized mechanisms for bistability just so that it can deal with the rare cases of deeply ambiguous stimuli (which are typically encountered only in the lab). Probably, bistability—and its implied principle of mutual exclusivity—occurs as a result of brain architecture that evolved to deal with the far more common situations of "weak ambiguity" present in many sensory stimuli. Normally, a wealth of cues in the environment renders one interpretation much more likely than others, but the fact that competing interpretations are seldom experienced (outside the lab) is nevertheless not obvious a priori.

How the brain achieves this uniqueness of perception requires explanation, and bistability may offer a window to the underlying mechanisms. As we observed, there are some commonalities between the dynamics of bistability in plaids and those reported in other domains (mainly binocular rivalry). These commonalities led us to hypothesize the existence of general principles governing how the brain implements mutual exclusivity. In more concrete terms, then, our second goal is to study the commonalities—as well as the differences—of bistability in plaids and other domains, and how they constrain models of the underlying mechanisms.

## CONSTANCY OVER TIME OF THE AVERAGE DURATION OF BISTABLE ALTERNATIONS

Do the average durations of coherence and transparency epochs during plaid perception show any consistent trends over time? There are two reasons to ask this question. First, there have been many references in the literature to "adaptation" or "satiation" as playing a role in plaid perception (e.g., Adelson and Movshon, 1982; Wallach, 1935). One might therefore expect to find some fingerprint of adaptation in the dynamics of alternations—for example, a slowing down of the alternations in prolonged observations. (Weakening the competing stimuli leads to slower alternations in binocular rivalry; if adaptation has the effect of weakening the perceived interpretation, a consequent slowing down of the alternations might be expected.)

The second reason to examine how the average durations behave is methodological: if they are stable over time, this would facilitate deriving dynamics-based measures of the strength of the coherence and transparency percepts. We therefore examined the periods spent perceiving coherence and transparency over very long observation times. Observers watched a moving plaid for 5 min and reported what they perceived ("coherence" or "transparency") continually by pressing one of two mouse buttons (see figure 8.1B; see Hupé and Rubin, 2003, for details of experimental procedures). This procedure was repeated ten times with the same stimulus, but with very long breaks between consecutive trials: there were at most two trials per day (one in the morning and one in the evening).

Figure 8.2 shows scatter plots of epoch durations, separated into coherence (left) and transparency (right) epochs. While there is wide variability between the durations of the epochs in each trial, when all trials are superimposed, a clear picture emerges: the average durations of the coherent and transparent epochs are very stable over time[3] (for more data supporting this observation, see Hupé and Rubin, 2003). There is one exception to this statement: the average duration of the very first epoch, which was always coherent,[4] was longer than that of subsequent coherent epochs. This singularity of the first epoch may be why researchers had a subjective impression that the epochs shorten over time (e.g.,

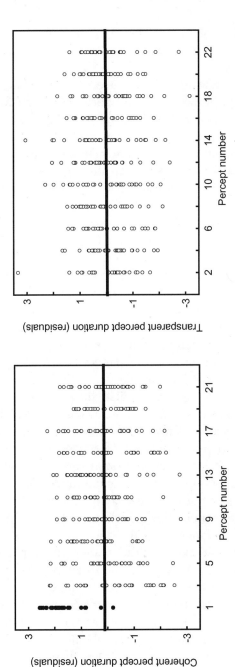

**Figure 8.2**  Duration of coherence (left) and transparency (right) epochs in bistable alternations of a single plaid stimulus viewed for multiple trials of 5 min each (three observers; data present residual variance after removing intersubject variability). The durations are plotted as a function of their ordinal positions within each trial. Best-fitting linear trends indicate no significant drift up or down (i.e., the average durations are constant over time, excluding the first coherent epoch; see text). For stimulus parameters and sample scatter plots of individual observers, see Hupé and Rubin (2003).

Wallach, 1935; J. A. Movshon, personal communication), and why they conjectured about the role of adaptation (or "satiation"; Wallach, 1976) in the alternations.

However, our data indicate that this subjective impression is misleading, created solely by the first singular epoch. When the first epoch is excluded, the best-fit linear trends show a zero slope for both coherence and transparency. This means that we can really talk of a steady-state phase of bistable alternations in plaids, which sets in immediately after the first epoch and consists of epochs that, although variable in duration, are drawn from distributions with stationary means and variances.

The stability of the average durations over time has both methodological and theoretical implications. Methodologically, it means that we can derive measures of the relative strengths of the coherent and transparent percepts from dynamics data, without concern that those measures may change due to arbitrary factors such as observation time. Specifically, if we denote the average durations spent reporting coherence and transparency by C and T, respectively, then $C/[C + T]$ is the steady-state probability of perceiving the coherent percept, which gives a measure of its relative strength. (Note: the first coherence percept is excluded from C; it will be treated separately in the section "Dynamics-Based Measures.") This measure is analogous to that used in binocular rivalry studies, the relative time spent perceiving one of the monocular stimuli $(R/[R + L])$, which is known to vary with stimulus strength (e.g., by changing contrast; Levelt, 1968). Indeed, in the next section we show that $C/[C + T]$ varies systematically with manipulations of plaid parameters. Moreover, the dynamics-based measure is sensitive to parametric variations even in regimes where brief-presentation methods suffer from "ceiling" and "floor" effects.

From a theoretical point of view, the stability of the average durations imposes significant constraints on models of bistability. Many models assume some form of adaptation of the dominant percept as the main factor that leads to alternations. If such adaptation indeed plays a role, our data suggest that it has to be short-lived and its effects cannot accumulate over time. Otherwise, the average durations would change over time (as they change with stimulus strength). Given the clear results we obtained in plaids, it is interesting to pose the same question for binocular rivalry stimuli: Do the average durations of bistable alternations change over time? Previously, there had been reports of lengthening of the durations over time. Lehky (1988) proposed that this may be an indirect result of adaptation to contrast (decreased effective contrast leads to weaker stimuli, which lead to longer bistable durations).

Nava Rubin and Jean-Michel Hupé

If Lehky's conjecture is correct, then binocular rivalry stimuli that are not affected by contrast should show stable average durations, as we found for plaids. This is not a hypothetical statement: although contrast often affects the rate of rivalry alternations (see chapter 1 in this volume), for some stimuli, contrast is not a major factor. To test this directly, we used a stimulus introduced by Bossink, Stalmeier, and De Weert (1993), consisting of fields of random dots moving in orthogonal directions in the two eyes. For this stimulus, speed has a major effect on the monocular stimulus strength, whereas contrast has only a minor effect. Figure 8.3 shows scatter plots of the dominance durations for the left-eye and right-eye stimuli for ten repetitions of 5-min trials (each trial was well separated in time from the others, as before). The results suggest that when extraneous factors (such as contrast adaptation) are eliminated, the average durations of perceptual alternations in binocular rivalry, as for plaids, are stable over time. (Similar results were obtained from two naive observers; data not shown.) This in turn suggests that whatever role adaptation plays in causing perceptual alternations, the mechanisms may be similar in different bistability domains.

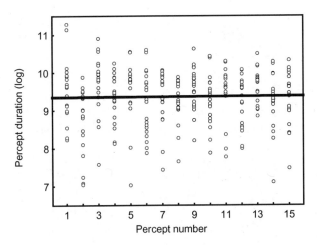

**Figure 8.3** Durations of monocular epochs in bistable alternations of a binocular rivalry stimulus viewed for multiple trials of 5 min each (two observers). The stimuli consisted of random dot surfaces moving in orthogonal directions in the two eyes (see Bossink, Stalmeier, and De Weert, 1993; epochs were computed in "compound" method—see Mueller and Blake, 1989). The average durations of perceptual alternations are constant over time. In contrast to bistability in plaids, there is no tendency for the first epoch in binocular rivalry to be longer.

Dynamics of Perceptual Bistability

Another way to ask about possible adaptation effects is to check whether there is a correlation between the durations of a given coherence epoch and the subsequent transparency epoch, and between a given coherence epoch and the next coherence epoch (and similarly for a given transparency epoch). Figure 8.4 presents scatter plots for the four pairs. Denoting the $i$th coherence epoch by $C_i$ and the following transparency epoch by $T_i$, the data for $\{T_i \to C_{i+1}\}$ and $\{T_i \to T_{i+1}\}$ show no correlation at all, while $\{C_i \to T_i\}$ and $\{C_i \to C_{i+1}\}$ show significant but weak correlations (slight tendency for longer $C_i$'s to be followed by longer $T_i$'s and then by shorter $C_{i+1}$'s). Overall, the data suggest that the length of one epoch has little effect on the following epochs. Lehky (1995) performed a similar analysis for binocular rivalry data and found no correlations between the lengths of successive epochs. This suggests that if adaptation is involved in bistability, its influence does not carry over from one epoch to another, since if it did, one should observe systematic trends, such as long $T_i$ epochs followed by longer than average $C_{i+1}$ epochs and shorter

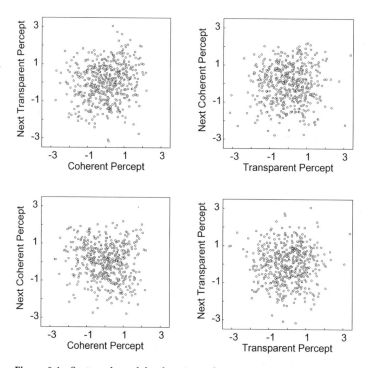

**Figure 8.4** Scatter plots of the durations of successive epochs (top, between-type; bottom, within-type). The length of one epoch has little or no effect on the length of the following epochs (see text).

Nava Rubin and Jean-Michel Hupé

than average $T_{i+1}$ epochs (due to the increased accumulated adaptation of $T$ in epoch $i$).

## THE DISTRIBUTION OF BISTABILITY DURATIONS

Next, we examined the distributions of coherence and transparency durations, and the relations between them. Figure 8.5 shows a histogram of the coherence durations as a function of duration length. As observed in other domains of bistability, the distribution resembles a skewed Gaussian, peaking at intermediate values and falling off slowly, with a long tail. In other domains of bistability (most notably binocular rivalry), gamma distributions have typically been used to fit the histograms of bistable durations (e.g., Leopold, and Logothetis, 1996; Levelt, 1968; Logothetis, Leopold, and Sheinberg, 1996). For our plaid data, we found that log-normal distributions provide as good a fit, and often better. For the data in figure 8.5, for example, the best fit log-normal yielded $p < 0.07$, whereas the best-fit gamma yielded $p < 0.2$. Interestingly, Lehky (1995) reported that for his binocular rivalry data, when compared directly (for the same data set), log-normal distributions provided an as good or a better fit than gamma distributions.

The idea that the log-normal function provides a better fit to bistable alternations data is intriguing, because it suggests that the logarithms of

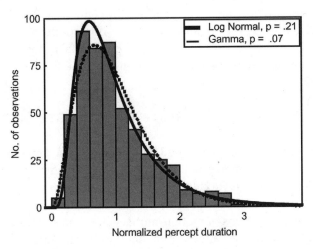

**Figure 8.5** Histogram of the durations of coherent periods is better fit by a log-normal than a gamma distribution. Data from repeated 5-min trials with a single stimulus and three observers (as in figure 8.2). Data from individual observers were normalized to each observer's mean before pooling.

Dynamics of Perceptual Bistability

duration of each percept are normally distributed, which has consequences for what might be the underlying mechanisms of the perceptual switches. It is, however, not trivial to obtain data that would clearly and strongly point to one functional form over another. Pooling data across observers, or even across trials with different stimulus parameters, leads to mixing of values that are drawn from different distributions (i.e., distributions that have different parameters, though the same functional form). To address this problem, researchers often normalize data to observers' individual means before pooling (as we did in figure 8.5). But as long as the underlying distributions generating the data are not well understood, it is also not clear what effect this procedure has on the subsequent ability to make strong statements about what functional form best fits the data. Furthermore, while normalizing data per observer is common, in most studies the data from trials with different stimulus parameters are pooled with no adjustment procedures.

We addressed this issue in analyzing data from our experiments with plaids. We collected dynamics data for a large stimulus set, systematically varying plaid parameters that affect the tendency for coherence, and then performed an ANOVA with all parametric manipulations (as well as observer identity) taken into account. The analysis revealed two important points: first, that transforming the raw data to log values led to models with excellent fit to the parametric effects, and second, that the residual variances distributed normally (Hupé and Rubin, 2003). The latter point provides strong support for the claim that the log of durations is indeed normally distributed. In turn, this supports the use of log-normal distributions to fit histograms of perceptual durations. Theoretical work is needed to assess the implications of these findings for models of bistability.

## DYNAMICS-BASED MEASURES OF THE STRENGTH OF COHERENCE

In a series of experiments, we used the dynamics-based measure $C/[C + T]$ to test the effect of manipulating various plaid parameters on the relative strength of coherence. (Recall that this measure gives the relative time spent perceiving coherence out of the entire observation time.) The angle between the gratings' directions of motion, alpha, has the most dramatic effect (figure 8.6). As alpha is changed from small to large, perception shifts from being dominated by coherence to being dominated by transparency.

The importance of the angular separation between motion signals as a strong cue for motion segmentation has a clear ecological basis, since

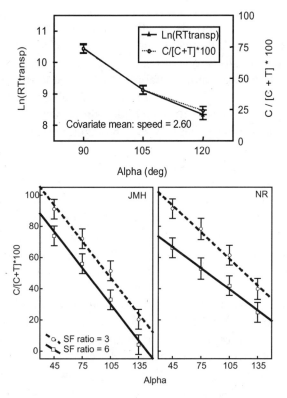

**Figure 8.6** The dynamics-based measure $C/[C + T]$ shows a linear relationship to alpha (the angle between gratings' directions of motion) in a wide range of plaid parameter spaces. (*A*) Rectangular-wave plaids, four observers. (*B*) Sine-wave plaids, data from individual observers. For stimulus parameters, see Hupé and Rubin (2003).

different objects tend to move in independent directions. The effect of alpha on the probability of perceiving coherence was observed previously, with brief-presentation methods. However, those methods yielded sigmoid-shaped curves with rapid transitions between 100% responses "coherence" and 100% responses "transparency," flanked by wide ranges of alpha where the responses were constant at those extreme values (e.g., Kim and Wilson, 1993). In contrast, the dynamics-based measure $C/[C + T]$ reveals a near-linear transition from 0% to 100%, indicating a gradual—not abrupt—change in relative strength between coherence and transparency.

In a detailed analysis elsewhere, we showed that the sigmoid curves found with brief-presentation methods resulted from "ceiling" and "floor" artifacts inherent to this paradigm (Hupé and Rubin, 2003).

Essentially, the brief trials used there (~1 sec) reflect only what happens in the initial observation periods, and those tend to be dominated repeatedly by the same percept (either coherence or transparency), leading to stimuli classified categorically as one or the other. However, when more observation time is allowed (~1 min), bistability is observed even when one of the two percepts is strongly dominant in short observations. Thus, the dynamics approach reveals the true underlying effect of increasing alpha, which is to decrease the relative strength of coherence in a gradual, near-linear manner.[5]

In the section "Constancy over Time" we noted that for plaids composed of rectangular-wave gratings, the first epoch was always coherent, and its mean duration was longer than that of subsequent coherent epochs. Interestingly, a long initial epoch of coherence was observed even for stimuli that were subsequently dominated by the transparency percept—that is, for which $C/[C + T]$ was less than 0.5 (e.g., for large alpha values). This asymmetry between the two competing percepts, coherency, and transparency, may be unique to plaids. Preliminary findings suggest the asymmetry may be further unique to stimuli where there is ambiguity about the relative depth of the two constituent gratings, so that the transparent percept is in fact comprised of two possible percepts which alternate over time (first one of the gratings is seen in front, and then the other). It could be that this further "splitting" of one of the competing percepts (transparency) is what breaks the symmetry between it and coherence, but more research is needed to test this hypothesis further.

Whatever the reason for the prolonged first coherent percept in rectangular-wave plaids, we have been able to use it as an additional measure of the relative strength of coherence. The mean duration of the first epoch can be extracted from the same experiments where observers continually indicate their percept in trials of 1–2 min (for measuring $C/[C + T]$; recall that the first coherent epoch is excluded from the calculation of $C/[C + T]$, and therefore the two measures are methodologically independent). It can also be collected more efficiently, in a paradigm where observers are asked to press a button as soon as they see the plaid separate into two transparent gratings, terminating the trial. We termed this measure $RT_{transp}$ (response time to report transparency; note, however, that this is not a speeded-reaction task: observers were asked not to "try" to see more of one percept or the other, that is, "passive" viewing instructions). In both cases we found that $RT_{transp}$ shows the same gradual, linear decrease with alpha, in agreement with the gradual decrease in the relative strength of coherence revealed by $C/[C + T]$ (Hupé and Rubin, 2003).

Nava Rubin and Jean-Michel Hupé

The gradual effect of alpha on the strength of coherence has important implications for models of motion integration and segmentation, since it suggests that there is not a "critical" value of alpha where the system switches from one interpretation to the other. Several existing models of plaid perception implement a "decision" between coherence and transparency with a switch at such a critical value, mirroring the rapid transition from all-coherence to all-transparency found with brief presentations (see, e.g., Wilson and Kim, 1994). However, our dynamics data indicated that the underlying transition is actually gradual. This behavior resembles what is found in binocular rivalry: a gradual change in $R/[R + L]$ as the contrast of one of the monocular stimuli is changed. This type of behavior is explained well by models of binocular rivalry, which assume a continual competition between the two rivaling stimuli, with mutual inhibition ensuring that only one is allowed to prevail at any given moment (Blake, 1989; Laing and Chow, 2002; Lehky, 1988). This type of model can be adapted to motion segmentation and integration, and will naturally give rise to the gradual changes in the relative strength of coherence and transparency in plaids that we observed. We elaborate on this in the next section.

## LEVELT'S SECOND PROPOSITION IN BINOCULAR RIVALRY AND IN PLAID PERCEPTION

No comparison with the dynamics of perceptual alternations in binocular rivalry would be complete without reference to Levelt's second proposition (Levelt, 1968). We have already mentioned that changing the strength of one of the monocular stimuli (e.g., by changing its contrast) affects the relative time spent perceiving that stimulus (see also chapter 1 in this volume). The change is in the direction one would expect intuitively: when one stimulus is strengthened (while the other is kept unchanged), the relative time spent perceiving it increases. Levelt examined more closely how this increase took place, by studying what happened to the absolute durations of epochs perceiving each of the two monocular stimuli. (Recall that while the lengths of the bistable epochs vary stochastically from one alternation to the other, their means are stable over time, for a given stimulus. One may therefore study the effect of stimulus manipulations on the lengths of those mean durations.)

One might intuitively expect that increasing the strength of one stimulus would lead to an increase in its mean dominance duration, and possibly that there would also be a decrease in the mean dominance duration of the other (competing) stimulus. But when Levelt (1968) tested this, he found, surprisingly, that the changes in absolute durations were restricted to those of the other stimulus (the one whose strength was not changed). He summarized this result in what has become known as Levelt's second proposition: "Increase of the stimulus strength in one eye will not affect $t^-$ [the mean dominance durations] for the same eye . . . $t_r^-$ [the mean dominance durations of the right-eye stimulus] can only be affected by $\lambda_1$ [the left-eye stimulus strength], not $\lambda_r$."[6]

Why is Levelt's second proposition surprising? What implicit assumptions does this finding challenge? To answer this, let us consider the simplest model of how the perceptual switches might arise. Assume that the dominant (perceived) stimulus undergoes gradual adaptation (i.e., some form of weakening of the neural activity representing it). At some point the competing percept would become (relatively) stronger and consequently take over. In this simple model, a strengthening of stimulus A would be expected to increase its dominance duration—because it would take longer for the adaptation to bring it to a level low enough for B (the competing stimulus) to take over. Moreover, this simple model provides no mechanism for the strength of stimulus A to affect the mean dominance durations of B at all—let alone affect primarily those durations.

There is wide agreement about the crucial ingredients of a model that would account for Levelt's second proposition. Such a model must allow some form of coupling between the neural representations of the two percepts. Indeed, most modern models of binocular rivalry use an architecture of reciprocal inhibition between two neuronal populations that represent the rival percepts (Blake, 1989; Laing and Chow, 2002; Lehky, 1988). As a consequence, increasing the strength of one stimulus also increases the inhibition it exerts on the competing stimulus, and it is via this inhibitory coupling that one stimulus affects the dominance durations of the competing stimulus.

Levelt's second proposition had significant impact on how binocular rivalry is understood, because it suggested that the bistability results from an active process of continual competition between the two monocular stimuli. But the view of bistability as an active process of competition remained largely confined to binocular rivalry. In other domains (e.g., ambiguous figures) the view that perceptual alternations result from passive adaptation (fatigue) of the dominant percept is still common. This is also the case for plaids, where models generally implement a "decision" between the two possible interpretations. The concept of a continual,

Nava Rubin and Jean-Michel Hupé

active competition between the two possible interpretations is virtually absent from the literature.

But the parallels we observed between the dynamics of perceptual alternations in binocular rivalry and in plaids led us to hypothesize that the bistable alternations in plaid perception may also arise from an active competition between the coherence and transparency interpretations. Drawing on the analysis of what Levelt's second proposition implied for binocular rivalry, we reasoned that if one observed a similar phenomenon for plaids, it would be strong evidence for our hypothesis. We therefore asked: If we could change the strength of only one (say the transparent) interpretation, without affecting the other (coherent) interpretation, what would be the effect of this manipulation on the mean dominance durations of the two interpretations?

In binocular rivalry, changing the strength of one of the competing stimuli without affecting the other is most often done by changing the contrast of one monocular stimulus. But in the case of plaids, it is not obvious how to affect only the transparent (or coherent) interpretation. Since the two stimulus interpretations are mediated by the same external image, manipulation of a parameter such as contrast would obviously affect both the transparent percept and the coherent percept. The present lack of thorough understanding of the mechanisms underlying motion integration and segmentation further complicates the task of establishing that we affected only one interpretation. Nevertheless, we were able to find a manipulation that quite certainly changed the strength of only the transparent percept, without affecting the coherent percept. Without going into the details here, it involved switching the depth relationship between the two constituent gratings (by varying the intersections' luminance, not their stereoscopic disparity; Hupé and Rubin, manuscript in preparation). When we checked the effect, we found that the average dominance duration of transparency did not change. Instead, when the transparent interpretation was strengthened, coherence durations decreased markedly. This result is, in effect, a generalization of Levelt's second proposition to the domain of plaid perception.

The finding that an analogue of Levelt's second proposition can be observed for plaids supports our hypothesis that in the domain of motion perception, too, bistable alternations are caused by active competition between the two interpretations—here, the coherent and transparent percepts. Transferring the ideas prevalent in binocular rivalry to motion integration and segmentation, this would suggest an architecture where the neural representations of the coherent and transparent interpretations mutually inhibit one another in a struggle for perceptual dominance. These ideas represent a significant departure from the view common at present, which assumes that integration requires global processing, while segmentation is obtained directly via the responses of local motion detectors (Adelson and Movshon, 1982; Movshon et al., 1985). Models that implement this approach typically involve a feedforward stage of "decision" whether or not to integrate the local cues (e.g., Wilson and Kim, 1994). In such models, a need for competition does not arise naturally.

There is, however, evidence that motion segmentation also requires global processing (see Braddick, 1993). Indeed, some authors have postulated independence of integration and segmentation mechanisms—for example, Liden and Pack (1999) proposed to "subdivide the second stage into two parallel computations, one for integration and the other for segmentation." In such a model, implementing competition between the two mechanisms is a natural way to reach a decision between the two possible outcomes (see also Yuille and Grzywacz, 1998). This would lead to a situation where only one interpretation, integration or segmentation, can prevail at any given moment, as is observed perceptually, but would also offer a natural mechanism for the dynamics of bistability we have observed, including the plaid-motion analogue of Levelt's second proposition.

More generally, our findings point to the need to revise how other bistable phenomena are understood as well. The perceptual alternations observed for virtually every ambiguous stimulus may reflect not just passive adaptation but also a general strategy adopted by the brain, implementing mutual inhibition between competing interpretations of sensory stimuli. This idea, which may appear radical at first glance, is in fact consistent with known brain architecture, which is rich in reciprocal connections and inhibitory synapses. Research in other domains of perceptual bistability may offer new insights on whether this architecture is related to general computational principles.

**NOTES**

1. Under certain conditions, "mixture states" (i.e., percepts that are a superposition of the competing stimuli) are reported. But those are fairly rare, such as the "fusion" observed at very low contrast in binocular rivalry (Burke, Alais, and Wenderoth, 1999; Liu, Tyler, and Schor, 1992). The "patchy" percepts sometimes observed in binocular rivalry are not mixture states in this sense, since in every spatial location only one monocular image is perceived.

2. According to this view, "mixture states," which are exceptions to the mutual exclusivity principle, may reflect imperfections in how mutual exclusivity is implemented by the brain.

3. Von Grunau and Dubé (1993) reported a shortening of the perceptual epochs over time, but this conclusion was most likely due to a methodological problem in how the average durations were computed; see Hupé and Rubin (2003).

4. The first epoch was always coherent only for rectangular-wave plaids. For sinusoidal-grating plaids, the first percept could be either coherent or transparent, and its average duration did not differ from that of subsequent epochs of the same type (see also the section "Dynamics-Based Measures," and Hupé and Rubin, 2003).

5. Ceiling/floor effects, which are the only sources of deviations from linearity in the effect of alpha, can also be observed with the dynamics approach; they occur only at the extremes. For very small alpha values, coherence is so strong that the entire observation time, albeit long, may still not yield a single transparent epoch. Consequently, $C/[C + T]$ hits the ceiling value of 1, breaking the linear (middle) portion of the curve. Similarly, for very large alpha values transparency may dominate to the extent that $C/[C + T]$ hits the floor value of 0.

6. Subsequent work has shown that Levelt's second proposition is somewhat overstated: in many cases, changing the strength of one eye's stimulus will also affect the dominance durations of that eye (Bossink, Stalmeier, and De Weert, 1993). However, it is generally the case that changing stimulus strength in one eye has a much more pronounced effect on the dominance durations of the other eye (Leopold and Logothetis, 1996; Logothetis, Leopold, and Sheinberg, 1996; Mueller and Blake, 1989).

## REFERENCES

Adelson, E. H., and Movshon, J. A. (1982). Phenomenal coherence of moving visual patterns. *Nature, 300*, 523–525.

Blake, R. (1989). A neural theory of binocular rivalry. *Psychological Review, 96*, 145–167.

Bossink, C. J., Stalmeier, P. F., and De Weert, C. M. (1993). A test of Levelt's second proposition for binocular rivalry. *Vision Research, 33*, 1413–1419.

Braddick, O. (1993). Segmentation versus integration in visual motion processing. *Trends in Neurosciences, 16*, 263–268.

Burke, D., Alais, D., and Wenderoth, P. (1999). Determinants of fusion of dichoptically presented orthogonal gratings. *Perception, 28*, 73–88.

Hupé, J. M., and Rubin, N. (2003). The dynamics of bi-stable alternation in ambiguous motion displays: A fresh look at plaids. *Vision Research, 43*, 531–548.

Kim, J., and Wilson, H. R. (1993). Dependence of plaid motion coherence on component grating directions. *Vision Research, 33*, 2479–2489.

Laing, C. R., and Chow, C. C. (2002). A spiking neuron model for binocular rivalry. *Journal of Computational Neuroscience, 12*, 39–53.

Lehky, S. R. (1988). An astable multivibrator model of binocular rivalry. *Perception, 17*, 215–228.

Lehky, S. R. (1995) Binocular rivalry is not chaotic. *Proceedings of the Royal Society of London, B, 259*, 71–76.

Leopold, D. A., and Logothetis, N. K. (1996). Activity changes in early visual cortex reflect monkeys' percepts during binocular rivalry. *Nature*, 379, 549–553.

Levelt, W. J. M. (1968). *On Binocular Rivalry*. The Hague and Paris: Mouton.

Liden, L., and Pack, C. (1999). The role of terminators and occlusion cues in motion integration and segmentation: A neural network model. *Vision Research*, 39, 3301–3320.

Liu, L., Tyler, C. W., and Schor, C. M. (1992). Failure of rivalry at low contrast: Evidence of a suprathreshold binocular summation process. *Vision Research*, 32, 1471–1479.

Logothetis, N. K., Leopold, D. A., and Sheinberg, D. L. (1996). What is rivalling during binocular rivalry? *Nature*, 380, 621–624.

Movshon, J. A., Adelson, E. H., Gizzi, M. S., and Newsome, W. T. (1985). The analysis of moving visual patterns. In *Pattern Recognition Mechanisms*, C. Chagas, R. Gattas, and C. Gross, eds., 117–151. New York: Springer-Verlag.

Mueller, T. J., and Blake, R. (1989). A fresh look at the temporal dynamics of binocular rivalry. *Biological Cybernetics*, 61, 223–232.

Von Grunau, M., and Dubé, S. (1993). Ambiguous plaids: Switching between coherence and transparency. *Spatial Vision*, 7, 199–211.

Wallach, H. (1935). Über visuell wahrgenommene Bewegungsrichtung. *Psychologische Forschung*, 20, 325–380.

Wallach, H. (1976). *On Perception*. New York: Quadrangle.

Wilson, H. R., and Kim, J. (1994). A model for motion coherence and transparency. *Visual Neuroscience*, 11, 1205–1220.

Wuerger, S., Shapley, R., and Rubin, N. (1996). "On the visually perceived direction of motion" by Hans Wallach: 60 years later. *Perception*, 25, 1317–1367.

Yuille, A. L., and Grzywacz, N. M. (1998). A theoretical framework for visual motion. In T. Watanabe, ed., *High-Level Motion Processing*, 187–211. Cambridge, Mass.: MIT Press.

# 9 Interocular Grouping in Binocular Rivalry: Basic Attributes and Combinations

Thomas V. Papathomas, Ilona Kovács, and Tiffany Conway

One of the most interesting questions currently under debate is what rivals during binocular rivalry (for excellent reviews on this question, see Blake, 2000). There is a wide spectrum of possibilities between two extreme theories on this issue. At one end, there are eye-based theories of binocular rivalry. In their pure form, these theories posit that rivalry is the result of mostly bottom-up-driven inhibition among monocular neurons (Wolfe, 1986; Blake, 1989). Experimental evidence favoring such theories is provided by psychophysical studies, including the eye-swapping paradigm of Blake, Westendorf, and Overton (1980), the stimulus change procedure (Blake, et al., 1998), and Shimojo and Nakayama's (1990) study on the relationship between occlusion, eye of origin, and binocular rivalry. In more recent work, Alais and Blake (1998) have revised the pure form of the theory to include feedback from higher-level areas in the brain and neural interactions through lateral connections between cortical hypercolumns (Alais and Blake, 1999).

At the other extreme are stimulus-based theories, which, in their pure form, posit that it is coherent perceptual representations which compete during binocular rivalry, independently of the eye of origin. Although there is no experimental evidence supporting such a pure form of the theory, evidence for some role of stimulus coherence has been provided by psychophysical studies (e.g., Stirling, 1901; Diaz-Caneja, 1928, translated by Alais et al., 2000; Creed, 1935; Whittle, Bloor, and Pocock, 1968; Logothetis, Leopold, and Sheinberg, 1996; Kovács et al., 1996; Alais and Blake, 1999; Suzuki and Grabowecky, 2002) and neurophysiological findings (e.g., Logothetis and Schall, 1989; Leopold and Logothetis, 1996; Sheinberg and Logothetis, 1997).

Kovács et al. (1996) studied the phenomenon of interocular grouping (IOG) of color extensively. They used displays in which each eye's image contained elements of two different colors (red and green) against an equi-luminant yellow background. Each pair of elements was placed in the two eyes in identical locations (with respect to the fixation mark), but they were of opposite color, thus eliciting chromatic binocular rivalry. Even though each eye contained elements of both colors, Kovács et al. obtained evidence for stable and relatively long percepts in which all the elements appeared to be of one color (all-red or all-green). This was strong evidence that color was able to produce IOG.

Is color unique in this ability to form coherent perceptual representations? In this study we report on results of psychophysical experiments that were designed to assess the roles of both stimulus coherence and eye of origin in binocular rivalry. We studied the ability of four basic attributes (color, orientation, spatial frequency, and motion), as well as some of their combinations, to form coherent perceptual organizations. In the main experiment, we used two distinct rivaling types of elements, type A and type B, placed randomly in the display; as an example, type A and type B elements could be Gabor patches oriented at $+45°$ and $-45°$, respectively. There were two configurations. In the conventional one, all the type-A elements were in one eye's display, and the rivaling type-B elements were placed in the corresponding locations of the other eye. Eye competition and stimulus competition are confounded in this type of display. In the patchwork configuration, these two factors are deconfounded: the stimulus of one eye is composed of both type A and type B; the other eye's stimulus contains the complementary rivaling elements, types B and A, in the corresponding locations, resulting in local rivalry for every element.

Stimulus coherence can be assessed by noting how often observers obtain percepts where all elements appear to be of type A (or all of type B) in the patchwork configuration. Ideally, if an attribute can be organized into a coherent perceptual form by grouping all similar elements independently of eye of origin, observers would obtain the all-A or all-B percepts most of the time. In the case of color, observers do obtain the all-red or all-green percepts with frequencies that are significantly above chance-level performance, even though each monocular image contains mixed-color elements (Kovács et al., 1996).

On the other hand, rivalry could be due only to eye-of-origin factors, such as bottom-up-driven, mutually inhibitory interactions between monocular neurons (to suppress the other eye's input), or excitatory interactions between same-eye monocular neurons (to propagate one eye's dominant region). One must note that "eye" rivalry really refers to what is rivaling in a given region (or receptive field) of the visual field, not what is rivaling

T. V. Papathomas, I. Kovács, and T. Conway

throughout the entire visual field. The strength of eye-of-origin factors can be assessed by comparing performances in the conventional configuration (where all elements are identical in each eye's image) and the patchwork configuration (where both types of elements are present in each eye's image). If eye-of-origin factors played the major role in rivalry, then observers would rarely obtain the all-A or the all-B percepts in the patchwork configuration. Certainly, observers would obtain the all-A and all-B percepts more frequently in the conventional than in the patchwork configuration. The rest of this chapter presents details on the methods and results of these experiments, and concludes with a discussion of the main findings.

## METHODS

To assess the roles of both stimulus coherence and eye of origin in binocular rivalry, we studied rivalry using four basic attributes: color (C), spatial frequency (F), motion (M), and orientation (O). For these four attributes, there are a total of 11 possible combinations: six pairs, four triplets, and one quartet combination. In addition to testing IOG for each basic attribute (C, F, M, and O), we limited the study to the following six combinations: FM (spatial frequency and motion), FO, OM, FOM, FOC, and FOMC.

For each basic attribute, we used two distinct rivaling "values," A and B, to produce the type-A and type-B elements for that attribute; for example, for the motion attribute, A and B are downward and upward direction of motion, respectively (see details below). The values were selected so as to elicit binocular rivalry when they were shown in corresponding retinal locations in the two eyes. The parameters were selected to balance the strength of the type-A and type-B stimuli, namely, to make the relative predominances of type-A and type-B elements approximately equal. The predominance of a stimulus is the proportion of the total viewing time that the stimulus dominates.

The background had a uniform luminance of $9.1 \text{ cd}/\text{m}^2$. The chromaticity for the "unique" yellow color of the background was obtained separately for each observer (see below). In the color condition, the stimuli were colored circular patches ($C_A$ = red, $C_B$ = green), the chromaticity of which varied with a Gaussian profile ($\sigma = 53$ min of arc) from pure red (or green) at the center of the patch, progressing toward the unique yellow of the background away from the center.

For spatial frequency, rivaling stimuli were horizontally oriented Gabor patches with $F_A$ = low spatial frequency (2.60 cycles per degree: cpd) and

$F_B$ = high spatial frequency (10.87 cpd), with balanced contrasts between $F_A$ and $F_B$. The high and low values had a frequency difference of more than two octaves; also, the high spatial frequency was a noninteger multiple of the low spatial frequency, to minimize coincidences of peaks and troughs in the images of the two eyes.

Rivaling motion stimuli were horizontally oriented Gabor patches, the contours of which moved in the directions $M_A$ = downward and $M_B$ = upward at a constant velocity of 0.7°/sec. Finally, rivaling orientation stimuli were Gabor patches at orientations of $F_A = -45°$ and $F_B = +45°$. All the patches had a Gaussian envelope ($\sigma = 53$ min of arc). The Gaussian envelope was truncated at a radius of 1.36° to blend with the uniform background.

When rivaling stimuli differed in only one attribute, all other attributes were kept at a neutral value N. This value was between the rivaling A and B settings of the attribute. The following were the neutral values of the single attributes: the neutral value $C_N$ for color was yellow; horizontal stationary Gabor patches provided the neutral stimulus for motion ($M_N$ = stationary) as well as for orientation ($O_N = 0°$); the geometric average of the two rivaling frequencies was the neutral value for spatial frequency ($F_N = 5.32$ cpd).

When multiple attributes were combined, the two rivaling stimuli (the type-A and type-B stimuli) were composed of combinations of all the individual A and B values of the constituent attributes; as before, the non-involved attributes were assigned their neutral values N. For example, the stimuli for the FO condition were A stimulus = $-45°$-oriented low-frequency Gabor patch; B stimulus = $+45°$-oriented high-frequency Gabor patch. A schematic of this stimulus, with only six elements, is shown in figure 9.1. As another example, the stimuli for the FOM condition were A stimulus = $-45°$-oriented low-frequency Gabor patch, moving downward (in the southwest direction); B stimulus = $+45°$-oriented high-frequency Gabor patch, moving upward (in the northeast direction).

Each eye's stimulus consisted of eight nonoverlapping elements on a uniform, unique yellow background, located randomly around a central fixation mark within a 5.75° × 5.75° frame. Elements in the right and left eyes occupied corresponding retinal positions but were of opposite type (A and B), thereby inducing local rivalry by virtue of the single attribute (or combination of attributes) being tested.

Under binocular rivalry conditions, three stable percepts were possible: (1) "strictly uniform A" and (2) "strictly uniform B" percepts, when all eight elements appeared to be of type A or type B, respectively, and (3) "mixed" percept, when both types of elements were visible.

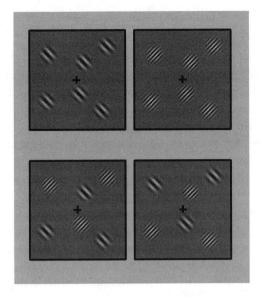

**Figure 9.1** A schematic diagram of the stimuli for the combination of spatial frequency and orientation (these are not actual stimuli used in the experiment). Top panel: conventional configuration; bottom panel: patchwork configuration.

As evidenced in the final results, some attributes were much weaker than others in eliciting IOG. As a result, we needed to relax the requirement for strictly uniform percepts, in order to avoid floor effects and to afford as meaningful a comparison of weak attributes as possible. Accordingly, we asked observers to report percepts in which at least seven of the elements appeared the same, and this is what we denote as "uniform A" or "uniform B" percepts.

Observers were instructed to press one of four buttons as soon as the percept changed, where the button corresponded to the newly obtained percept. For each trial, the average lengths of perceptual dominance, as well as cumulative durations of dominance for each percept, were computed and used as the dependent variables.

Two stimulus configurations were used for each of the ten conditions for single attribute or combinations of attributes.

1. In the conventional configuration (figure 9.1, top), all elements of type A were placed in one eye, and all the rivaling B elements were placed in the other eye; all the A elements were presented to either the left eye or the right eye.

2. In the patchwork configuration (figure 9.1, bottom), there were exactly four elements of type A and four elements of type B in one eye, with the rivaling elements in the other eye.

We used the predominances of the two uniform percepts (uniform A and uniform B) as a measure of the ability of an attribute to produce coherent percepts. Comparing the above measures in the conventional configuration, where eye of origin plays a role, against the patchwork configuration, where it does not play any role, could assess the strength of the eye-of-origin factor.

As mentioned earlier, the values of A and B of each attribute needed to be balanced for relative predominance. Some balancing values were obvious, and required no additional experiments. For example, the values $O_A = -45°$ and $O_B = +45°$ were assumed to have equal strengths for orientation; similarly, it is reasonable to expect the values $M_A = $ motion downward and $M_B = $ motion upward to be balanced. These expectations were confirmed in the actual experiments. Other balancing values required some preliminary experiments to obtain the equiluminant setting for the red and green colors, the unique yellow background value, and the balancing contrasts for the two values of spatial frequencies that were used in the main experiment.

**Equiluminant Settings**

To isolate the effect of color on binocular rivalry alternations, the luminance of each element needed to be equal to that of the background to ensure that only the chromatic attribute was contributing to the alternations. We employed the reverse-phi motion method of Gorea, Papathomas, and Kovács (1993a, 1993b), which obtains a luminance setting for a patch of color which must be equiluminant to that of the background.

**Unique Yellow**

We next adjusted the chromaticity of the yellow background to make the values of the color attribute, $C_A = $ red and $C_B = $ green, equally salient (i.e., chromatically equidistant from the resulting background, which is called "unique yellow") (Raaijmakers and De Weert, 1975; Papathomas, Gorea, et al., 1999). This procedure, which was run separately for each observer, was designed to produce balanced colors $C_A$ and $C_B$, and the results of the main experiment indicate that we succeeded in this task.

T. V. Papathomas, I. Kovács, and T. Conway

**Spatial Frequency**

The task was to balance the strengths of the elements with $F_A$ = low and $F_B$ = high spatial frequency. In this preliminary experiment, we used a single low-spatial-frequency Gabor patch in one eye, and a high-spatial-frequency patch in the other eye. We randomly assigned the values of the frequency to the left or right eye. The contrast of the $F_B$ patch was fixed at 86%, and we recorded its average predominance for four values of contrast for the $F_A$ patch. We obtained the point of subjective equality by fitting psychometric curves to the data.

**RESULTS**

The results of the main experiment are shown in figure 9.2A for the conventional configuration, and 9.2B for the patchwork configuration, respectively. Both graphs plot the predominances of the uniform A and B percepts (i.e., the percentages of the total viewing time that the respective percepts dominated). The ten attribute conditions are shown along the horizontal axis. For each condition, the light and dark bars indicate the predominances of the uniform percepts for the corresponding A and B stimuli. The predominances of the A and B stimuli indicate the percentage of time that the uniform percepts are experienced. Obtaining balanced parameters separately for each observer in the preliminary experiments was time-consuming but justified. Indeed, a look at the results of figure 9.2A and 9.2B shows that the predominances of the A and B stimuli were rather well balanced.

As stated before, comparing performances under the same attribute conditions in figures 9.2A and 9.2B can assess the role of the eye of origin in binocular rivalry. A one-tailed t-test comparing performances with the conventional and patchwork rivalry stimuli separately for the "uniform A" and "uniform B" predominances showed differences below the 5% significance level for all but the FOC "uniform B" condition. This comparison reveals that the eye of origin is indeed an important factor in determining predominance in all attribute conditions, since the cumulative predominance of coherent stimuli in patchwork conditions was less than in conventional conditions. The same pattern of results was evident in the study by Kovács et al. (1996).

To evaluate the strength of individual attributes and their combinations, let us obtain the probability of achieving the uniform percepts (i.e., at least seven elements of the same type) purely by chance. If we assume that each

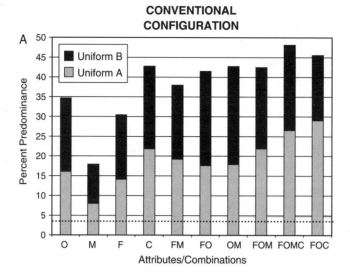

**CONVENTIONAL CONFIGURATION**

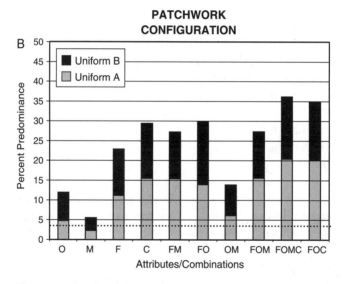

**PATCHWORK CONFIGURATION**

**Figure 9.2** Results of the experiment with (*A*) conventional configuration and (*B*) patchwork configuration. Stimulus conditions are shown along the horizontal axis. The light and dark bars show the relative predominances of the uniform percepts for stimuli A and B, respectively (i.e., the percentages of the total viewing time that the respective percepts dominated). The solid horizontal line just below 5% indicates chance-level performance. See text for more details on stimulus conditions.

T. V. Papathomas, I. Kovács, and T. Conway

element has an equal probability of being perceived as either A or B, independently of the eye of origin, then the probability of at least seven elements being of type A is approximately 3.516% $(= 0.5^8 + 8 \times 0.5^8)$, where the first term in parentheses is the probability of a strictly uniform A percept, and the second term is the probability of the eight different cases where only one of the elements is perceived to be of type B. If we further assume that the cumulative duration of a state, as a ratio of the entire time of observation, is proportional to the probability of that state, then the predominance of the "uniform A" or "uniform B" percepts, as predicted by pure chance, is 3.516%;[1] the dotted lines in figures 9.2A and 9.2B indicate this chance-level performance. Thus, for an attribute to be considered as a potent factor for eliciting IOG, the attribute's percentages of uniform percepts for A and B must exceed 3.516%, and their sum must exceed 7.032% for the patchwork configuration. (Performance in the conventional configuration is not relevant for assessing the attribute's ability to elicit IOG, because it is confounded with eye-of-origin influences.) All attributes, except for O, M, and their combination, OM, had IOG indices above 3.516%, at the 95% confidence interval.

A first look at the data shows that motion does not appear to contribute to IOG, and that orientation is a weak contributor, but these conclusions hold only for the particular geometrical arrangement used in this experiment (see "Discussion" for other studies that have used global arrangements and provided evidence for stronger influences of motion and orientation in binocular rivalry).

The pattern of results across conditions appears very similar in the conventional and the patchwork configurations. In particular, color and motion appear to be, respectively, the strongest and weakest attributes in eliciting IOG in both configurations. Also, in general, combinations of attributes tend to produce stronger IOGs than those produced by the constituent attributes in both configurations. Thus, the percentages of uniform percepts for FM are larger than those for either F or M; the same is true for FO and OM, although the latter is marginal in the patchwork configuration.

## DISCUSSION

The main finding of our study is that both stimulus coherence and eye of origin play a role in binocular rivalry, and point to a theory that lies somewhere in the middle of the spectrum between the two extreme forms of eye-based[2] and stimulus-based theories of binocular rivalry. The results from the present experiment have confirmed our earlier finding (Kovács et al., 1996) that the coherence of the stimuli plays a significant role in binocular rivalry, in addition to the role played by the eye of origin. Ooi and He (2003), working with a Kanizsa-square display consisting of four pairs of rivaling colored corners, obtained data that support a similar conclusion.

We next examine the strength of the attributes in eliciting IOG by referring to figure 9.2B. Numerous studies have confirmed that color is a potent attribute for producing IOG (Treisman, 1962; Kulikowski, 1992; Kulikowski and Walsh, 1995; Kovács et al., 1996; Ooi and He, 2003). Our study indicates that color's ability to group same-type elements across the rivaling eyes is significantly stronger than that of the other attributes. In an effort to explain this ability, Van Lier and De Weert's (2003) experiments deal with the interesting issue of how the activation of a particular color patch in one eye, hitherto suppressed by a binocularly rivaling high-contrast patch, propagates the activation of same-color patches in different locations of the same, as well as of the contralateral, eye. Their psychophysical method enables the study of intra- and interocular color activations and interactions. It would be interesting to see their method extended to investigate the intra- and interocular interactions of other attributes, such as spatial frequency and orientation.

Our results also indicate that spatial frequency was a potent factor in eliciting IOG, indicating that it is capable of forming coherent perceptual representations. On the contrary, orientation was barely effective, and motion was ineffective with the stimuli used in this experiment. However, one must be careful in drawing generalized conclusions about the ability of orientation and motion to form coherent perceptual organizations. The only conclusion that can be drawn is that orientation and motion were not effective in eliciting IOG for the particular random arrangement of Gabor patches used in this experiment.

The reason for being so cautious is that the arrangement used in our experiment is quite inappropriate for orientation-based contour formation. More appropriate arrangements can elicit stronger IOG. For example, Fehér, Kovács, and Papathomas (1997) used a more pertinent arrangement of oriented Gabor patches that emphasized orientation-based contours and obtained evidence for interocular grouping of contours. Suzuki and Grabowecky (2002) also obtained evidence for the role of global shape in single-eye dominance as well as mixed-eye dominance. Similarly, for motion, Alais and Blake (1998) provided evidence for stronger global influences of motion with a more appropriate global arrangement that enabled motion and orientation to form coherent perceptual organizations. Further experiments with strategically designed stimuli are needed to investigate the strength of orientation and motion as factors of stimulus coherence in binocular rivalry.

Finally, a major question on stimulus-based influences in binocular rivalry concerns the involvement of top-down processes. Namely, is stimulus coherence driven purely by bottom-up mechanisms, or are schema-driven mechanisms involved that use the bottom-up signals to construct and test coherent perceptual representations in an attempt to achieve a meaningful stable percept (Andrews and Purves, 1997; Papathomas, Kovács, et al., 1999)? Earlier studies that presented evidence for top-down influences (Walker, 1978, provides a thorough review of this early literature) may be subjected to alternative interpretations, because they used subjective reports of percepts. One early study which used objective criteria is that by Neisser and Becklen (1975), who reported a highly significant role of selective attention in binocular rivalry. Paradoxically, this study has rarely been cited in the recent literature on binocular rivalry, even though the companion experiment with two spatially superimposed competing episodes, reported in the same article, is one of the most frequently cited works on selective attention.

More recent evidence for attentional modulation in binocular rivalry was provided by Ooi and He (1999) and Sasaki and Gyoba (2002). Neurophysiological evidence (see Logothetis, 1998, for a review), obtained through single-cell recordings in monkeys, indicates that cell activity correlates better at higher visual stages (but see Polonsky et al., 2000, for fMRI evidence with humans that rivalry-driven neural fluctuations were about the same in areas V1, V2, V3, V3a, and V4v). As argued by Ooi and He (1999), the fact that neural activity in higher stages is modulated by attention, coupled with the view that these stages are involved in rivalry, may explain the effect of attention on binocular rivalry. Except for the evidence for the role of stimulus coherence and attention, there is no recent objectively obtained evidence for high-level influences, such as meaning and attitude, that was reported in early studies (Walker, 1978).

In summary, our findings suggest that the eye-based theories of binocular rivalry must be revised to include the role of stimulus coherence and percept competition. One possible model may include spatial domains of monocular dominance that are organized according to some rules of perceptual organization and stimulus coherence. Blake and Logothetis (2002) underscored the distinction between influences on dominance by such factors as context, and influences on suppression by stimulus strength. Finally, there is a definite need to study the role that high-order processes play in taking advantage of the coherence of the stimulus.

## ACKNOWLEDGMENTS

The authors wish to thank Akos Fehér for stimulating discussions and suggestions, and for developing the programs for the experiments with John Szatmary. We are grateful to David Alais and Randolph Blake for the invitation to the workshop on binocular rivalry in June 2002 and for editing this volume.

## NOTES

1. This stochastic analysis does not take into account other factors that may contribute to integrating a coherent percept out of patched image fragments. For example, Lee and Blake (2002) showed observers animations, each frame of which was a collage of random patches from two different coherent images; the animation of these patched frames obeyed the empirical gamma distributions that were obtained under binocular rivalry. Interestingly, these animations produced coherent "wholes" at a rate that significantly exceeded the rate predicted by chance alone.

2. We must emphasize that this version of an eye-based theory is an extreme form that no researcher endorses.

## REFERENCES

Alais, D., and Blake, R. (1998). Interactions between global motion and local binocular rivalry. *Vision Research, 38*, 637–644.

Alais, D., and Blake, R. (1999). Grouping visual features during binocular rivalry. *Vision Research, 39*, 4341–4353.

Alais, D., O'Shea, R. P., Mesana-Alais, C., and Wilson, I. G. (2000). On binocular alternation. *Perception, 29*, 1437–1445.

Andrews, T. J., and Purves, D. (1997). Similarities in normal and binocularly rivalrous viewing. *Proceedings of the National Academy of Sciences of the United States of America, 94*, 9905–9908.

Blake, R. (1989). A neural theory of binocular rivalry. *Psychological Review, 96*, 145–167.

Blake, R. (2001). A primer on binocular rivalry, including current controversies. *Brain and Mind, 2*, 5–38.

Blake, R., Westendorf, D. H., and Overton, R. (1980). What is suppressed during binocular rivalry? *Perception, 9*, 223–231.

Blake, R., Yu, K., Lokey, M., and Norman, H. (1998). Binocular rivalry and motion perception. *Journal of Cognitive Neuroscience, 10*, 46–60.

T. V. Papathomas, I. Kovács, and T. Conway

Blake, R., and Logothetis, N. K. (2002). Visual competition. *Nature Reviews: Neuroscience,* 3, 13–21.

Creed, R. S. (1935). Observations on binocular fusion and rivalry. *Journal of Physiology,* 84, 381–392.

Diaz-Caneja, E. (1928). Sur l'alternance binoculaire. *Annales d'Oculistique,* 165 (October): 721–731.

Fehér, A., Kovács, I., and Papathomas, T. V. (1997). Contour continuity can drive interocular grouping during binocular rivalry. *Investigative Ophthalmology and Visual Science,* 38, S642.

Gorea, A., Papathomas, T. V., and Kovács, I. (1993a). Two motion systems with common and separate pathways for color and luminance. *Proceedings of the National Academy of Sciences of the United States of America,* 90, 11197–11201.

Gorea, A., Papathomas, T. V., and Kovács, I. (1993b). Motion perception with spatiotemporally matched chromatic and achromatic information reveals a "slow" and a "fast" motion system. *Vision Research,* 33, 2515–2534.

Kovács, I., Papathomas, T. V., Yang, M., and Fehér, A. (1996). When the brain changes its mind: Interocular grouping during binocular rivalry. *Proceedings of the National Academy of Sciences of the United States of America,* 93, 15508–15511.

Kulikowski, J. J. (1992). Binocular chromatic rivalry and single vision. *Ophthalmic and Physiological Optics,* 12, 168–170.

Kulikowski, J. J., and Walsh V. (1995). Demonstration of binocular fusion of color and texture. In *Early Vision and Beyond,* T. V. Papathomas, C. Chubb, A. Gorea, and E. Kowler, eds., 27–32. Cambridge, Mass.: MIT Press.

Lee, S. H., and Blake, R. (2002). Local eye rivalry can yield global, interocular dominance (abstract), *Journal of Vision,* 2, 463a.

Leopold, D. A., and Logothetis, N. K. (1996). Activity changes in early visual cortex reflect monkeys' percepts during binocular rivalry. *Nature,* 379, 549–553.

Logothetis, N. K. (1998). Single units and conscious vision. *Philosophical Transactions of the Royal Society of London,* B353, 1801–1818.

Logothetis, N. K., Leopold, D. A., and Sheinberg, D. L. (1996). What is rivalling during binocular rivalry? *Nature,* 380, 621–624.

Logothetis, N. K., and Schall, J. D. (1989). Neuronal correlates of subjective visual perception. *Science,* 245, 761–763.

Neisser, U., and Becklen, R. (1975). Selective looking: Attending to visually specified events. *Cognitive Psychology,* 7, 480–494.

Ooi, T. L., and He, Z. J. (1999). Binocular rivalry and visual awareness: The role of attention. *Perception,* 28, 551–574.

Ooi, T. L., and He, Z. J. (2003). A distributed intercortical processing of binocular rivalry: Psychophysical evidence. *Perception,* 32, 155–166.

Papathomas, T. V., Gorea, A., Fehér, A., and Conway, T. E. (1999). Attention-based texture segregation. *Perception and Psychophysics,* 61, 1399–1410.

Papathomas, T. V., Kovács, I., Fehér, A., and Julesz, B. (1999). Visual dilemmas: Competition between eyes and between percepts in binocular rivalry. In *What Is Cognitive Science?*, E. LePore and Z. Pylyshyn, eds., 263–294. Malden, Mass.: Basil Blackwell.

Polonsky, A., Blake, R., Braun, J., and Heeger, D. J. (2000). Neuronal activity in human primary visual cortex correlates with perception during binocular rivalry. *Nature Neuroscience*, 3, 1153–1159.

Raaijmakers, J. G. W., and De Weert, C. M. M. (1975). Linear and nonlinear opponent color coding. *Perception and Psychophysics*, 18, 474–480.

Sasaki, H., and Gyoba, J. (2002). Selective attention to stimulus features modulates interocular suppression. *Perception*, 31, 409–419.

Sheinberg, D. L., and Logothetis, N. K. (1997). The role of cortical temporal areas in perceptual organization. *Proceedings of the National Academy of Sciences of the United States of America*, 94, 3408–3413.

Shimojo, S., and Nakayama, K. (1990). Real world occlusion constraints and binocular rivalry. *Vision Research*, 30, 69–80.

Stirling, W. (1901). An experiment on binocular color vision with half-penny postage-stamps. *Journal of Physiology* (London), 27, 1901–1902.

Suzuki, S., and Grabowecky, M. (2002). Evidence for perceptual "trapping" and adaptation in multistable binocular rivalry. *Neuron*, 36, 143–157.

Treisman, A. (1962). Binocular rivalry and stereoscopic depth perception. *Quarterly Journal of Experimental Psychology*, 14, 23–37.

Van Lier, R. J., and De Weert, C. M. M. (2003). Intra- and interocular colour-specific activation during dichoptic suppression. *Vision Research*, 43, 1111–1116.

Walker, P. (1978). Binocular rivalry: Central or peripheral selective processes? *Psychological Bulletin*, 85, 376–389.

Whittle, P., Bloor, D. C., and Pocock, S. (1968). Some experiments on figural effects. *Perception and Psychophysics*, 4, 183–188.

Wolfe, J. M. (1986). Stereopsis and binocular rivalry. *Psychological Review*, 93, 269–282.

# 10  Binocular Rivalry and the Perception of Depth

Ian P. Howard

It is tempting to dismiss binocular rivalry as a laboratory artifact associated with dissimilar stimulation of the two eyes. In fact, however, the stimulus conditions producing rivalry occur in two conditions in the natural environment. First, dissimilar monocular stimulation occurs when there are objects located at depths far from the plane of fixation and convergence. And second, it happens along an off-horizontal step in depth associated with viewing one far object that is partially occluded by a nearer one. In this chapter I review evidence that potentially rivalrous stimulation under this second condition is involved in depth perception.

In his *Optics*, Euclid (323–285 B.C.) described how a far object occludes a near object by an extent that varies with the position of the objects with respect to the horizon and their distances from the eye (see Burton, 1945). He also explained how two eyes see more of a sphere or cylinder than either eye alone when the object is smaller than the interocular distance. He was thus aware that the two eyes obtain different views of a solid object. Leonardo da Vinci noticed the same thing in the fifteenth century. He drew the diagrams shown in figure 10.1A to illustrate occlusion zones on a surface viewed through an aperture. He suggested that occlusion zones could create impressions of depth (Strong, 1979). Nakayama and Shimojo (1990) suggested that depth created this way be called da Vinci stereopsis. Thus, it was suggested that zones visible to only one eye play a role in depth perception long before anyone suggested that disparity between corresponding images had anything to do with depth perception. After Wheatstone demonstrated the role of disparity in depth perception (see chapter 2 in this volume), people forgot about the potential importance of monocular zones. Interest in this factor was rekindled only in the last few decades.

Next to a vertical edge of an opaque object seen by both eyes lies a region of a far surface that is visible to only one eye, as in figure 10.1B. This

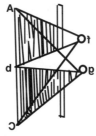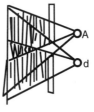

(A)

Left-eye
monocular zone   Binocular occlusion zone   Right-eye
monocular zone

Opaque object

(B)

Far object

Near object

(C)

(D)

is a *monocular occlusion zone* (Howard and Rogers, 2002). A region visible only to the left eye is a left monocular zone, and a region visible only to the right eye is a right monocular zone.

An object lying in front of a surface with similar texture and luminance may not be visible. In figure 10.1C, the near object is camouflaged to the left eye because its image is superimposed on a matching far surface, but the right eye sees it because this eye sees the object against a different background. This is an unpaired monocular image due to *monocular camouflage.*

I will review evidence that these unpaired images affect binocular rivalry, modify impressions of depth created by binocular disparity, and generate impressions of depth in their own right. We will see that the sign of perceived depth relations created by unpaired images conforms to simple geometrical rules. However, the magnitude of depth is ambiguous because the observer does not know how far an occluded object extends behind the occluder or how far a camouflaged image is displaced from the edge of the far object. I will introduce a new type of display that removes the ambiguity of depth magnitude inherent in monocular occlusion and camouflage. In this display, an impression of depth is created by an object that can be seen by only one eye even though it is not occluded or camouflaged to the other eye. I call this effect monocular transparency. Finally, I will describe how depth impressions can be created by binocular rivalry between occlusion zones.

## MONOCULAR OCCLUSION AND RIVALRY

Monocular occlusion and camouflage obey the following geometrical rules:

1. A monocular occlusion zone seen by a given eye is on the temporal side of the near binocular object. Thus, a left-eye monocular occlusion zone

◄ **Figure 10.1** Monocular zones. (*A*) Drawings made by Leonardo da Vinci of occlusion zones created by looking through an aperture. Note Leonardo's use of mirror writing. (Adapted from Strong, 1979). (*B*) Monocular zones created by a near opaque object. Each zone is on the temporal side of the eye that sees it. (*C*) The near object is not visible to the left eye because the near and far surfaces are similar. The near object is visible to the right eye because that eye sees it against a different background. The monocular image is on the nasal side of the far object. (*D*) With convergent fusion, the black disk appears in front of the background. The monocular crescent on the appropriate (temporal) side appears in the plane of the background. The crescent on the inappropriate (nasal) side engages in binocular rivalry with the background. (Adapted from Shimojo and Nakayama, 1990.)

Binocular Rivalry and the Perception of Depth

occurs on a left-facing occluding edge and a right monocular zone occurs on a right-facing occluding edge. An unpaired image due to camouflage is on the nasal side of the far binocular object against which the near object is camouflaged.

2. A monocular occlusion zone is more distant than the binocular object, while a monocular image due to camouflage is nearer than the binocular object against which the near object is camouflaged.

3. Although unpaired images due to occlusion or camouflage do not have matching images in the other eye, they may be superimposed on distinct images from the other eye. The two sets of images should engage in rivalry.

With convergent fusion of the stereogram of figure 10.1D, the black disk appears in front of the background. Monocular zones occur on both sides of the black disk. The monocular zone on the left side that would be created by a near black disk survives binocular rivalry with the dots of the background and appears to be part of the far textured surface. The monocular zone on the right side is on the wrong side for monocular occlusion and engages in binocular rivalry with the dot pattern in the other eye.

We can conclude, as did Shimojo and Nakayama (1990), that binocular rivalry is strongly modified by whether or not differences between two images could arise naturally from surfaces at different distances.

## INTERACTIONS BETWEEN MONOCULAR OCCLUSION AND DISPARITY

With crossed fusion of the stereogram in figure 10.2A, the vertical grating appears beyond the diamond frame on the right (Anderson, 1999). This interpretation is supported by the fact that monocular zones created by the disparity conform to the occlusion configuration. On the left, the white bars separate from the black bars and appear to come out of the plane of the diamond and extend over the background. This interpretation is supported by the fact that the monocular zones of the white bars conform to the camouflage configuration. In figure 10.2B, the black bars come forward on the left because only they can be interpreted as being camouflaged against the black background. Figure 10.2C does not produce an impression of depth on the left because the intermediate luminance of the background does not support either an occlusion or a camouflage interpretation.

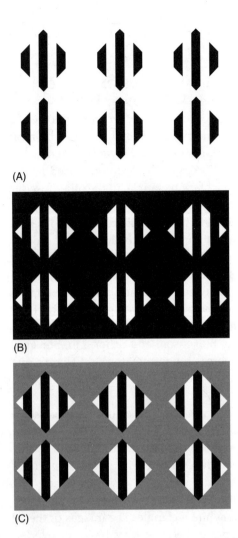

(A)

(B)

(C)

**Figure 10.2** Effects of background on occlusion/camouflage. (*A*) With crossed fusion, in the right fused image both white and black bars of the grating appear beyond the diamond frames because monocular zones conform to the occlusion configuration. In the left fused image, the white bars come forward and extend over the background because only they can be interpreted as camouflaged against the white background. (*B*) In the left fused image, black bars come forward and extend over the background because only they are seen as camouflaged against the black background. (*C*) The left fused image does not create a definite impression of depth because the background does not support either an occlusion or a camouflage interpretation. The right fused image supports an occlusion configuration.

Binocular Rivalry and the Perception of Depth

Anderson and Nakayama (1994) reviewed the role of monocular occlusion in stereoscopic vision.

## DEPTH FROM MONOCULAR OCCLUSION ALONE

The most interesting question is whether impressions of depth can be created when the only information is that supplied by monocular occlusion or monocular camouflage. Liu, Stevenson, and Schor (1994) used the stereograms shown in figure 10.3A. In one fused image, a white rectangle stands out from a black rectangle. In the other fused image, a white rectangle appears through a hole in the black rectangle. There are no corresponding lateral edges in the white rectangle to generate horizontal disparity. The proximal stimulus is equivalent to that produced by a white rectangle partially occluding or seen beyond a larger black rectangle.

There are two possible artifacts in Liu, Stevenson, and Schor's display. First, disparities exist between the inner horizontal boundaries (Gillam, 1995). A simple line stereogram consisting of only horizontal lines with these same disparities, as in figure 10.3B, creates the same relative depth as that created by Liu, Stevenson, and Schor. Liu, Stevenson, and Schor (1997) argued that whereas the terminators in Gillam's display have the same luminance polarity, those in their display have opposite luminance polarity.

The second artifact is misconvergence on the black shapes due to the asymmetry of the images. It is as if edges with opposite luminance polarity repel each other. Any misconvergence is indicated by the separation of the nonius lines. This induces a disparity into the images of the partially occluded black rectangle—a crossed disparity when the black shape appears nearer than the white rectangle, and an uncrossed disparity when it appears beyond the white rectangle. The images of the white rectangle do not acquire a disparity because they have no overlapping vertical edges. The white rectangle defaults to the plane of convergence (zero disparity). The depth effect could therefore arise from an illusory depth of the black shape relative to the white rectangle. In figure 10.3C the separation of the nonius lines increases with the perceived depth of the white rectangle, as predicted by the vergence account of the depth effect.

Gillam and Nakayama (1998) designed stereograms that are free of disparity artifacts, in which the depth must arise from monocular occlusion only. Gillam, Blackburn, and Nakayama (1999) constructed the display shown in figure 10.4A. Each eye sees a gap where the other eye sees only a black surface. The real 3-D display that would produce

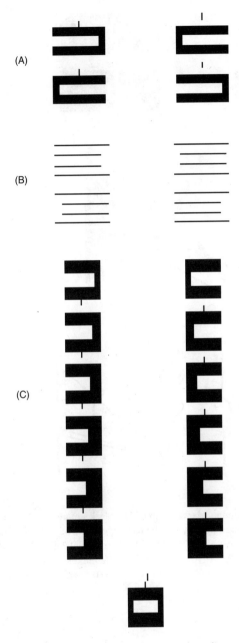

**Figure 10.3** Stereopsis with no corresponding vertical edges. (*A*) One fused stereogram appears as a white rectangle in front of a black rectangle. The other image appears as a white rectangle seen through a black rectangle. The nonius lines are offset in opposite directions in the two cases, showing that the eyes are misconverged. (Adapted from Liu, Stevenson, and Schor, 1994.) (*B*) The horizontal boundaries extracted from (*A*) contain disparities that create the same depth impressions as those in (*A*). (Redrawn from Gillam, 1995.) (*C*) Convergent fusion of the six stereograms creates the display at the bottom, in which a white rectangle appears to stand out. Depth and nonius offset increase down the set.

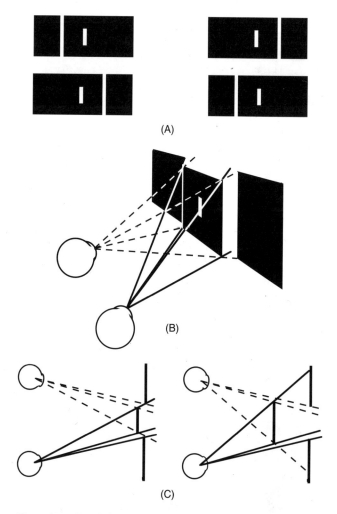

(A)

(B)

(C)

**Figure 10.4**  Depth from monocular occlusion. (*A*) A black square appears in front of a black rectangle in one fused image and beyond the rectangle in the other fused image. (Adapted from Gillam, Blackburn, and Nakayama, 1999.) (*B*) An actual 3-D display that creates the images of the stereograms in (*A*). (*C*) Plan views of different displays that produce the same images in the two eyes. The occluding object is closer to the occluded surface in one display than it is in the other.

these images is depicted in figure 10.4B, and this is the impression created. The wider the gap, the greater the perceived depth separation between the squares. It is as if the visual system partitions the black region seen in one eye into two halves and matches each half with one of the squares in the other eye.

These stereograms seem to be free of artifacts, and we may therefore conclude that monocular occlusion can create an impression of depth in the total absence of other cues to depth.

However, while the sign of depth is unambiguous in these displays, the magnitude of depth is unspecified. For example, in figure 10.4C, the external stimuli are different but the images they create are the same. The observer has no way of knowing how far an occluded object extends behind the occluder or how far a camouflaged object is displaced from the edge of the far object. Nevertheless, impressions of depth may vary systematically with the size of the gaps in figure 10.4A if the observer makes the default assumption that the vertical edges of the near square just abut the edges of the far squares.

## DEPTH FROM MONOCULAR TRANSPARENCY

While trying to design a stereogram based on monocular zones that provides unambiguous information about depth magnitude, I discovered a new type of stimulus, which I call monocular transparency. One version of the stereogram is shown in figure 10.5A. The key idea is that a square has the same color as a background. For one eye, the square just fills a gap in the background so that its lateral edges are not visible. For the other eye, the square is displaced relative to the gap. For this eye, the square is totally visible because it or the background is depicted as being transparent. When the square is displaced one way, it appears transparent and in front of the background. When the square is displaced the other way, it appears beyond a transparent surface. The effect is not due to monocular occlusion but rather to monocular transparency. The full width of the square is visible to one eye and must be assumed to fill the gap for the other eye. If it did not fill the gap, a region of transparency would be visible. Thus, the magnitude of depth created by monocular transparency is unambiguous if the observer uses the available information. When the images in figure 10.5A are fused, one square appears in front of the background and the other appears beyond the background.

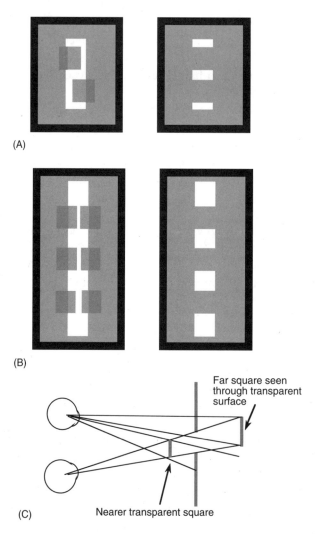

(A)

(B)

Far square seen
through transparent
surface

Nearer transparent square

(C)

**Figure 10.5** Depth from monocular transparency. (*A*) Crossed fusion creates an impression of a square beyond a transparent surface, and uncrossed fusion, of a transparent square in front of a surface. (*B*) The magnitude of depth increases with the extent of displacement of the monocular square relative to the vertical bar. (Redrawn from Howard and Duke, 2003.) (*C*) The physical arrangement that creates the depth effects in (*A*).

There are no conventional disparities in this display. The effect cannot be due to vergence because both images are symmetrical and depth occurs in both directions at the same time. The greater the displacement of the squares relative to the slit, the greater the perceived depth, as can be seen in figure 10.5B. Figure 10.5C shows the physical arrangement that would give rise to the effects produced in figure 10.5A.

We measured the depth produced by the monocular transparency display shown in figure 10.6A relative to a disk-shaped depth probe (Howard and Duke, 2003). The two images were generated on computer monitors and presented in a mirror stereoscope. The monocular square was offset relative to the gap at each of several visual angles between 0° and 4.2°. I will refer to these offsets as pseudo disparities. Subjects adjusted the disparity of the depth probe until the probe appeared at the same depth as the square in the test display. For six of ten subjects the pseudo disparity of the square in the transparency display was set equal to the actual disparity of the depth probe over the whole range of pseudo disparities. There was little variability in the depth settings. Thus, for these subjects, monocular transparency was just as good a depth cue as binocular disparity (figure 10.7). We made the same measurements with an actual disparity added to the monocular transparency display, as shown in figure 10.6B. This did not improve the accuracy of the depth settings, as can be seen in figure 10.7. Thus, the magnitude of depth produced by monocular transparency alone is just as accurate as that produced by monocular transparency plus real disparity.

We then measured the depth produced by the display shown in figure 10.6C. With crossed fusion this corresponds to the camouflage configuration and creates the impression of a square in front of a surface with a gap. In this case, the width of the square, and hence the magnitude of depth, is not specified. For this display, pseudo disparities of up to about 0.5° produced as much depth as a real disparity. At these disparities, subjects must have assumed that the monocular square was just as wide as the gap. However, higher pseudo disparities produced progressively less depth than that created by real disparity or by pseudo disparity in the monocular transparency display, as can be seen in figure 10.7.

Depth in a monocular transparency display could possibly be due to (1) disparity between one edge of the square and a subjective contour created across the gap; (2) disparity between the corners of the square and the corners of the gap; or (3) disparity between the upper and lower edges of the squares and the upper and lower edges of the gap. We designed a display that controls for these possible artifacts.

Left-eye images       Right-eye images

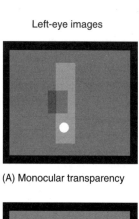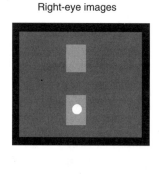

(A) Monocular transparency

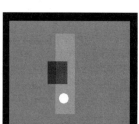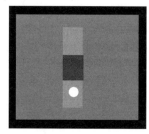

(B) Monocular transparency plus disparity

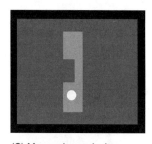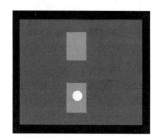

(C) Monocular occlusion

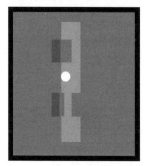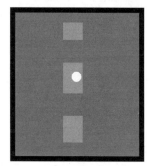

(D) Control. The two stereograms produce the same depth. If depth were due to disparity between the corners elements, depth in the lower stereogram would be twice that in the upper stereogram.

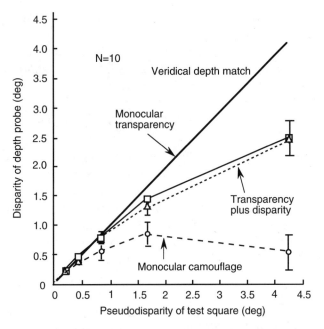

**Figure 10.7** Mean data for 10 subjects. The disparity of the depth probe producing the same impression of depth as the test square, plotted against the pseudo disparity of each of the three test squares. (Redrawn from Howard and Duke, 2003.)

Fusion of the upper images in figure 10.6D creates the standard monocular transparency effect. Depth magnitude is similar to that created by the equivalent disparity of the white disks. Fusion of the lower images in figure 10.6D creates similar depth effects. If depth were due to artifact (1) or (2), then depth in the lower stereogram should be much greater than that in the upper stereogram because the edges and corners of the monocular rectangle are further away from the subjective contour or corners of the gap. According to artifact (3) there should be no depth in the lower stereogram because the horizontal edges of the monocular rectangle no longer match the horizontal edges of the gap.

◄ **Figure 10.6** Stereograms used for testing monocular transparency. (*A*) Depth from monocular transparency. (*B*) Depth from monocular transparency plus real disparity. (*C*) Depth from monocular camouflage. (*D*) Cross fusion should create two rectangles standing out in depth. If depth were determined by disparity between the corners of the monocular element and corners in the other eye, the depth of the lower rectangle would be twice that of the upper rectangle.

For each display, subjects adjusted the disparity of the white depth probe to match the depth of the test square for each of several pseudo disparities of the test square.

Binocular Rivalry and the Perception of Depth

We have shown that monocular transparency can produce depth over a wide range of pseudo disparities which is similar to that created by real disparity. Although the depth created by monocular camouflage varies with the magnitude of pseudo disparity, it falls well short of that created by a real disparity as disparity is increased.

## DEPTH FROM RIVALRY BETWEEN OCCLUSION ZONES

I have shown that depth with unambiguous sign can be created by binocular rivalry between rivalrous monocular zones (Howard, 1995). If one views a surface covered with black and white patches through a hole in a near surface, as in figure 10.8A, one eye may see a black patch where the other eye sees a white patch. These two monocular zones have opposite luminance polarity and therefore undergo binocular rivalry.

In the stereogram shown in figure 10.8B, the image for one eye consists of a set of black circular rims filled with white or filled with black. The image for the other eye is the same except that corresponding disks have opposite luminance polarities. For most observers this creates the impression of a black-and-white dotted surface seen through black-rimmed holes in a nearer surface. I called this the sieve effect. There are no disparities between any of the edges in the display. The magnitude of disparity indicated by the sieve effect is not specified, except that it should be at least as large as that created by a disparity equal to the diameter of the disks. Tsai and Victor (2000) asked subjects to set the disparity of a patch in a random-dot display so that its perceived depth matched that produced by the sieve effect. Although quite variable, the disparity settings indicated that the contents of the rivalrous disks were perceived as more distant than the surrounding surface.

There are three depth effects, each described in the following paragraphs, to which the sieve effect could be related.

A random-dot stereogram with a central square of binocularly uncorrelated dots set in a surround of correlated dots, produces fluctuating depth even though there is no disparity between the uncorrelated regions (Julesz, 1960; Frisby and Mayhew, 1978). O'Shea and Blake (1987) dubbed this rival depth. They found that the direction of depth is a function of the direction of fixation disparity. This suggests that subjects were responding to the disparity between the images of the surround regions induced by fixation disparity, relative to the undefined disparity in the inner square. This effect cannot account for the sieve effect because the depth of sieve effect has a definite sign, even without misconvergence.

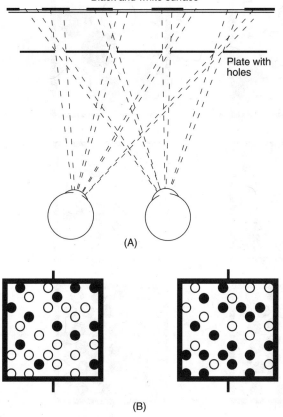

Black and white surface

Plate with holes

(A)

(B)

**Figure 10.8**    The sieve effect. (*A*) A black-and-white surface seen through holes in a near surface creates a pattern of binocular rivalry without disparity. (*B*) For most people, fusion of
these images creates an impression of a surface with holes, with a black-and-white surface
seen through the holes. (From Howard, 1994.)

The sieve effect can be explained as follows. Rivalry within a small area
shows exclusive dominance in which one image or another is seen at any
one time. Therefore, at any instant, the contents of each fused disk are seen
as either white or black. Over the whole pattern, the contents of some
elements will appear black and some, white. A surface with black and
white patches seen through holes in a near surface creates this same proximal stimulus, as illustrated in figure 10.8A.

When the disks subtend more than about 1°, as in figure 10.9A, the
rivalrous contents appear as a silvery sheen at an indeterminate depth, an
effect known as binocular luster. This is because luminance rivalry in large

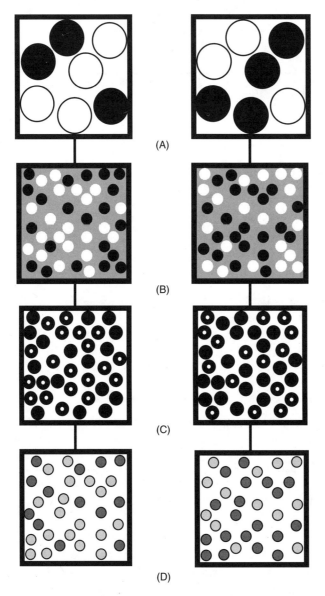

**Figure 10.9** Factors that destroy the sieve effect. (*A*) Disks subtending more than about 1°
create binocular luster rather than the sieve effect. (*B*) Removal of the rims around the white
disks abolishes the sieve effect. (*C*) As the white disks are reduced to dots, they no longer
rival the black disks but appear as a set of white dots. The dots appear in front of or behind
the surrounding area, according to the state of vergence. (*D*) The sieve effect is less impres-
sive when contrast between the rivalrous disks is reduced. (From Howard, 1995.)

areas shows not exclusive dominance but, rather, mosaic dominance, which creates binocular luster.

The sieve effect is replaced by indeterminate depth when there are no binocular rims, as in figure 10.9B. This is probably because there is no longer an impression of rimmed portholes through which the rivalrous surface is seen (Matsumiya and Howard, 2001).

When the white disks are reduced to small spots in a larger black disk, as in figure 10.9C, the spots appear to float in depth, sometimes nearer than the background and sometimes beyond it. The white spots are always visible because there are no nearby contours in the other eye to compete with them. The lack of a good fusion lock for the monocular white dots produces instability of vergence. This causes each dot sometimes to come closer to that edge of the black disk with which it has an uncrossed disparity and, at other times, to come closer to the edge with which it has a crossed disparity. The depth created by small dots is not due to rivalry but to disparities induced in the rims of the disks by vergence.

When the contrast between the rivalrous disks is decreased, as in figure 10.9D, the sieve effect is reduced or absent. This could be because, for small rivalrous regions of low contrast, exclusive rivalry is replaced by luminance mixture (Liu, Tyler, and Schor, 1992).

### SUMMARY

Leonardo da Vinci was correct when he suggested that monocular occlusion could serve as a cue to depth. Monocular occlusion zones may produce depth in the absence of other depth cues. Although the sign of depth created by monocular occlusion stereograms is unambiguous, the magnitude of depth is not uniquely specified. I designed monocular transparency stereograms that contain unambiguous information about depth magnitude. The depth they create is similar in magnitude to that created by real disparity. I also showed that depth can be created by rivalry between occlusion zones of opposite luminance. Thus, stimuli that resemble those which generate binocular rivalry or which actually generate binocular rivalry can provide information about relative depth. Stimuli of this kind occur at many locations in most natural scenes.

### REFERENCES

Anderson, B. L. (1999). Stereoscopic surface perception. *Neuron,* 24, 919–928.

Anderson, B. L., and Nakayama, K. (1994). Towards a general theory of stereopsis: Binocular matching, occluding contours, and fusion. *Psychological Review,* 101, 414–445.

Burton, H. E. (1945). The optics of Euclid. *Journal of the Optical Society of America*, 35, 357–372.

Frisby, J. P., and Mayhew, J. E. W. (1978). The relationship between apparent depth and disparity in rivalrous texture stereograms. *Perception*, 7, 661–678.

Gillam, B. (1995). Matching needed for stereopsis. *Nature*, 37, 202–204.

Gillam, B., Blackburn, S., and Nakayama, K. (1999). Stereopsis based on monocular gaps: Metrical encoding of depth and slant without matching contours. *Vision Research*, 39, 493–502.

Gillam, B., and Nakayama, K. (1998). Quantitative depth for a phantom surface can be based on cyclopean occlusion cues alone. *Vision Research*, 39, 109–112.

Howard, I. P. (1995). Depth from binocular rivalry without spatial disparity. *Perception*, 24, 67–74.

Howard, I. P., and Duke, P. A. (2003). Monocular transparency generates quantitative depth. *Vision Research*, 43, 2615–2621.

Howard, I. P., and Rogers, B. J. (2002). *Seeing in Depth*. Vol. 2, *Depth Perception*. Toronto: I. Porteous.

Julesz, B. (1960). Binocular depth perception of computer generated patterns. *Bell System Technical Journal*, 39, 1125–1162.

Liu, L., Stevenson, S. B., and Schor, C. M. (1994). Quantitative stereoscopic depth without binocular correspondence. *Nature*, 367, 66–69.

Liu, L., Stevenson, S. B., and Schor, C. M. (1997). Binocular matching of dissimilar features in phantom stereopsis. *Vision Research*, 37, 633–644.

Liu, L., Tyler, C. W., and Schor, C. M. (1992). Failure of rivalry at low contrast: Evidence of a suprathreshold binocular summation process. *Vision Research*, 32, 1471–1479.

Matsumiya, K., and Howard, I. P. (2001). Relation between depth produced by the sieve effect and frequency of binocular rivalry. *Investigative Ophthalmology and Visual Science*, 42, S403.

Nakayama, K., and Shimojo, S. (1990). Da Vinci stereopsis: Depth and subjective occluding contours from unpaired image points. *Vision Research*, 30, 1811–1825.

O'Shea, R. P., and Blake, R. (1987). Depth without disparity in random–dot stereograms. *Perception and Psychophysics*, 42, 205–214.

Shimojo, S., and Nakayama, K. (1990). Real world occlusion constraints and binocular rivalry. *Vision Research*, 30, 69–80.

Strong, D. S. (1979). *Leonardo on the Eye*. New York: Garland.

Tsai, J. J., and Victor, J. D. (2000). Neither occlusion constraint nor binocular disparity accounts for the perceived depth in the "sieve effect." *Vision Research*, 40, 2265–2276.

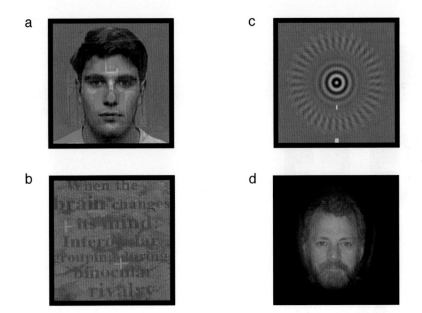

**Plate 1** Four examples of pairs of dissimilar images that, when viewed through red/green glasses, trigger binocular rivalry. (*a*) House/human face rival targets used by Frank Tong and colleagues to study brain activation during dominance and suppression phases of rivalry (work detailed in chapter 4). (*b*) Monkey/jungle scene targets used by Kovács et al. (1996) to examine spatial grouping in binocular rivalry (work described in chapter 6). (*c*) Concentric radial grating and spiral grating used by Wilson et al. (2001) to measure the spread of dominance at the time of rivalry transitions (work described in chapter 17). (*d*) Photographs of different individuals that, when viewed dichoptically, yield binocular rivalry despite similarities in global facial structure; in reality, the two individuals pictured here experience stable friendship, with their differences of view resolved harmoniously. See chapter 1.

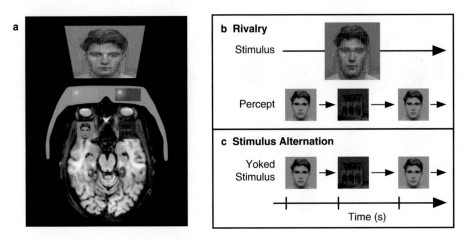

**Plate 2** (*a*) Schematic illustration of the binocular rivalry display and extrastriate areas of interest superimposed on a transverse MRI slice. The fusiform face area (FFA; right hemisphere) and parahippocampal place area (PPA; bilateral) are shown. During rivalry scans, a face and house were continuously presented to different eyes (using red/green filter glasses). Observers reported alternately perceiving only the face or the house for a few seconds at a time, as illustrated in (*b*). (*c*) On stimulus alternation scans, the physical stimulus alternated between the face image and the house image, using the same temporal sequence of alternations reported in a previous rivalry scan. (Modified, with permission, from Tong et al., 1998.) See chapter 4.

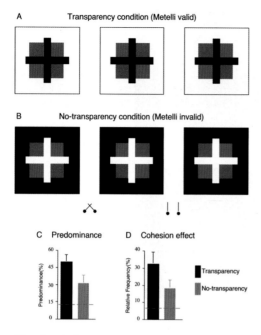

**Plate 3** (*A*) Transparent surface condition (Metelli valid). (*B*) No-transparency condition (Metelli invalid). For both displays, the smaller colored squares have crossed disparity with respect to the cross. Convergent fusers should free-fuse the left and middle half-images. (*C, D*) Averaged predominance and averaged cohesion indices (n = 6) for both conditions are above the chance level (12.5% and 6.25%, respectively; dashed lines). Most significantly, the predominance and cohesion indices for perceiving same-color transparent surfaces (black bars) are higher. See chapter 7.

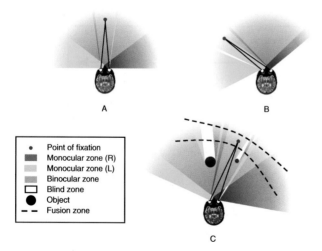

**Plate 4** Monocular and binocular regions of the visual field are mixed during natural vision. (*A*) During normal viewing of an object, a portion of each eye's view is blocked by the nose. For straight-ahead viewing, this results in a binocular field of roughly 114° visual angle centered on the object of interest. In addition to the unpaired temporal crescents, each eye's blind spot adds a monocular region nearer to the center of gaze. (*B*) A gaze shift (version) results in a smaller binocular visual field due to enhanced obstruction from the nose. Shown here is a large version in which the center of gaze is itself monocular. (*C*) Cluttered scenes lead to a highly inhomogeneous field of monocular, binocular, and blind zones, even in Panum's fusional area (dashed lines). See chapter 13.

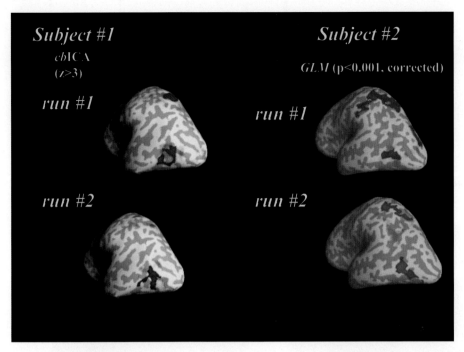

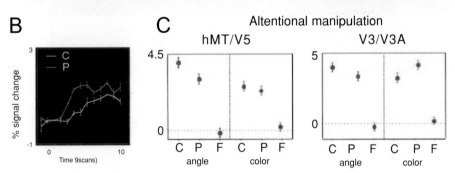

**Plate 5** (*A*) The sensorimotor network activated by perceptual switches of ambiguous plaids includes hMT[+]/V5 and the hand motor area (perceptual reports were indicated by finger button presses). This network is revealed both by GLM (general linear model) and cortex-based ICA (independent component analysis). Note the similar dynamics across subjects and across runs, regardless of whether GLM or ICA analysis was applied. (*B*) Motion responses in hMT[+]/V5 to an ambiguous stimulus as compared to a common rest baseline (nonrest baselines suffer from possible buildup of adaptation phenomena, as well as from the occurrence of irregular perceptual switches). The response associated with perception of component motion is significantly higher than the response associated with the perception of pattern motion ($p < 0.0001$, paired t-test) (adapted from Castelo-Branco et al., 2002). (*C*) Average group activity in hMT[+]/V5 and V3/V3A in an experiment that included different tasks manipulating attention (color and angle tasks). In the angle task, which requires subjects to pay equal attention to both pattern and component conditions, the response to component motion in hMT[+]/V5 was significantly higher than the response to pattern motion (ANOVA and post hoc tests, $p = 0.02$, for comparison between component and pattern motion response). C, component stimulus; P, pattern stimulus; F, fixation. See chapter 14.

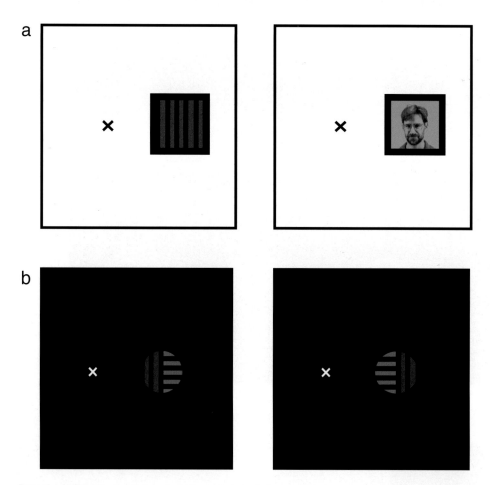

**Plate 6** (*a*) Stimuli presented, one to each eye, to test whether rivalry between complex stimuli, similar to those used by Lumer et al. (1998), might yield differences between JW's hemispheres. No qualitative differences were found (O'Shea and Corballis, 2001). (*b*) Example of Diaz-Caneja-type rivalry stimuli. Occasionally, perception is of a red vertical grating alternating with a green horizontal grating, showing that visual grouping can operate across the eyes to yield coherence rivalry. JW reported similar coherence rivalry from his two hemispheres (similar to that of intact-brain observers) (O'Shea and Corballis, 2003b). See chapter 16.

# 11 From Contour to Object-Face Rivalry: Multiple Neural Mechanisms Resolve Perceptual Ambiguity

Timothy J. Andrews, Frank Sengpiel, and Colin Blakemore

In constructing a representation of the visual world, the brain has to cope with the fact that any given two-dimensional retinal image could be the projection of countless object configurations in the three-dimensional world (Helmholtz, 1924). As we move about, or as the ambient illumination changes, the size, shape, intensity, and spectral quality of the images on the retina also change. To be useful, perception cannot simply represent the physical quality of images. Rather, it must take into account the context in which a stimulus appears.

Although in most situations this inherent ambiguity is resolved by the visual system, there are occasions when human vision alternates between different perceptions of a stimulus. Common examples of such bistable stimuli include figure–ground reversals (Rubin, 1915)[1], transparent three-dimensional objects (Necker, 1832; Wheatstone, 1838; Purves and Andrews, 1997), and binocular rivalry (Blake, 1989). Although fascinating in their own right, bistable stimuli offer a potentially fruitful paradigm for understanding how the brain routinely resolves ambiguity in the retinal image. This is because the physical nature of the stimulus does not change; therefore, any shifts in awareness presumably are mirrored only by stages of visual processing that are tightly linked to a perceptual decision.

A number of recent reports using one particular paradigm, binocular rivalry, have provoked a lively debate over the stage in visual processing at which signals access perception (Andrews, 2001; Blake and Logothetis, 2002). Two general theories have emerged. One possibility is that visual information is suppressed by inhibitory interactions prior to or at the stage of monocular confluence. In this concept, changes in perception would be mediated by shifts in the balance of suppression between neurons selective for one or another monocular image. Since these interactions must occur early in the visual pathway (e.g., the lateral geniculate nucleus or layer 4 of primary visual cortex), any changes in the activity of neurons in higher visual areas would be explained by a loss of input, perhaps equivalent to closing one eye. The alternative hypothesis is that rivalry reflects a competition between different stimulus representations. This would be comparable to the viewing of other bistable stimuli, such as the vase-face stimulus, and as such would be relevant to the resolution of ambiguity in normal viewing.

In this chapter, we argue that it is misleading to imagine that there is a single mechanism underlying binocular rivalry. Rather, it is likely that the neural events that underlie binocular rivalry (and other bistable stimuli) occur at multiple stages throughout the visual system (see also chapters 3 and 7 in this volume). First, we show that contour rivalry involves inhibitory or suppressive interactions between binocular neurons in primary visual cortex. Second, we suggest that the neural events that underlie contour rivalry can occur independently of binocular interactions for motion. Finally, we show that the neural events involved in resolving ambiguity in another bistable stimulus (the vase-face illusion) occur in visual areas within the temporal lobe.

## THE SITE AND MECHANISM OF CONTOUR RIVALRY

The episodic perceptual suppression of one eye's image during binocular rivalry is a compelling phenomenon that should be reflected in the firing pattern of single neurons at some stage in the visual system (Barlow, 1972). The apparent "competition" between the two eyes could be construed to imply that the interactions underlying rivalry occur at a stage where information about the eye of origin is still preserved. Indeed, most traditional models of binocular rivalry assume that this phenomenon is based on alternating dominance and suppression of the two eyes' inputs into V1 (Blake, 1989; Lehky and Blake, 1991).

Here we describe the stimulus dependence of interocular interactions in both the lateral geniculate nucleus (LGN) and striate cortex (V1) of normal cats, and evaluate the role that the suppressive behavior seen in V1 may play in binocular rivalry. We recorded from single neurons in the LGN and V1 of anesthetized cats that viewed dichoptically presented drifting gratings. These represent classic examples of stimuli evoking contour rivalry (Du Tour, 1760; Wheatstone, 1838; Lejeune, 1956).[2]

We recorded from 17 LGN cells in laminae A and A1 (12 X cells and 5 Y cells), all monocularly driven by conventional stimuli. To test for binocular interaction, we employed a procedure that we found best reveals

T. J. Andrews, F. Sengpiel, and C. Blakemore

suppressive effects (Sengpiel and Blakemore, 1994): the receptive field in one (the dominant) eye was stimulated continuously with an optimal "conditioning" grating, and at intervals, gratings of various orientations were presented to the other (nondominant) eye. This stimulus paradigm mimics "flash suppression": when one views a grating monocularly for a few seconds, and an orthogonal grating is then introduced to the other eye, the first grating will not be seen at all for some time (Wolfe 1984; see chapter 12 in this volume). The advantage of this paradigm is that one can safely predict the perceptual outcome without having tested it directly (which of course is not possible in anesthetized animals).

In seven LGN cells (including both X and Y cells; 41% of those tested) the binocular responses differed significantly from those through the dominant eye alone. In all these cases, the interaction was entirely inhibitory: we never saw significant augmentation of the response even when the stimuli were identical in the two eyes. More important, binocular inhibition was essentially independent of the orientation of the gratings shown to the nondominant eye, such that it occurred even when the grating shown to the nondominant eye was identical in orientation to that presented to the dominant eye. But since we know that in rivalry, alternating suppression occurs only when the stimuli are dissimilar in the two eyes, and not when stimuli are fusible, it seems reasonable to exclude the possibility that the perceptual conflict is resolved at that level of monocular representation. This conclusion is supported by single-cell recording from macaque LGN (Lehky and Maunsell, 1996).

In layer 4 of cat V1 many of the cells are monocular, and also orientation selective. We therefore reasoned that they might be involved in the interactions that underlie contour rivalry. Of the five monocular neurons we studied, four showed significant interocular suppression. However, as in the LGN, there was no evidence of any orientation-selective suppression that one might expect to find if these cells were mediating rivalry, and suppression occurred with both very similar (fusible) and dissimilar (rival) orientations present in the two eyes (see figure 11.1B).

Only binocularly driven neurons outside layer 4 exhibited effects that did seem to correlate with binocular contour rivalry (and fusion). In over 90% of binocular neurons, we observed the expected facilitation of the dominant eye's response when the other eye was simultaneously stimulated with a grating of optimal orientation and optimal relative spatial phase. In perception, fusion of contours depends on the similarity of spatial frequency. For example, vertical gratings of slightly different spatial frequency in the two eyes are perceived as tilted in depth around

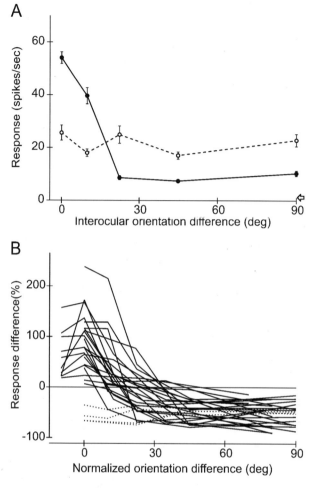

**Figure 11.1** Orientation dependence of binocular interactions in an individual complex cell (*A*) and for 27 cortical neurons (*B*), modified from Sengpiel, Blakemore, and Harrad (1995). (*A*) Results of the binocular stimulation protocol for a layer 2/3 complex cell. A "conditioning" grating of optimal orientation and direction of drift was presented continuously to the dominant, ipsilateral eye, and gratings of various orientations were shown intermittently to the contralateral eye. Filled circles plot mean responses (± SEM) during binocular stimulation against the difference in orientation of the gratings in the two eyes, and unfilled circles show the mean responses during the immediately preceding periods of monocular stimulation. The arrow indicates the mean level of spontaneous discharge. (*B*) Binocular interaction functions for 27 cortical cells, plotting the difference between binocular and monocular responses as a function of the interocular difference in orientation. These functions show the range of variability in the depth of suppression and in the threshold interocular orientation difference for the transition between facilitation and suppression. All tuning curves with maximum facilitation at an orientation difference other than zero have been shifted to peak at zero. Included are the four monocular units recorded in layer 4 (data plotted as dotted lines), where suppression was essentially independent of interocular difference in orientation.

the vertical axis, as expected from the geometry of actual rotated surfaces. But fusion and the perception of tilt break down at an interocular difference of about 0.4 octave (Blakemore, 1970). Concordant with these findings, we observed that dichoptic gratings of different spatial frequency, but identical orientation, demonstrate facilitation over a similarly narrow range of spatial frequency difference. Furthermore, a transition to suppression occurs when spatial frequency differs by more than 0.5 octave between the two eyes (figure 11.2A; Sengpiel, Freeman, and Blakemore, 1995).

These binocular neurons exhibited interocular suppression *selectively* for stimuli that also cause binocular contour rivalry in humans. When the nondominant eye was stimulated with a high-contrast grating oriented orthogonal to the optimal orientation being shown to the dominant eye, 56% of the binocular neurons showed statistically significant suppression, reducing the mean spike rate by between 15% and 90% of the monocular response through the dominant eye. The suppression with orthogonal stimulation did not vary convincingly with the spatial phase of the grating in the nondominant eye.

Among all the cells that exhibited iso-orientation facilitation and cross-orientation suppression, the transition between the two occurred at between 5° and 70° from the peak; for most it was between about 15° and 35°, with a mean of 22°. This value is in reasonable agreement with the finding that fusion gives way to binocular rivalry at an interocular orientation difference of about 30° in human observers (Braddick, 1979). Figure 11.1A illustrates the orientation dependence of interocular interactions for a representative complex cell recorded in layer 2/3; pooled results for 27 cortical cells are displayed in figure 11.1B. Cells with narrower orientation tuning tended to be suppressed at smaller interocular orientation differences and to have stronger suppression than did cells with broader orientation tuning.

A key characteristic of contour rivalry is that once a grating is perceptually suppressed, suppression persists despite changes in stimulus parameters, particularly orientation (Blake and Lema, 1978). We found that the interocular suppression of binocular neurons in V1 caused by the presentation of rival contours was also independent of the parameters of the contours. For example, suppression could be elicited by a range of spatial frequencies to which the cell was not sensitive. When suppression was exerted by gratings with spatial frequencies that were too high to elicit an excitatory response from the cell in question, suppression became independent of orientation (Sengpiel, Freeman, and Blakemore, 1995). Moreover, in strabismic cats, which lack the normal facilitation for binocularly

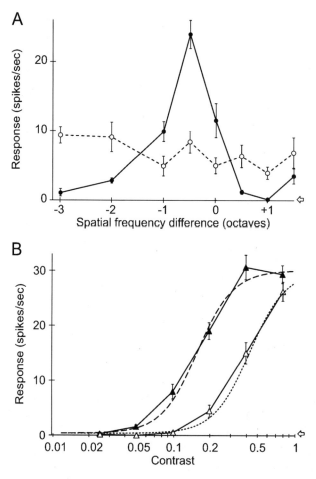

**Figure 11.2** Spatial frequency dependence of binocular interactions (*A*) and effect of interocular suppression on the contrast–response function (*B*). (*A*) Binocular responses of a layer 5 complex cell as a function of the spatial frequency presented to the nondominant eye (modified from Sengpiel, Freeman, and Blakemore, 1995). The dominant eye was stimulated continuously with a grating of optimum orientation and spatial frequency (1.13 c/deg) while a grating of the same orientation but varied in spatial frequency was presented intermittently to the nondominant eye. Filled circles plot mean responses (± SEM) during binocular stimulation against the difference in spatial frequency of the gratings in the two eyes, and unfilled circles show the mean responses during the immediately preceding periods of monocular stimulation. The abscissa is plotted in octaves relative to the spatial frequency of the grating shown to the dominant eye. The arrow represents the mean spontaneous discharge. (*B*) Effects of interocular suppression on the contrast–response function of a layer 2/3 complex cell (modified from Sengpiel et al., 1998). Mean responses (± SEM) are plotted against effective Michelson contrast of the (optimally oriented) test grating in the dominant eye, in the presence and absence of a grating of the orthogonal orientation placed in the

T. J. Andrews, F. Sengpiel, and C. Blakemore

matched stimuli, interocular suppression occurs with any stimulus orientation, even when the gratings shown to the two eyes have the same spatial frequency (Sengpiel et al., 1994). This virtual absence of selectivity for orientation at the neuronal level resembles pathological suppression in strabismic humans (see Holopigian, Blake, and Greenwald, 1988).

Finally, we examined the strength of interocular suppression in terms of its effect on neuronal contrast thresholds. In human rivalry, the contrast increment needed to break suppression and render the suppressed stimulus visible is about 0.3–0.5 log unit (Fox and Check, 1966, 1968; Wales and Fox, 1970). We found that in cat V1, contrast-response functions for an optimal grating in one eye are shifted to the right by an average 0.17 log unit in the presence of an orthogonal grating in the other eye (figure 11.2B; Sengpiel et al., 1998).

These results demonstrate that interactions between binocular neurons in V1 may contribute toward the changes in perception during contour rivalry. However, in one important respect, interocular suppression falls short of what one would expect of a direct neural correlate of binocular rivalry: it does not exhibit any significant waxing and waning over time. When orthogonal gratings were presented to the two eyes for up to 30 sec, suppression was generally strongest over the initial 1–3 sec, with slight recovery to a tonic level, which was then sustained over the remainder of the period of binocular stimulation. For most cells, spike trains from individual trials revealed no obvious variation of suppression over time, nor did the overall depth of suppression vary substantially from trial to trial. Since our study was concerned with single-neuron responses, we did not examine whether synchronization of activity between groups of cells was affected by the nature of the stimuli or whether it varied in time with presentation of rival stimuli (see chapter 14 in this volume).

corresponding region in the nondominant eye (contrast, 0.9). Contrast–response data obtained under the control, unsuppressed condition were fitted by a hyperbolic ratio function,

$$R = R_{\max} \cdot c^n / \left( c_{50}^n + c^n \right) + b,$$

where $R_{\max}$ is the maximum attainable response, $c_{50}$ is the contrast that elicits the half-maximal response, and $b$ is the cell's spontaneous activity. Filled triangles plot unsuppressed responses; the dashed line represents the best fit ($R_{\max} = 29.69$ spikes/sec, $c_{50} = 0.16$, $n = 2.93$). Open triangles show suppressed responses; the dotted line represents the best fit under the assumption that $R_{\max}$ and $n$ are unaffected ($c_{50} = 0.43$). This corresponds to a threshold elevation by 0.43 log unit.

What is the substrate of interocular suppression in V1? We hypothesize that it derives from a network of inhibitory connections between binocular neurons in neighboring ocular dominance (OD) columns (Sengpiel and Blakemore, 1994, 1996). We suggest that the response properties of binocular neurons in V1 can be explained by a combination of both suppressive and facilitative mechanisms. Thus, the binocular facilitation for matched stimuli, thought to underlie fusion and stereopsis, is superimposed on nonselective inhibitory interaction between the two eyes. In that sense, binocular rivalry/interocular suppression may be the "default" outcome of binocular vision (see Blake and Camisa, 1978).

A possible anatomical substrate for the excitatory and inhibitory binocular interactions postulated above is schematically illustrated in figure 11.3A. Thin lines symbolize excitatory, and thick lines, inhibitory, connections. Excitatory intrinsic connections tend to be clustered (Rockland and Lund, 1982; Gilbert and Wiesel, 1983) and more frequently link regions of similar than dissimilar orientation preference (Ts'o, Gilbert, and Wiesel, 1986; Kisvárday et al., 1997): they may mediate disparity-sensitive binocular facilitation. Connectivity between sites of oblique or orthogonal orientation preference is provided mainly by projections to intercluster regions (Kisvárday et al., 1997). Long-range inhibitory connections are much more diffuse and more uniformly distributed across orientation and ocular dominance columns (Somogyi et al., 1983; Kisvárday and Eysel, 1993).

One possible implementation of interocular suppression is reciprocal inhibition between cells dominated by the two eyes that lie in neighboring OD columns. Since the majority of excitatory synapses on neurons in area 17 derive from closely neighboring cells rather than from thalamic afferents (Kisvárday et al., 1986; Douglas and Martin, 1991; Nicoll and Blakemore, 1993), the responses of cortical neurons are likely to depend crucially on "amplification" of input from the thalamus operating through this local excitatory circuitry (Douglas, Martin, and Whitteridge, 1989; Douglas and Martin, 1991). Perhaps inhibitory interactions between adjacent OD columns, responsible for suppressive interocular interactions, modulate the gain of this local excitatory circuitry (figure 11.3B). The resultant interocular suppression will be overcome by binocular facilitation when the images in the two eyes are sufficiently similar.

Since adjacent ocular dominance columns tend to represent very similar regions of visual space, one would therefore predict that the interocular suppression field in one eye should be of similar location and extent as the classical, excitatory receptive field of a neuron in the other eye. We

T. J. Andrews, F. Sengpiel, and C. Blakemore

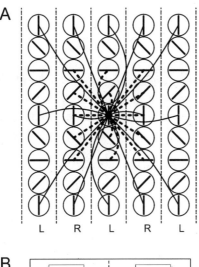

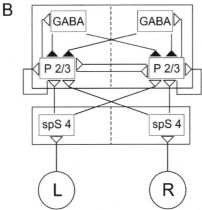

**Figure 11.3** Schematic diagrams of intrinsic horizontal connections (*A*) and of within- and between-columns signal processing (*B*) that might underlie binocular interaction in cat V1. (*A*) Surface view of orientation and ocular dominance domains with horizontal connections (modified from Sengpiel and Blakemore, 1996). Parallel slabs or "columns" marked L and R represent left-eye and right-eye OD columns, respectively. Columns of cells with similar orientation preference are depicted as circles with an oriented line inside. Thin lines represent excitatory projections that selectively connect neurons of similar orientation preference within and between neighboring OD columns; while thick dashed lines show widespread nonselective inhibitory connections. (*B*) Diagram of a cortical microcircuitry in V1 that could generate binocular responses of the type we observed. Circles marked L and R represent left- and right-eye inputs, respectively, to spiny stellate cells in layer 4 of V1 (spS 4). Layer 2/3 pyramidal cells are indicated as P 2/3, and GABA-ergic interneurons as GABA. Open and filled triangles represent excitatory and inhibitory synapses, respectively. Vertical dashed lines separate cells with predominantly left-eye excitatory input from those with predominantly right-eye input.

From Contour to Object-Face Rivalry

mapped suppression fields using small circular grating patches (Sengpiel et al., 2001). We found that the suppression field of V1 neurons is generally centered on the same position in space and is slightly larger (by a factor of 1.3) than the minimum response field, measured through the same eye. These results are in agreement with the observation by Blake, O'Shea, and Mueller (1992) that the size of grating patches engaging in whole-stimulus rather than piecemeal rivalry is scaled with stimulus eccentricity in a way that reflects the cortical magnification factor in V1 (Hubel and Wiesel, 1974). In other visual areas, where responses are less dependent on stimulus size and location, these findings might not have been expected.

Altogether, our results support the hypothesis that contour rivalry arises from mutual inhibition between pools of neurons dominated by either the left or the right eye within retinotopically confined areas in V1. However, the proposed link between interocular suppression and the OD columnar architecture (see also Sengpiel et al., 2001) should not be misinterpreted to imply that it is monocular neurons which interact. As we and others have shown, suppression during contour rivalry is much more likely to involve binocular rather than monocular cells in V1. However, it is not clear whether a similar neural mechanism is used to resolve rivalry for other aspects of vision.

## INDEPENDENT RIVALRY FOR CONTOUR AND MOTION

Although binocular rivalry has been most commonly studied with orthogonal gratings (contour rivalry), it can also be elicited when the monocular images are distinguished by other attributes of vision, such as color or motion. In this section, we review evidence that rivalry for different aspects of vision can involve independent visual processes. Specifically, we present data which show that a visual stimulus whose contours are rendered literally invisible through binocular rivalry can nevertheless contribute to the perception of movement.

A moving surface covered with stripes of a single orientation, viewed through a circular aperture, is usually seen as drifting in a direction orthogonal to the grating's orientation, whatever the actual direction of surface movement (Wallach, 1976). The ambiguity of a moving grating is resolved, however, if other features are added to the surface. A simple demonstration of such "pattern" motion is provided by the superimposition of two drifting gratings, orthogonal to one another. While each grating presented alone would appear to move in its own "component" direction, orthogonal to its contours, the two fuse together, forming a

T. J. Andrews, F. Sengpiel, and C. Blakemore

"plaid" that drifts along an axis that usually corresponds to the vector average of the two components (Adelson and Movshon, 1982). Thus both gratings contribute to the direction of pattern motion as well as to the perceived form of the stimulus.

To determine whether the system responsible for the awareness of movement could integrate component motion signals delivered separately to the two eyes, we presented human subjects with orthogonal moving gratings (4° diameter) that were viewed dichoptically. Even when the two gratings were identical in color, spatial frequency, and temporal frequency, they never fused to form a plaid, as they do when viewed through both eyes simultaneously. For periods of a few seconds at a time, totaling about half the entire 1-min viewing period, one or the other of the two monocular gratings appeared to fill the entire field. During these epochs of apparently pure monocular perception, the grating almost always appeared to drift orthogonal to its orientation, just as it would if the other grating were not present.

Rarely, with these large fields, did direct and complete transitions occur between one eye's view and the other's. Usually, after a few seconds of apparently monocular perception, the grating broke up into a fluid mosaic consisting of contiguous patches of grating of the two different orientations (usually termed "piecemeal rivalry"), the boundaries of which could shift slowly. Eventually the patchy mosaic was replaced for a few seconds by the other completely monocular view. In the fluid mosaic, which was seen for about half the entire viewing period, the individual patches were typically about one-third of the diameter of the entire patch (i.e., about 1° or more across). Again, only one orientation was seen within each individual patch. Nevertheless, the entire mosaic usually appeared to move coherently, as if on a single surface, in the pattern-motion direction, appropriate to the combination of velocities of the two monocular gratings (see figure 11.4A).

One might imagine that when the mosaic is seen during dichoptic viewing, the perceived direction is simply determined by integration of directional information from the visible single-grating patches, rather than through the integration of motion information from a grating whose orientation information is suppressed from perception (see Alais et al., 1998). To test for this possibility, we used orthogonal grating patches that were so small (< 1° diameter), and presented for such a short time (1.5 sec), that on most trials, one orientation dominated completely over the entire area for the whole period of exposure (Blake, O'Shea, and Mueller, 1992). The two gratings were always of oblique orientation and each could move in one of

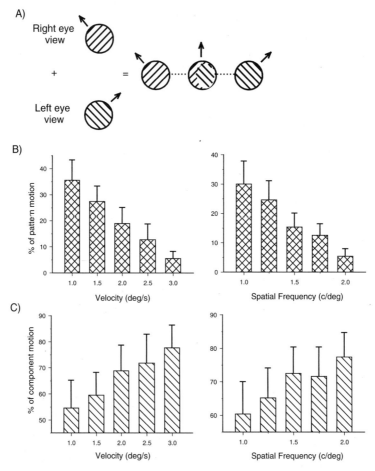

**Figure 11.4** Integration of motion information during contour rivalry (modified from Andrews et al., 2002). (*A*) During the transitions between exclusive dominance of one grating to dominance by the other, a fluid mosaic of contiguous patches of the two gratings is often seen. The grating patches within this mosaic are usually seen to move together, in the direction of pattern motion. Thus, the motion signals in the two eyes are combined while orientation signals continue to rival. (*B*) The grating in one eye (the standard) was kept unaltered while the grating presented to the other eye was gradually changed. The proportion of dichoptic pattern motion decreased as the gratings were made more different from one another in velocity or spatial frequency. (*C*) In contrast, the periods of exclusive perceptual dominance increased in duration as the stimulus characteristics of the two gratings were made more dissimilar. The columns represent the mean from four observers. Error bars show 1 SEM.

T. J. Andrews, F. Sengpiel, and C. Blakemore

the two possible component directions. The orientations and directions were all randomized from trial to trial, producing four possible combinations (Andrews and Blakemore, 1999). Randomly interleaved with these conflicting presentations were nonrivalrous control stimuli, in which the oblique grating patches shown to the two eyes were identical in orientation and direction of drift. With such small patches and brief presentations, the subjects were usually unaware of whether the stimulus was binocularly fused or rivalrous. They simply had the impression of a single, drifting grating.

For the nonrivalrous stimuli, as expected, subjects reported the grating moving in the appropriate component direction. For the rivalrous stimuli, whichever grating dominated consciousness also seemed to move orthogonal to its orientation (the expected component direction) on about 50% of trials. However, for fully half of the presentations, the single perceived grating appeared to drift in the direction of pattern motion predicted from the combination of movements in the two eyes, just as if the two gratings were actually superimposed (Andrews and Blakemore, 1999).

Evidence that the same mechanism underlies pattern motion in dichoptic and normal binocular viewing was apparent when the component gratings were made progressively more different from one another. We observed a similar decrease in the incidence of normal and dichoptic pattern motion when the difference in color, direction of motion, contrast, velocity, or spatial frequency between gratings was increased (figure 11.4B; Andrews and Blakemore, 2002). Moreover, as the stimulus properties of the gratings presented to the two eyes were made more different, there was a complementary increase in the amount of time that one grating or the other dominated perception over the whole patch (figure 11.4C). These results suggest that the dicohoptic combination of moving gratings occurred in a manner similar to that observed in normal binocular vision (Adelson and Movshon, 1982; Stoner, Albright, and Ramachandran, 1990; Krauskopf and Farell, 1990).

This phenomenon, in which perceived movement is influenced by an apparently invisible grating, is compatible with other findings that show stimuli rendered invisible during binocular rivalry can nevertheless contribute either to the perception of apparent motion (Wiesenfelder and Blake, 1991) or to the motion aftereffect (Lehmkuhle and Fox, 1975). Previous reports also suggest that when stimuli of different colors are presented to the two eyes, chromatic rivalry can occur independently of binocular interaction between the shapes or movements of the targets (Creed, 1935; Carney, Shadlen, and Switkes, 1987; see also chapter 5 in this volume).

Can we draw any conclusions about the neural correlates of this phenomenon? Most neurons in primary visual cortex (V1) of monkey respond selectively to bars and gratings at particular orientations (Hubel and Wiesel, 1968). During contour rivalry, these neurons exhibit significant interocular suppression (see above). Direction-selective responses are also apparent in the activity of neurons in V1 (Hubel and Wiesel, 1968). However, these neurons respond only to component motion. When shown plaids moving in various directions, they fire only when one of the components has an orientation close to the optimum for the receptive field, as if they are blind to the other grating (Movshon et al., 1985). Clearly such activity cannot account for pattern motion perception. Direction-selective neurons in V1 send signals, directly and indirectly, to the extrastriate area MT (Dubner and Zeki, 1971). A significant fraction of cells in MT are selective for pattern motion: they have the same preferred direction for drifting plaids as they do for single gratings (Movshon et al., 1985). Such cells, which presumably combine component motion signals from earlier stages of analysis (such as the local motion elements in piecemeal rivalry), appear to encode the perceived direction of pattern motion. Indeed, the activity of neurons in MT has been shown to covary with the changes in perceived direction of motion during binocular rivalry (Logothetis and Schall, 1989).

## NEURAL CORRELATES OF PERCEPTUAL AMBIGUITY

The spontaneous alternation in perception that occurs when different images are presented to the two eyes (binocular rivalry) has many features in common with that experienced when viewing other ambiguous stimuli (Logothetis, Leopold, and Sheinberg, 1996; Andrews and Purves, 1997). A number of reports have suggested that activity in relatively "high" areas of visual cortex correlates with changes in perception that occur during binocular rivalry in both monkeys (Leopold and Logothetis, 1996; Sheinberg and Logothetis, 1997) and humans (Tong et al., 1998). However, recent evidence suggests that the simple rivalry between contours of different orientation depends on inhibitory or suppressive interactions occurring in primary visual cortex (Polonsky et al., 2000; Tong and Engel, 2001), as suggested earlier by Sengpiel and Blakemore (1994; see above). Interestingly, modulations of BOLD signals from V1 also correlate with rivalry state when the rival targets are more complex (Lee and Blake, 2002).

This recent controversy suggests that the mechanism underlying rivalry might be quite different, in nature and location, from that causing shifts in the perception of other ambiguous figures. In a recent study, we investigated human cortical activity while subjects were viewing the vase-face illusion, where different stimulus interpretations (faces and vase) were clearly competing (Andrews et al., 2002).

We took advantage of the fact that inanimate objects and faces are known to be analyzed in different areas of extrastriate visual cortex. Using fMRI, we localized regions of visual cortex selective for unambiguous faces in the fusiform gyrus and the superior temporal sulcus (Kanwisher, McDermott, and Chun, 1997). Object-selective areas were localized in the parahippocampal gyrus (Epstein and Kanwisher, 1998) and the lateral occipital lobe (LOC) (Malach et al., 1995). However, the selectivity of neural responses to these different classes of stimuli does not in itself demonstrate that the conscious perception of a face or an object is made explicit in these visual areas. It could be that this activity represents a divergence of processing before the level at which percepts arise. Indeed, it is also possible that explicit representations of faces and objects cannot be localized to particular areas in the brain, but are widely distributed (Haxby et al., 2001).

To determine whether the perception of faces and objects is made explicit in these areas, in the sense that activity correlates with conscious perception regardless of the physical stimulus, we monitored activity when subjects viewed the ambiguous vase-faces stimulus. We hypothesized that a cortical area which makes "explicit" in its activity the interpretation of a face would show more activity for a perceptual transition from vase to faces than for a shift from faces to vase. Conversely, areas directly involved in or leading to the awareness of inanimate objects ought to display an opposite pattern of activity. We further posited that if an area is involved in a specific aspect of visual awareness, the trial-by-trial variation in activity should correlate with the subjects' perceptual responses.

Since the frequency of spontaneous perceptual change was too rapid to be followed by the underlying BOLD response, we devised the procedure of adding local contrast gradients to emboss the edges of the ambiguous stimulus (figure 11.5A), and thus prolong perception of either the vase or the face after a perceptual transition. The activity of face-selective voxels in the fusiform gyrus did indeed discriminate between the alternative perceptions of the stimulus in this paradigm (figure 11.5B). Greater activity was detected following vase-to-faces transitions than during faces-to-vase changes.

These results are consistent with an earlier fMRI study of binocular rivalry in which complex objects (houses) and faces were presented independently to the two eyes and house-to-face changes in perception were

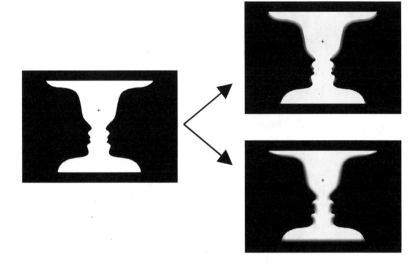

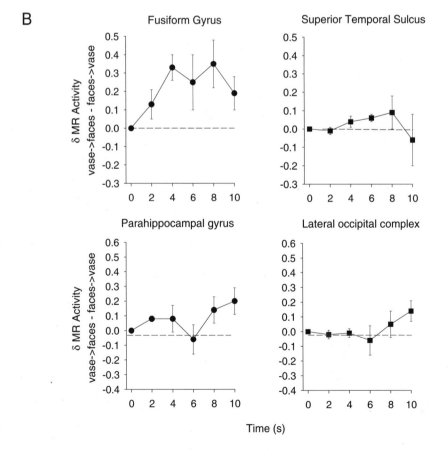

associated with increased activity in the fusiform gyrus (Tong et al., 1998). However, the authors also reported that face-to-house changes resulted in a decrease in MR signal, while we did not find a systematic decrease following perceptual switches to the nonpreferred (vase) percept. Kleinschmidt et al. (1998) also report increases in activity in the fusiform gyrus during changes in perception only when subjects viewed the vase–faces stimulus, although they did not discriminate the direction of perceptual changes. This leads us to speculate that the competitive inter-actions underlying binocular rivalry between complex figures might, in some circumstances, employ a mechanism different from that involved in the interpretation of conventional ambiguous figures (see Andrews, 2001).

Activity in voxels in the superior temporal sulcus that were selective for unambiguous faces were not statistically significant predictors for the two perceptual interpretations of the vase-faces image (figure 11.5B). One explanation for area being able to distinguish between photographs of faces and objects, but not able to discriminate between the vase and faces in the ambiguous stimulus, is the paucity of explicit detail in the latter. It is possible that areas in the superior temporal sulcus are more concerned with the details of facial structure, such as eye gaze, expression, and lip movement (Perrett et al., 1985; Hasselmo, Rolls, and Baylis, 1989; Calvert et al., 1997; Haxby, Hoffman, and Gobbini, 2000). Consistent with these findings, lesions to the superior temporal sulcus in nonhuman primates do not impair face recognition (Heywood and Cowey, 1992).

Areas selective for unambiguous inanimate objects were similarly unable to discriminate the direction of perceptual change when view-ing the vase-faces stimulus (figure 11.5B). Perceptual transitions to the preferred percept (faces-to-vase) did not produce more activity than shifts to the nonpreferred percept (vase-to-faces) in either the parahippocampal

◄ **Figure 11.5** Activity in face- and object-selective areas when viewing the vase–faces stimulus. (*A*) An event-related paradigm was employed in which the sudden onset of per-ception of either the faces or the vase was prolonged by adding subtle local contrast gradi-ents (embossing) to one edge of the figure–ground boundary. Thus, following a vase-to-faces transition, the standard image was replaced by an embossed-face version of the same stimu-lus (top), whereas subsequent to a faces-to-vase change, an embossed vase version (bottom) replaced the standard. (*B*) Face-selective voxels in the fusiform gyrus, but not the superior temporal sulcus, reflected the perceptual interpretation of faces in the Rubin figure when prolonged by the embossing technique. Object-selective voxels in the parahippocampal gyrus and lateral occipital complex did not show selectivity for the perceptual interpretation of the vase. Each curve represents a mean time course from three subjects. Error bars show 1 SEM.

gyrus or the lateral occipital lobe. Again, the most parsimonious explanation for this result is that the vase representation is a less salient percept than the photographs of objects that were used to define this area.

The observation that activity in the fusiform gyrus was selective for the different conscious interpretations of the vase–faces stimulus when prolonged by embossing does not alone imply that the perception of a face is made explicit in this area. It could be, for example, that this activity simply reflects differential responsiveness to the relatively unambiguous embossed image rather than to the initial spontaneous switch to perception of faces (see also Hasson et al., 2001). To control for the change in the stimulus, we compared activity in the fusiform gyrus when the sequence of stimuli was identical but perception was different (figure 11.6A). We found that even when the physical stimulation remained the same, more activity was recorded in the fusiform gyrus when a vase-to-faces transition preceded the presentation of an embossed face compared to when a faces-to-vase switch was initially reported (figure 11.6B). Moreover, using an analysis of choice probability (Britten et al., 1996), we found that the face-selective area in the fusiform gyrus was statistically predictive of the subjects' responses on a trial-by-trial basis (figure 11.6C). The implication is that activity in the fusiform gyrus could make a decision which leads directly to the perception of a face.

Our results are consistent with other studies which have shown that the responses of regions within the temporal lobe are modulated by selective attention to faces (O'Craven, Downing, and Kanwisher, 1999) or when a degraded image of a face becomes recognizable after the subject views a photographic version of the same image (Dolan et al., 1997). More generally, it could be that this area is directly involved in the awareness of a broader range of specialized object categories (Tarr and Gauthier, 2000). Together these results strongly suggest that activity in the fusiform gyrus "face area" reflects the perceived rather than merely the retinal stimulus.

## CONCLUSION

Results from three lines of investigation lead us to believe that there is no single mechanism underlying binocular rivalry (and the perception of other ambiguous stimuli). Intuitively, the visual system must first determine whether the images in the two eyes should fuse or rival. Given the parallel nature of visual processing (Felleman and Van Essen, 1991), we suggest that the level at which competitive interactions occur will vary with the submodality of vision which is explicit in different bistable

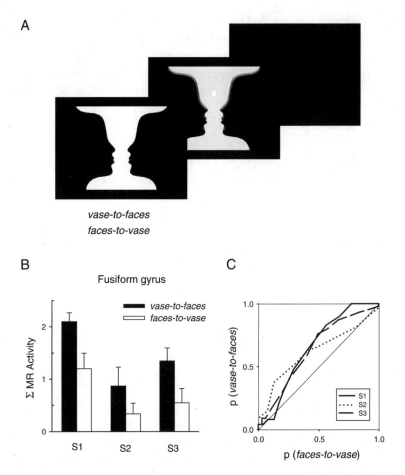

**A**

*vase-to-faces*
*faces-to-vase*

**B**

Fusiform gyrus

■ *vase-to-faces*
□ *faces-to-vase*

Σ MR Activity

2

1

0

S1    S2    S3

**C**

p (*vase-to-faces*)

1.0

0.5

0.0

0.0    0.5    1.0

p (*faces-to-vase*)

—— S1
······ S2
– – S3

**Figure 11.6** Activity in the fusiform gyrus predicted conscious perception of the vase–faces stimulus (modified from Andrews et al., 2002). (*A*) Responses were selected for all sequences in which a change of perception ("vase-to-faces" and "faces-to-vase") for the standard Rubin's stimulus, signaled by a button press, was followed by embossing of the face contours, thus biasing subsequent perception toward the faces percept and, therefore, "confirming" or "charging" the initial percept. (*B*) Each bar represents the integrated MR response for 6 sec after the spontaneous shift of perception. The sequence of physical images was identical in both conditions, yet more activity occurred when the perception of faces in the ambiguous figure was confirmed by the embossing than when it was changed. (*C*) To assess whether the activity of the fusiform gyrus could predict perception when viewing the ambiguous stimulus on a trial-by-trial basis, we calculated the proportion of trials in which the MR activity correctly (hits) and incorrectly (false alarms) predicted the direction of perceptual change. Analysis of the data showed significant choice probabilities were apparent in the fusiform gyrus for each subject.

stimuli. Second, if it has determined that the images are incompatible, the visual system must then have a mechanism to suppress one monocular image and render the other image dominant. It is quite conceivable that this process occurs independently of the process that is involved in registering whether the two images are compatible (see Blake, 2001).

## ACKNOWLEDGMENTS

We are very grateful to Denis Schluppeck, Tobe Freeman, and Richard Harrad for their collaboration in this work.

## NOTES

1. Although the vase–face illusion is generally attributed to Rubin (1915), similar pictorial ambiguities were used in paintings by artists such as Pierre Crussaire in the eighteenth century (see chapter 2 in this volume).

2. Although Ptolemy (ca. 150) made the first reference to contour rivalry, Wheatstone was the first to systematically describe this phenomenon (Wade, 1998).

## REFERENCES

Adelson, E. H., and Movshon, J. A. (1982). Phenomenal coherence of moving visual patterns. *Nature*, 300, 523–525.

Alais, D., Van der Smagt, M. J., Van den Berg, A. V., and Van de Grind, W. A. (1998). Local and global factors affecting the coherent motion of gratings presented in multiple apertures. *Vision Research*, 38, 1581–1591.

Andrews, T. J. (2001). Binocular rivalry and visual awareness. *Trends in Cognitive Sciences*, 10, 407–409.

Andrews, T. J., and Blakemore, C. (1999). Form and motion have independent access to consciousness. *Nature Neuroscience*, 2, 405–406.

Andrews, T. J., and Blakemore, C. (2002). Integration of motion information during binocular rivalry. *Vision Research*, 42, 301–309.

Andrews, T. J., and Purves, D. (1997). Similarities in normal and binocularly rivalrous viewing. *Proceedings of the National Academy of Sciences of the United States of America*, 94, 9905–9908.

Andrews, T. J., Schluppeck, D., Homfray, D., Matthews, P., and Blakemore, C. (2002). Activity in the fusiform gyrus predicts conscious perception of Rubin's vase-face illusion. *Neuroimage*, 17, 890–901.

Barlow, H. B. (1972). Single units and sensation: A neuron doctrine for perceptual psychology? *Perception*, 1, 371–394.

T. J. Andrews, F. Sengpiel, and C. Blakemore

Barlow, H. B., Blakemore, C., and Pettigrew, J. D. (1967). The neural mechanism of binocular depth discrimination. *Journal of Physiology*, 193, 327–342.

Blake, R. (1989). A neural theory of binocular rivalry. *Psychological Review*, 96, 145–167.

Blake, R. (2001). Primer on binocular rivalry, including controversial issues. *Brain and Mind*, 2, 5–38.

Blake, R., and Camisa, J. (1978). Is binocular vision always monocular? *Science*, 200, 1497–1499.

Blake, R., and Lema, S. A. (1978). Inhibitory effect of binocular rivalry suppression is independent of orientation. *Vision Research*, 18, 541–544.

Blake, R., and Logothetis, N. K. (2002). Visual competition. *Nature Reviews: Neuroscience*, 3, 13–21.

Blake, R., O'Shea, R. P., and Mueller, T. J. (1992). Spatial zones of binocular rivalry in central and peripheral vision. *Visual Neuroscience*, 8, 469–478.

Blakemore, C. (1970). A new kind of stereoscopic vision. *Vision Research*, 10, 1181–1199.

Braddick, O. J. (1979). Binocular single vision and perceptual processing. *Proceedings of the Royal Society of London*, B204, 503–512.

Britten, K. H., Newsome, W. T., Shadlen, M. N., Celebrini, S., and Movshon, J. A. (1996). A relationship between behavioral choice and the visual responses of neurons in macaque MT. *Visual Neuroscience*, 13, 87–100.

Calvert, G. A., Bullmore, E., Brammer, M. J., Campbell, R., Iversen, S. D., Woodruff, P., McGuire, P., Williams, S., and David, A. S. (1997). Silent lipreading activates the auditory cortex. *Science*, 276, 593–596.

Carney, T., Shadlen, M., and Switkes, E. (1987). Parallel processing of motion and colour information. *Nature*, 328, 647–649.

Creed, R. S. (1935). Observations on binocular fusion and rivalry. *Journal of Physiology*, 84, 381–392.

Dolan, R. J., Fink, G. R., Rolls, E., Booth, M., Holmes, A., Frackowiak, R. S. J., and Friston, K. J. (1997). How the brain learns to see objects and faces in an impoverished context. *Nature*, 389, 596–599.

Douglas, R. J., and Martin, K. A. C. (1991). A functional microcircuit for cat visual cortex. *Journal of Physiology*, 440, 735–769.

Douglas, R. J., Martin, K. A. C., and Whitteridge, D. (1989). A canonical microcircuit for neocortex. *Neural Computation*, 1, 480–488.

Dubner, R., and Zeki, S. M. (1971). Response properties and receptive fields of cells in an anatomically defined region of the superior temporal sulcus in the monkey. *Brain Research*, 35, 528–532.

Du Tour, E.-F. (1760). Pourquoi un objet sur lequel nous fixons les yeux paroit-il unique? *Mém. Math. Phys. Acad. Roy. Sci. Paris*, 3, 514–530.

From Contour to Object-Face Rivalry

Epstein, R., and Kanwisher, N. (1998). A cortical representation of the local visual environment. *Nature, 392,* 598–601.

Felleman, D. J., and Van Essen, D. C. (1991). Distributed hierarchical processing in the primate cerebral cortex. *Cerebral Cortex, 1,* 1–47.

Fox, R., and Check, R. (1966). Forced-choice form recognition during binocular rivalry. *Psychonomic Sciences, 6,* 471–472.

Fox, R., and Check, R. (1969). Detection of motion during binocular rivalry suppression. *Journal of Experimental Psychology, 78,* 388–395.

Gilbert, C. D., and Wiesel, T. N. (1983). Clustered intrinsic connections in the cat visual cortex. *Journal of Neuroscience, 3,* 1116–1133.

Hasselmo, M. E., Rolls, E. T., and Baylis, G. C. (1989). The role of expression and identity in the face-selective responses of neurons in the temporal visual cortex of monkey. *Behavioral Brain Research, 32,* 203–208.

Hasson, U., Hendler, T., Bashat, D. B., and Malach, R. (2001). Vase or face? A neural correlate of shape-selective grouping processes in the human brain. *Journal of Cognitive Neuroscience, 13,* 744–753.

Haxby, J. V., Gobbini, M. I., Furey, M. L., Ishai, A., Schouten, J. L., and Pietrini, P. (2001). Distributed and overlapping representations of faces and objects in ventral temporal cortex. *Science, 293,* 2425–2430.

Haxby, J. V., Hoffman, E. A., and Gobbini, M. I. (2000). The distributed human neural system for face perception. *Trends in Cognitive Sciences, 4,* 223–233.

Helmholtz, H. von. (1924). *Helmholtz's Treatise on Physiological Optics,* J. P. C. Southall, trans. Dover: New York.

Heywood, C. A., and Cowey, A. (1992). The role of the "face-cell" area in the discrimination and recognition of faces by monkeys. *Philosophical Transactions of the Royal Society of London,* B335, 31–37.

Holopigian, K., Blake, R., and Greenwald, M. J. (1988). Clinical suppression and amblyopia. *Investigative Ophthalmology and Visual Science, 29,* 444–451.

Hubel, D. H., and Wiesel, T. N. (1968). Receptive fields and functional architecture of macaque visual cortex. *Journal of Physiology, 195,* 215–243.

Hubel, D. H., and Wiesel, T. N. (1974). Uniformity of monkey striate cortex: A parallel relationship between field size, scatter, and magnification factor. *Journal of Comparative Neurology, 158,* 295–305.

Kanwisher, N., McDermott, J., and Chun, M. M. (1997). The fusiform face area: A module in extrastriate cortex specialized for face perception. *Journal of Neuroscience, 17,* 4302–4311.

Kisvárday, Z. F., and Eysel, U. T. (1993). Functional and structural topography of horizontal inhibitory connections in cat visual cortex. *European Journal of Neuroscience, 5,* 1558–1572.

Kisvárday, Z. F., Martin, K. A. C., Freund, T. F., Maglóczky, Z., Whitteridge, D., and Somogyi, P. (1986). Synaptic targets of HRP-filled layer III pyramidal cells in the cat striate cortex. *Experimental Brain Research, 64,* 541–552.

T. J. Andrews, F. Sengpiel, and C. Blakemore

Kisvárday, Z. F., Tóth, E., Rausch, M., and Eysel., U. T. (1997). Orientation-specific relationship between populations of excitatory and inhibitory lateral connections in the visual cortex of the cat. *Cerebral Cortex*, 7, 605–618.

Kleinschmidt, A., Buchel, C., Zeki, S., and Frackowiak, R. S. (1998). Human brain activity during spontaneously reversing perception of ambiguous figures. *Proceedings of the Royal Society of London*, B265, 2427.

Krauskopf, J., and Farell, B. (1990). Influence of colour on the perception of coherent motion. *Nature*, 348, 328–331.

Lee, S. H., and Blake, R. (2002). V1 activity is reduced during binocular rivalry. *Journal of Vision*, 2, 618–626.

Lehky, S. R., and Blake, R. (1991). Organization of binocular pathways: Modeling and data related to rivalry. *Neural Computation*, 3, 44–53.

Lehky, S. R., and Maunsell, J. H. R. (1996). No binocular rivalry in the LGN of alert macaque monkey. *Vision Research*, 36, 1225–1234.

Lehmkuhle, S. W., and Fox, R. (1975). Effect of binocular rivalry suppression on the motion aftereffect. *Vision Research*, 15, 855–859.

Lejeune, A. (1956). *L'Optique de Claude Ptolémée dans la version Latine d'après l'Arabe de l'Émir Eugène de Sicile*. Louvain: Université de Louvain.

Leopold, D. A., and Logothetis, N. K. (1996). Activity changes in early visual cortex reflect monkeys' percepts during binocular rivalry. *Nature*, 379, 549–553.

Logothetis, N. K., Leopold, D. A., and Sheinberg, D. L. (1996). What is rivalling during binocular rivalry? *Nature*, 380, 621–624.

Logothetis, N. K., and Schall, J. D. (1989). Neuronal correlates of subjective visual perception. *Science*, 245, 761–763.

Löwel, S., and Singer, W. (1992). Selection of intrinsic horizontal connections in the visual cortex by correlated neuronal activity. *Science*, 255, 209–212.

Malach, R., Reppas, J. B., Kwong, K. K., Jiang, H., Kennedy, W. A., Ledden, P. J., Brady, T. J., Rosen, B. R., and Tootell, R. B. H. (1995). Object-related activity revealed by functional magnetic resonance imaging in human occipital cortex. *Proceedings of the National Academy of Sciences of the United States of America*, 92, 8135–8138.

Movshon, J. A., Adelson, E. H., Gizzi, M. S., and Newsome, W. T. (1985). The analysis of moving visual patterns. In *Pattern. Recognition Mechanisms*, C. Chagas, R. Gattass, and C. Gross, eds., 117–151. New York: Springer-Verlag.

Necker, L. A. (1832). Observations on some remarkable phenomena seen in Switzerland; and an optical phenomenon which occurs on viewing a figure of a crystal or geometrical solid. *London and Edinburgh Philosophical Magazine and Journal of Science*, 1, 329–337.

Nicoll, A., and Blakemore, C. (1993). Patterns of local connectivity in the neocortex. *Neural Computation*, 5, 665–680.

O'Craven, K. M., Downing, P. E., and Kanwisher, N. (1999). FMRI evidence for objects as the units of attentional selection. *Nature*, 401, 584–587.

Perrett, D. I., Smith, P. A. J., Potter, D. D., Mistlin, A. J., Head, A. S., Milner, A. D., and Jeeves, M. A. (1985). Visual cells in the temporal cortex sensitive to face view and gaze direction. *Proceedings of the Royal Society of London,* B223, 293–317.

Polonsky, A., Blake, R., Braun, J., and Heeger, D. J. (2000). Neuronal activity in human primary visual cortex correlates with perception during binocular rivalry. *Nature Neuroscience,* 3, 1153–1159.

Purves, D., and Andrews, T. J. (1997). The perception of transparent three-dimensional objects. *Proceedings of the National Academy of Sciences of the United States of America,* 94, 6517–6522.

Rockland, K. S., and Lund, J. S. (1982). Widespread periodic intrinsic connections in the tree shrew visual cortex. *Science,* 215, 1532–1534.

Rubin, E. (1915). *Synsoplevede Figurer.* Copenhagen: Gyldenalske.

Sengpiel, F., Baddeley, R. J., Freeman, T. C. B., Harrad, R., and Blakemore, C. (1998). Different mechanisms underlie three inhibitory phenomena in cat area 17. *Vision Research,* 38, 2067–2080.

Sengpiel, F., and Blakemore, C. (1994). Interocular control of neuronal responsiveness in cat visual cortex. *Nature,* 368, 847–850.

Sengpiel, F., and Blakemore, C. (1996). The neural basis of suppression and amblyopia in strabismus. *Eye,* 10, 250–258.

Sengpiel, F., Blakemore, C., and Harrad, R. (1995). Interocular suppression in the primary visual cortex: A possible neural basis of binocular rivalry. *Vision Research,* 35, 179–195.

Sengpiel, F., Blakemore, C., Kind, P. C., and Harrad, R. (1994). Interocular suppression in the visual cortex of strabismic cats. *Journal of Neuroscience,* 14, 6855–6871.

Sengpiel, F., Freeman, T. C. B., and Blakemore, C. (1995). Interocular suppression in cat striate cortex is not orientation selective. *NeuroReport,* 6, 2235–2239.

Sengpiel, F., Freeman, T. C. B., Bonhoeffer, T., and Blakemore, C. (2001). On the relationship between interocular suppression in the primary visual cortex and binocular rivalry. *Brain & Mind,* 2, 39–54.

Sheinberg, D. L., and Logothetis, N. K. (1997). The role of temporal cortical areas in perceptual organization. *Proceedings of the National Academy of Sciences of the United States of America,* 94, 3408–3413.

Somogyi, P., Kisvárday, Z. F., Martin, K. A. C., and Whitteridge, D. (1983). Synaptic connections of morphologically identified and physiologically characterized large basket cells in the striate cortex of the cat. *Neuroscience,* 10, 261–294.

Stoner, G. R., Albright, T. D., and Ramachandran, V. S. (1990). Transparency and coherence in human motion perception. *Nature,* 344, 153–155.

Tarr, M. J., and Gauthier, I. (2000). FFA: A flexible fusiform area for subordinate visual processing automatized by expertise. *Nature Neuroscience,* 3, 764–769.

Tong, F., and Engel, S. A. (2001). Interocular rivalry revealed in the human cortical blind-spot representation. *Nature*, 411, 195–199.

Tong, F., Nakayama, K., Vaughan, J. T., and Kanwisher, N. (1998). Binocular rivalry and visual awareness in human extrastriate cortex. *Neuron*, 21, 753–759.

Ts'o, D. Y., Gilbert, C. D., and Wiesel, T. N. (1986). Relationships between horizontal connections and functional architecture in cat striate cortex as revealed by cross-correlation analysis. *Journal of Neuroscience*, 6, 1160–1170.

Wade, N. J. (1998). *A Natural History of Vision*. Cambridge, Mass.: MIT Press.

Wales, R., and Fox, R. (1970). Increment detection thresholds during binocular rivalry suppression. *Perception and Psychophysics*, 8, 90–94.

Wallach, H. (1976). *On Perception*. New York: Quadrangle.

Wheatstone, C. (1838). Contributions to the physiology of vision.—Part the first: On some remarkable, and hitherto unobserved, phenomena of binocular vision. *Philosophical Transactions of the Royal Society of London*, B128, 371–394.

Wiesenfelder, H., and Blake, R. (1991). Apparent motion can survive binocular rivalry suppression. *Vision Research*, 31, 1589–1599.

Wolfe, J. M. (1984). Reversing ocular dominance and suppression in a single flash. *Vision Research*, 24, 471–478.

# 12 Responses of Single Neurons in the Human Brain During Flash Suppression

## Gabriel Kreiman, Itzhak Fried, and Christof Koch

### SINGLE NEURON RECORDINGS IN THE HUMAN BRAIN TO EXPLORE CONSCIOUS VISION

Patterns of visual information imaged on the two retinas are transformed into perceptual experiences through multiple hierarchical stages of neuronal processing. A large body of electrophysiological recordings has been concerned with correlating the neuronal responses with the visual input. However, psychophysical investigations have shown that our percepts can be dissociated from the incoming visual signal. The mechanisms of neuronal coding for conscious perception, as well as the whereabouts of the representation of percepts along the visual pathway, remain unclear. Assuming a hierarchical structure for the visual system (Felleman and Van Essen, 1991), the neuronal responses in early visual areas may reflect the incoming visual input, while the activity in at least some higher parts of cortex may strongly correlate with the subjective perceptual experience.

We took a unique opportunity to record the firing responses of neurons in the human brain and the relation of those responses to perception. Subjects were patients with pharmacologically intractable epilepsy who were implanted with depth electrodes to localize the seizure onset focus (Fried et al., 1999; Kreiman, Koch, and Fried, 2000a,b). The location and the number of recording electrodes were based exclusively on clinical criteria. The electrodes were implanted during surgery and could not be moved by the investigator until they were removed. Patients typically stayed in the hospital for approximately a week.[1]

A schematic representation of the electrodes we used is shown in figure 12.1A. Through the lumen of the electrodes, eight platinum/iridium microwires were inserted (Fried et al., 1999; Kreiman, 2002). The location of the electrodes was verified by structural magnetic resonance images

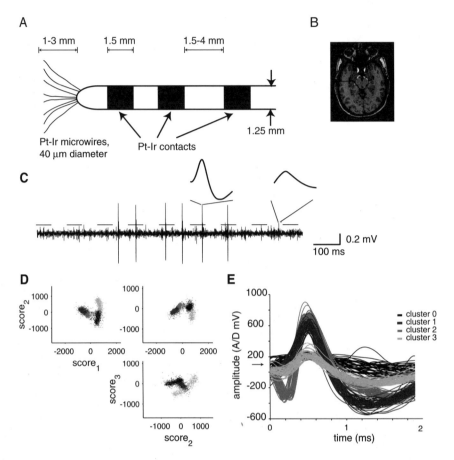

**Figure 12.1** Schematic of electrodes, sample of signals and waveforms. (*A*) Schematic of the type of electrode that was used (Fried et al., 1999; Kreiman, 2002). Broadband activity was monitored 24 hr per day from the platinum–iridium contacts along the electrode for clinical purposes. Single-unit data were acquired through the eight microwires. (*B*) Magnetic resonance image (1.5 tesla) showing the position of one electrode in the hippocampus. (*C*) Sample extracellular data obtained from one of the microwires after filtering and amplification. The activity of multiple units can be discriminated from the noise in extracellular recordings. (*D*) Spike sorting to isolated individual neurons was performed by separating the clusters in two-dimensional plots of several features of the waveforms. Here we illustrate only a subset of these features that includes the first three principal components of the data. Distinct gray tones correspond to different clusters. (*E*) Sample of the waveforms after spike sorting. Each cluster is shown as a separate gray tone.

G. Kreiman, I. Fried, and C. Koch

obtained before removing the electrodes and postoperatively (figure 12.1B and Fried, MacDonald, and Wilson, 1997; Kreiman, Koch, and Fried, 2000a,b). A sample of the data thus obtained is shown in figure 12.1C. Electrophysiological data were amplified, high-pass filtered (with a corner frequency of 300 Hz and digitally stored for off-line processing (Datawave, Denver, Colorado).

Individual neurons were discriminated from the extracellular recordings based on the height, width, and principal components of the waveforms (Datawave, Denver, Colorado), as shown in figure 12.1D–E.[2] In those microwires with neuronal recordings (a small fraction of the total as described in Kreiman (2002), we observed an average of 1.72 units per microwire. The information recorded from the depth electrodes during seizures was used to localize the seizure focus (Ojemann, 1997). While we should note that all the data come from epileptic patients, more than 80% of the recorded neurons were outside the areas of seizure focus. We did not observe any overall differences when comparing units within and outside the seizure onset focus in terms of their firing rates, visual selectivity, or waveform shape.

We investigated the extent to which the spiking activity from single neurons in the amygdala, hippocampus, entorhinal cortex, and parahippocampal gyrus of untrained subjects reflects retinal input versus perceptual experience. We observed that the activity of two-thirds of all visually selective neurons was tightly correlated with the perceptual alternations rather than the retinal input.

## FLASH SUPPRESSION PHENOMENON

Flash suppression constitutes a compelling phenomenon in which the same retinal inputs can give rise to distinct perceptual experiences (Sheinberg and Logothetis, 1997; Wolfe, 1984). It was originally described by Wolfe (1984) and was inspired by binocular rivalry. Flash suppression entails the perceptual suppression of a monocular image following the sudden onset of a different stimulus to the opposite eye (figure 12.2). Although two distinct images are presented to the left and right eyes during the "flash," subjects see only the flashed, novel stimulus. Such a dissociation provides an entry point for studying the neuronal correlates of visual consciousness (Blake and Logothetis, 2002; Crick and Koch, 1998; Logothetis, 1998; Myerson, Miezin, and Allman, 1981). The new stimulus is clearly and consistently observed, suppressing the stimulus previously shown monocularly (figure 12.2). It is important to emphasize that the same visual input

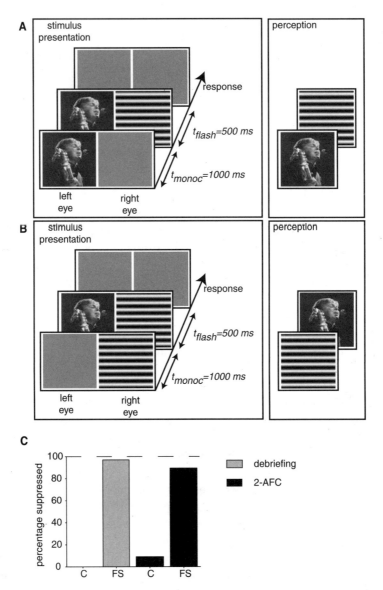

**Figure 12.2** Flash suppression phenomenon. (*A*) Flash suppression consists of the perceptual suppression of an image, previously shown monocularly, upon flashing a new stimulus to the contralateral eye. The left panel shows the stimulus presentation, and the right panel depicts the subjective perceptual report. In this example, a photograph of Paul McCartney was shown monocularly for 1000 msec, after which a horizontal grating was flashed onto the opposite eye for 500 msec while the same picture was shown to the original eye. Subjects were instructed to report their percept in a two-alternative, forced-choice manner after the disappearance of the flash. (*B*) Flash suppression test depicting the complementary condition to that in (*A*). During the flash period, the stimuli presented to the two eyes were the same as in (*A*). However, the subjective percept was exactly the opposite. (*C*) Percentage of suppression based on the 2AFC report (black bars) or debriefing (gray bars) for the flash suppression trials (FS) and the control trials (C).

can give rise to very different percepts, as can be seen by comparing figures 12.2A and 12.2B. In this example, during the flash period a photograph of Paul McCartney is shown to the left eye while a grating is presented to the right eye. Yet, depending on which image was already present monocularly, the subject reports seeing only Paul McCartney or only the grating during the flash.

Flash suppression is quite robust to several changes in the stimulation parameters. The monocular presentation time, $t_{monoc}$, can vary widely, and the effect is very strong for durations above 200 msec. A possible mechanism of suppression would be that the sudden change in stimulation to one eye could bias the competition between the two percepts due to a shift in attentional focus or to a motion/change signal. However, the effect can be observed after introducing a blank interstimulus interval (ISI) between the monocular and flash presentations. The suppression effect remains equally strong for ISIs less than 200 msec. A strong disruption (where subjects typically report observing a mixture of the two stimuli) is evident for ISIs longer than 500 msec. The flash duration, $t_{flash}$, can be as short as 10 msec. A long flash duration produces binocular rivalry (the contralateral stimulus is observed first and then alternation between the two stimuli takes place).

It seems unlikely that flash suppression can be explained as a form of forward masking or light adaptation because the luminance properties of the monocular stimulus do not affect the suppression and because the effect is invariant with parameter changes (Kreiman and Koch, 1999; Wolfe, 1984). A more recent version of flash suppression shows that the phenomenon can be generalized to elicit suppression in the absence of interocular conflict (Wilke, Leopold, and Logothetis, 2002).

Since the onset of perceptual transition is externally controlled, flash suppression allows finer temporal control and collection of more transitions than does binocular rivalry, in which fluctuations in perception are spontaneous and, therefore, unpredictable. Given the time constraints of the clinical environment, we focused on flash suppression. It seems legitimate, however, to ask whether the mechanisms of flash suppression coincide with those of binocular rivalry. At a global level, both binocular rivalry and flash suppression involve a competition between two alternative images. In both cases, the same visual input can give rise to two different percepts. One key difference is that the transitions are externally triggered in flash suppression, rather than internally induced as in rivalry. However, it is interesting to note that the minimum duration of $t_{monoc}$ coincides with the amount of time required to elicit binocular rivalry upon flashing different stimuli to the two eyes (Wolfe, 1984). Furthermore, the neuronal responses in the inferotemporal cortex visual area of the macaque brain during both phenomena are very similar (Sheinberg and Logothetis, 1997).

## NEURONAL ACTIVITY IN THE HUMAN BRAIN DURING FLASH SUPPRESSION

### Neurons That Followed the Percept

We recorded the activity of 428 single units in the human medial temporal lobe (MTL) while subjects reported their percept during flash suppression. The MTL typically constitutes one of the potential areas suspected to be part of the seizure onset focus. It receives direct input from the inferior temporal cortex, the highest purely visual area (Felleman and Van Essen, 1991; Suzuki, 1996; Cheng, Saleem, and Tanaka, 1997; Saleem and Tanaka, 1996), as well as from olfactory and auditory portions of the nervous system (Kandel, Schwartz, and Jessell, 2000). The MTL plays a prominent role in several explicit memory processes, including the storage and retrieval of information (Eichenbaum, 1997; Squire and Zola-Morgan, 1991; Zola-Morgan and Squire, 1993).

Of the 428 MTL neurons, 172 units were in the amygdala, 98 in the hippocampus, 130 in the entorhinal cortex, and 28 in the parahippocampal gyrus. The data reported here come from 14 patients (10 right-handed, 9 male, 24 to 48 years old).

Images were chosen from natural categories of stimuli and included faces of unknown actors portraying emotional expressions (Ekman, 1976), spatial layouts, famous people, animals, and abstract patterns (Kreiman, Koch, and Fried, 2000a). The two pictures in each flash-suppression trial were constrained to belong to different categories. Stimuli subtended a visual angle of approximately 3° and were presented separately to the right and left eyes by means of a pair of liquid crystal glasses that transmit light to one eye or the other in interlaced fashion (Crystal Eyes Stereographics, San Rafael, California).

Subjects were instructed to report their percept by pressing one button to indicate that the original image changed into a different picture or another button to indicate that it did not (and by verbal debriefing in 10% of trials). In approximately 10% of the trials, we presented only the monocularly shown image and a blank screen to the other eye during the flash as a control. The monocular stimulus was randomly delivered to either the

G. Kreiman, I. Fried, and C. Koch

left or the right eye. The suppression phenomenon is very strong, as is illustrated by the behavioral results in figure 12.2C.

The responses of a neuron located in the right amygdala showed a striking pattern of selectivity (figure 12.3A). This unit showed increased firing rate upon presentation of a black-and-white drawing of Curly, one of the characters of a well-known American TV comedy. On average, the unit changed its spiking activity from a rate of 1.7 spikes/sec during the baseline period to 7.9 spikes/sec (two-tailed t test, $p < 10^{-3}$). The neuron did not change its firing rate in response to other faces or to other black-and-white drawings. (We are not claiming that this is the only possible stimulus to which the neuron would respond—it simply was the only stimulus in our set of 47 pictures that enhanced its activity.) Other neurons changed their firing rates in response to more than one stimulus; still other neurons were broadly tuned, enhancing their activity upon presentation of several different pictures from one of the presented categories of stimuli (Kreiman, 2002; Kreiman, Koch, and Fried, 2000a).

Upon dichoptic presentation of the drawing of Curly, the neuronal response showed a strong dependence on perceptual state. When the picture of Curly was presented monocularly and an ineffective stimulus[3] perceptually suppressed the image of Curly during the flash, the neuron did not enhance its firing above background (figure 12.3B, left). However, when a different image was presented monocularly and the subject was presented with Curly as the flashed stimulus, the neuron showed a strong and transient response (figure 12.3B, right). The response during the flash, in other words, was similar to the response during the monocular presentation only when the subject reported seeing the preferred stimulus.

Figure 12.4 shows a summary of the responses of 12 neurons that responded selectively to one or a few individual images from our stimulus set.[4] These units showed a marked enhancement in firing rate in response to the monocular presentation of the stimulus (figure 12.4A); they did not respond beyond baseline during the binocular period when the effective stimulus was perceptually suppressed (figure 12.4A); and, finally, they showed a strong enhancement in their firing rate during the dichoptic period when the effective stimulus was consciously perceived (figure 12.4B).

Approximately 12% (a total of 51 units) of the recorded neurons showed visual selectivity with enough stimulus repetitions for analysis[5] during both the monocular presentation and the flash period. The majority (69%) of these neurons followed the perceptual report of the subjects. In other words, these neurons showed enhanced firing upon presentation of the

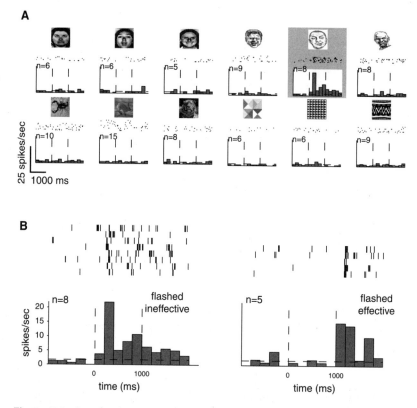

**Figure 12.3** Sample of neuronal responses. (*A*) Visual selectivity of a neuron in the right amygdala. Raster plots and post-stimulus time histograms are aligned to stimulus onset of the neuronal responses to a subsample of 12 pictures out of 47 presented pictures (Kreiman, 2002). The neuron enhanced its firing rate only upon presentation of the face of the comedian Curly, shown within a gray-shaded box. The horizontal dashed line shows the overall mean firing rate of this unit (1.7 Hz). Some of the stimuli were in color but are shown here in black and white. The number of presentations is indicated in the upper left corner of each histogram. Bin size: 200 msec. (*B*) Responses of the neuron during the flash-suppression test to the image of Curly. The format is the same as in (*A*). On the left, the neuronal responses were aligned to the onset of the monocular presentation of Curly (indicated by the first vertical dashed line). An ineffective stimulus was flashed (at the time indicated by the second vertical dashed line) and perceptually suppressed the image of Curly. On the right, an ineffective stimulus was shown monocularly. The image of Curly was flashed, and perceptually suppressed the ineffective stimulus.

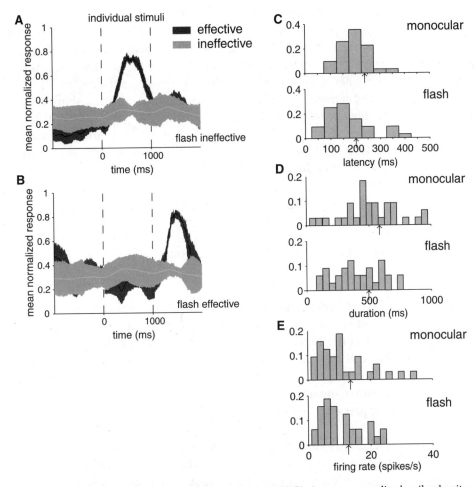

**Figure 12.4** Summary of neuronal responses. (*A–B*) Average normalized spike-density function obtained by convolving the spike train with a fixed Gaussian of 200 msec and dividing by the peak activity (n = 12 neurons selective to individual stimuli). (*A*) The dark gray trace corresponds to the responses aligned to the time of presentation of the monocular preferred stimulus; the light gray corresponds to the responses to all other stimuli. (*B*) The dark gray trace corresponds to the responses aligned to the onset of the flash of the preferred stimulus after a different stimulus had been presented monocularly; the light gray trace identifies all other presentations. The width of the shaded regions corresponds to 95% confidence intervals. The vertical dashed lines denote the monocular onset and the flash onset, respectively. (*C*) Distribution of response latencies during the monocular (top) and flash (bottom) presentations (n = 35 neurons). Bin size: 50 msec. (*D*) Distribution of response durations during the monocular and flash presentations. Bin size: 50 msec. (*E*) Distribution of the magnitude of the response during the monocular and flash presentations. Bin size: 2 spikes/sec.

preferred stimulus during the flash if and only if the image was consciously perceived. We observed neurons that followed the percept in all four areas of the MTL. Given the low number of neurons, it is difficult to draw any conclusion about possible distinctions across regions (the number of neurons that followed the percept ranged from 2 to 18).

The remaining third of the selective units did not show a statistically significant response during the flash period, regardless of the subject's percept (that is, in the presence of the two conflicting stimuli). It is unlikely that the lack of response of these neurons is due to the shorter presentation during the flash, given that the latencies of neurons in the MTL seem to be much shorter than $t_{flash} = 500$ ms (Kreiman, Koch, and Fried, 2000a). These neurons that did not respond during the flash showed only a weak response during the monocular presentation. It is possible that this weak response was not strong enough to be detected during the flash period. Alternatively, the conflicting presentation of two stimuli perhaps inhibited the response.

Importantly, we did not observe any neuron that responded when the preferred stimulus was not consciously perceived. Even though the preferred stimulus was physically present during the flash period, the neurons in the human MTL were oblivious to it unless the subject actually perceived the stimulus.

## Comparison of Neuronal Responses Between Perception and Suppression Phases

We directly compared the responses for those neurons which followed the percept during the two states in which the effective stimuli were subjectively perceived (i.e., when presented monocularly without contralateral stimulation and when presented and seen together with a contralateral stimulus). There was no significant difference in the distribution of the response latencies (figure 12.4C; two-tailed t-test, $p > 0.15$), durations (figure 12.4D, $p > 0.3$), or magnitudes evaluated by the total number of spikes (figure 12.4E, $p > 0.1$).[6] Therefore, in spite of the fact that there is a completely different stimulus present on one retina during the dichoptic period, the neuronal responses of these cells are very similar to those when the effective stimulus is presented monocularly. This supports the view that the neurons in the MTL primarily represent the percept rather than the visual input per se.

Given that the dichoptic period followed a monocular presentation, it is reasonable to ask whether the absence of response to the suppressed

G. Kreiman, I. Fried, and C. Koch

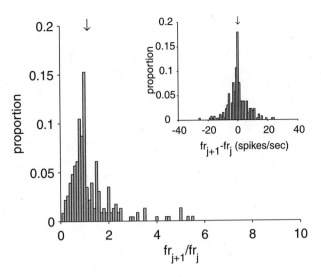

**Figure 12.5** Lack of change in response to consecutive presentation of the preferred stimuli. Distribution of the change in firing rate for consecutive presentations of preferred stimuli. For this figure we pooled data from several different experiments (Kreiman, Fried, and Koch, 2002; Kreiman, Koch, and Fried, 2000a, 2000b; n = 104 neurons). The main plot shows the ratio of firing rate in one presentation against that in the previous presentation (mean ratio = 1.23 ± 1.55, median ratio = 0.94). Bin size = 0.1 (only points with non-null firing rates were included here). The inset shows the difference in firing rates (all points included here; mean difference = −0.07 ± 4.84 spikes/sec). Bin size: 1 spike/sec.

stimulus is a consequence of adaptation of the neuronal response or a lack of response to consecutive presentations of the same preferred stimulus. To address this question, we pooled the neuronal responses from our entire data set (including previous experiments reported by Kreiman, Koch, and Fried, 2000a,b) and reanalyzed all the trials in which the preferred stimulus was presented in two consecutive trials. We did not observe any overall trend indicative of a reduction (or an enhancement) in the neuronal response (figure 12.5).[7]

**Correlation Between Neuronal Response and Percept**

How strong is the correlation between the single-neuron response and the percept? To learn the answer, we analyzed whether it was possible to predict the subject's percept based on the neuronal response. We performed an ROC signal detection analysis (Green and Swets, 1966) based on the spike counts at the single-trial level. This analysis yields a probability of

Responses of Single Neurons During Flash Suppression

misclassification of the neuron's preferred stimulus, $p_e$, ranging from 0 for perfect prediction to 0.5 for chance levels (since there are two possible choices). Figure 12.6A–B shows how $p_e$ decreases with increasing time windows used to compute the spike counts. The probability of misclassification during the monocular presentation was very similar to that during the flash period when the preferred stimulus was perceived. In contrast, when the preferred stimulus was perceptually suppressed, the performance of this classifier was basically at chance levels.

The number of errors of the classifier was quite high for integration windows of less than 200 msec at the level of single neurons. In order to attempt to extrapolate these results to how well small ensembles of neurons could reflect the subject's percept, we trained a support vector machine (SVM) (Vapnik, 1995) to classify the data into "perceived" and "not perceived" categories based on increasingly larger numbers of independent neurons.[8]

Figure 12.6C shows how the error rate decreased with increasing time windows and number of units. The gain in performance after offset of the flash (500 to 1000 msec after flash onset) is due to the continued response of some neurons beyond the disappearance of the stimuli. It is interesting to observe a slight saturation effect, whereby the increase in performance of the classifier decreases with time, indicating that quite accurate characterization of the percept can be obtained by analyzing 500 msec after flash onset. It should be noted that there are several assumptions here, including the independence of neuronal responses. It is conceivable that interactions such as synchronous firing could enhance even further the correlation with the percept for small ensembles of neurons.

## IN SEARCH OF THE NEURONAL REPRESENTATION OF THE PERCEPT

Models describing the perception of bistable images often propose a competition between distinct neuronal populations tuned to alternative representations of the external world (see chapters 3, 17, and 18 in this volume). Subjectively, one perceives the end result of this competition with one stimulus predominating over the other except during transition states or piecemeal states. Flash suppression constitutes a particularly strong variant where the transition duration is minimal (in most cases too brief to be noticed).

Our results suggest that the spiking activity of most of the visually selective neurons which we recorded in the medial temporal lobe

G. Kreiman, I. Fried, and C. Koch

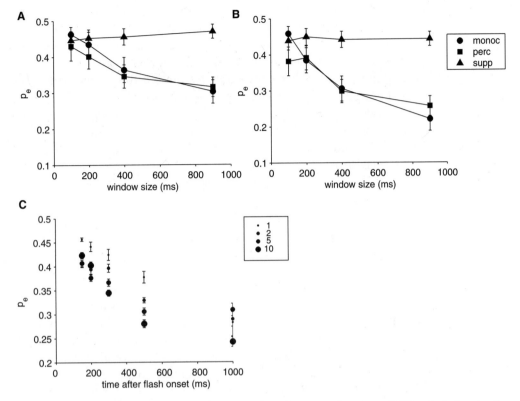

**Figure 12.6** Estimating the percept from the neuronal response. ROC analysis showing the probability of misclassifying the subject's perceptual report ($p_e$, $0 \leq p_e \leq 0.5$), based on the spike counts in different time windows. (*A*) 23 neurons broadly tuned to categories of natural stimuli. (*B*) 12 neurons selective to individual images. The time window starts 100 msec after stimulus or flash onset (circles: monocular stimulus; squares/triangles: perceived flash period and suppressed flash period, respectively). (*C*) Classification of the subject's perceptual report using a linear SVM (Vapnik, 1995) after pooling different numbers of broadly tuned, independently firing neurons. We used the implementation of SVM classifiers by Rifkin (2000) with the following parameters: linear cost per unit violation of the margin = 2; tolerance for the Karush–Kuhn–Tucker conditions = $10^{-4}$ (see Vapnik, 1995); equal weights for false alarms and miss errors; linear kernel with normalizer = 1. The x-axis denotes the time from onset of the flash.

In all cases, the data were split evenly and randomly between training and test sets (we tested leave-one-out cross validation in a random subset of 20% of the cases, and this yielded similar results). The normalized spike density function of each neuron was computed by convolving the spike train with a fixed-width Gaussian of 100 msec and dividing by the peak response. The normalized neuronal responses during the flash period of 1, 2, 5, or 10 neurons integrated over the indicated time windows were used as input to an SVM classifier with a linear kernel to discriminate between those trials in which subjects reported perceiving the preferred stimulus or the nonpreferred stimulus. The size of the marker indicates the number of neurons. For n = 1, we averaged over 20 possible selections of neurons. For n = 2, 5, and 10, we averaged over 50 random combinations of *n* neurons. As discussed in the text, it should be noted that there are many strong assumptions underlying this computation, including that the firing rates of these neurons are independent.

correlates well, at the single-trial level, with the visual conscious experience of the subject. These results parallel the observations made in the higher stages of the macaque visual system (Sheinberg and Logothetis, 1997). Similar to the data in the monkey inferior temporal cortex, we do not find any evidence for neurons that represent the perceptually suppressed image (i.e., the unconscious image) in the MTL.

While our data reflect the end result of the conflict between alternative percepts, they do not address the issue of where and how the competition is resolved. There is a strong projection from the inferior temporal cortex to the MTL structures in monkeys (Cheng, Saleem, and Tanaka, 1997; Logothetis and Sheinberg, 1996; Saleem and Tanaka, 1996; Suzuki, 1996; Tanaka, 1996); however, the detailed neuroanatomy is largely unknown in humans. Functional imaging, as well as neurological data, suggests a possible involvement of frontal areas during internally driven perceptual transitions (Lumer, Friston, and Rees, 1998; Ricci and Blundo, 1990).

Single-neuron studies in earlier visual areas of the macaque monkey reveal that a progressively higher proportion of neurons correlates with the subjective percept as one ascends the visual hierarchy from the LGN to V1 to V4/MT (Lehky and Maunsell, 1996; Leopold and Logothetis, 1996; Logothetis and Schall, 1989). (For a review, see Leopold and Logothetis, 1999). In higher areas, functional imaging also shows a correlation between BOLD measures of activation and perception (Tong et al., 1998).

Interestingly, in earlier visual areas, some neurons showed a response that was anticorrelated with the percept. This type of response was absent in monkey IT cortex as well as in our MTL recordings. Functional imaging shows that activity in V1 may correlate with the percept in binocular rivalry (Polonsky et al., 2000; Tong and Engel, 2001; Tononi et al., 1998). However, since the biophysical basis of the BOLD signal is not yet understood, great care should be exercised in identifying an increase in BOLD with an increase in firing frequency of neurons (Logothetis et al., 2001).

It has been suggested that overtraining in monkeys may influence the neuronal responses studied during binocular rivalry (Tononi et al., 1998). While it is known that training can modify the pattern of dominance during binocular rivalry (Leopold and Logothetis, 1999), our data show that strong neuronal modulation based on the percept can be found in naïve observers. It is plausible that the neuronal correlate of the percept is transferred from IT to MTL, where it might be involved in declarative memory storage processes (Eichenbaum, 1997; Kreiman, Koch, and Fried, 2000a; Rolls, 2000; Zola-Morgan and Squire, 1993). The proportion of

G. Kreiman, I. Fried, and C. Koch

human MTL neurons following the percept is smaller than the values reported for monkey IT cells (Sheinberg and Logothetis, 1997).

These differences could simply be due to the different criteria used to determine neuronal selectivity. They could also be due to differences between species. On the other hand, it is possible that the number of neurons which underlie and generate conscious visual perception peaks in intermediate areas of the brain, such as inferior temporal cortex, and is lower in medial temporal or prefrontal lobe structures (Crick and Koch, 2000; Jackendoff, 1987).

## ACKNOWLEDGMENTS

We would like to thank Geraint Rees, Nikos Logothetis, and John Allman for advice throughout this work; all patients for their participation; Ryan Rifkin for support with the SVM analysis; and Eve Isham, Charles Wilson, Tony Fields, and Eric Behnke for help with the recordings. This work was supported by grants from NIMH, NINDS, NSF, the Mettler Fund for Research Relating to Autism, the McDonnell-Pew Program in Cognitive Neuroscience, the W. M. Keck Foundation Fund for Discovery in Basic Medical Research, and a Whiteman Fellowship to GK. Parts of this chapter were described previously (Kreiman, 2002; Kreiman, Fried, and Koch, 2002).

## NOTES

1. All the experiments described here were conducted in the hospital. The studies conformed to the guidelines of the Medical Institutional Review Board at UCLA and were performed with the written consent of the subjects.

2. Similar results were obtained with a custom, semiautomatic spike-sorting algorithm based on a Bayesian approach (Kreiman, 2002).

3. A stimulus that did not cause a change in firing rate in this amygdala cell.

4. The same conclusions apply to 23 other neurons with broad selective responses (see Kreiman, Fried, and Koch, 2002, and figure 12.6A).

5. As we have reported previously, the majority of recorded neurons did not show visual selectivity. A possible reason for this observation is that many of these units may be nonvisual neurons. However, given that we presented only a small number of stimuli in a relatively short period of time, it is possible that in many cases we simply failed to find a visual stimulus that drove the cell.

6. In contrast, the responses to the effective stimulus when it was suppressed and when it was dominant were virtually independent, with a correlation coefficient of just 0.08.

7. It should be noted that in all these cases, the second presentation occurred at least 1000 msec after the first presentation and there was a behavioral response (button press) in between. In the present experiment, the flash period immediately followed the monocular presentation and there was no response in between these two periods.

8. For this purpose, we estimated the spike density function for each neuron and normalized it to the neuron's peak response (figure 12.4). The input to the SVM classifier with a linear kernel was the normalized neuronal response integrated over different time windows (figure 12.6C). The class for each entry was based on the subject's perceptual report. This analysis was restricted to the 23 broadly tuned neurons due to the very small number of repetitions available for training from the neurons selective to individual stimuli.

## REFERENCES

Blake, R., and Logothetis, N. K. (2002). Visual competition. *Nature Reviews: Neuroscience. 3*, 13–21.

Cheng, K., Saleem, K. S., and Tanaka, K. (1997). Organization of corticostriatal and corticoamygdalar projections arising from the anterior inferotemporal area TE of the macaque monkey: A *Phaseolus vulgaris* leucoagglutinin study. *Journal of Neuroscience, 17*, 7902–7925.

Crick, F., and Koch, C. (1998). Consciousness and neuroscience. *Cerebral Cortex, 8*, 97–107.

Crick, F., and Koch, C. (2000). The unconscious homunculus. *Neuro-Psychoanalysis 2*, 3–59.

Eichenbaum, H. (1997). How does the brain organize memories? *Science, 277*, 330–332.

Ekman, P. (1976). *Pictures of Facial Affect.* Palo Alto, Calif.: Consulting Psychologists Press.

Felleman, D. J., and Van Essen, D. C. (1991). Distributed hierarchical processing in the primate cerebral cortex. *Cerebral Cortex, 1*, 1–47.

Fried, I., MacDonald, K. A., and Wilson, C. (1997). Single neuron activity in human hippocampus and amygdala during recognition of faces and objects. *Neuron, 18*, 753–765.

Fried, I., Wilson, C. L., Maidment, N. T., Engel, J., Behnke, E., Fields, T. A., MacDonald, K. A., Morrow, J. M., and Ackerson, L. (1999). Cerebral microdialysis combined with single-neuron and electroencephalographic recording in neurosurgical patients. *Journal of Neurosurgery, 91*, 697–705.

Green, D., and Swets, J. (1966). *Signal Detection Theory and Psychophysics.* New York: Wiley.

Jackendoff, R. (1987). *Consciousness and the Computational Mind.* Cambridge, Mass.: MIT Press.

Kandel, E., Schwartz, J., and Jessell, T. (2000). *Principles of Neural Science,* 4th ed. New York: McGraw-Hill.

Kreiman, G. (2002). On the neuronal activity in the human brain during visual recognition, imagery and binocular rivalry. Ph.D. Thesis, California Institute of Technology.

Kreiman, G., Fried, I., and Koch, C. (2002). Single-neuron correlates of subjective vision in the human medial temporal lobe. *Proceedings of the National Academy of Sciences of the United States of America, 99*, 8378–8383.

Kreiman, G., and Koch, C. (1999). Flash suppression: Competition between eyes or patterns? *Investigative Opthalmology and Visual Science.* 40, S421.

Kreiman, G., Koch, C., and Fried, I. (2000a). Category-specific visual responses of single neurons in the human medial temporal lobe. *Nature Neuroscience,* 3, 946–953.

Kreiman, G., Koch, C., and Fried, I. (2000b). Imagery neurons in the human brain. *Nature,* 408, 357–361.

Lehky, S. R., and Maunsell, J. H. R. (1996). No binocular rivalry in the LGN of alert monkeys. *Vision Research,* 36, 1225–1234.

Leopold, D. A., and Logothetis, N. K. (1996). Activity changes in early visual cortex reflect monkeys' percepts during binocular rivalry. *Nature,* 379, 549–553.

Leopold, D. A., and Logothetis, N. K. (1999). Multistable phenomena: Changing views in perception. *Trends in Cognitive Sciences,* 3, 254–264.

Logothetis, N. K. (1998). Single units and conscious vision. *Philosophical Transactions of the Royal Society of London,* B353, 1801–1818.

Logothetis, N., Pauls, J., Augath, M., Trinath, T., and Oeltermann, A. (2001). Neurophysiological investigation of the basis of the fMRI signal. *Nature,* 412, 150–157.

Logothetis, N. K., and Schall, J. D. (1989). Neuronal correlates of subjective visual perception. *Science,* 245, 761–763.

Logothetis, N. K., and Sheinberg, D. L. (1996). Visual object recognition. *Annual Review of Neuroscience,* 19, 577–621.

Lumer, E. D., Friston, K. J., and Rees, G. (1998). Neural correlates of perceptual rivalry in the human brain. *Science,* 280, 1930–1934.

Myerson, J., Miezin, F., and Allman, J. (1981). Binocular rivalry in macaque monkeys and humans: A comparative study in perception. *Behavioral Analysis Letters,* 1, 149–159.

Ojemann, G. A. (1997). Treatment of temporal lobe epilepsy. *Annual Review of Medicine,* 48, 317–328.

Polonsky, A., Blake, R., Braun, J., and Heeger, D. J. (2000). Neuronal activity in human primary visual cortex correlates with perception during binocular rivalry. *Nature Neuroscience,* 3, 1153–1159.

Ricci, C., and Blundo, C. (1990). Perception of ambiguous figures after focal brain lesions. *Neuropsychologia,* 28, 1163–1173.

Rifkin, R. (2000). SvmFu. http://www.ai.mit.edu/projects/cbcl/software-datasets/index.html.

Rolls, E. (2000). Memory systems in the brain. *Annual Review of Psychology,* 51, 599–630.

Saleem, K. S., and Tanaka, K. (1996). Divergent projections from the anterior inferotemporal area TE to the perirhinal and entorhinal cortices in the macaque monkey. *Journal of Neuroscience,* 16, 4757–4775.

Sheinberg, D. L., and Logothetis, N. K. (1997). The role of temporal cortical areas in perceptual organization. *Proceedings of the National Academy of Sciences of the United States of America,* 94, 3408–3413.

Squire, L., and Zola-Morgan, S. (1991). The medial temporal-lobe memory system. *Science, 253*, 1380–1386.

Suzuki, W. A. (1996). Neuroanatomy of the monkey entorhinal, perirhinal and parahippocampal cortices: Organization of cortical inputs and interconnections with amygdala and striatum. *Seminars in the Neurosciences, 8*, 3–12.

Tanaka, K. (1996). Inferotemporal cortex and object vision. *Annual Review of Neuroscience, 19*, 109–139.

Tong, F., and Engel, S. A. (2001). Interocular rivalry revealed in the human cortical blind-spot representation. *Nature, 411*, 195–199.

Tong, F., Nakayama, K., Vaughan, J. T., and Kanwisher, N. (1998). Binocular rivalry and visual awareness in human extrastriate cortex. *Neuron, 21*, 753–759.

Tononi, G., Srinivasan, R., Russell, D. P., and Edelman, G. M. (1998). Investigating neural correlates of conscious perception by frequency-tagged neuromagnetic responses. *Proceedings of the National Academy of Sciences of the United States of America, 95*, 3198–3203.

Vapnik, V. (1995). *The Nature of Statistical Learning Theory.* New York: Springer-Verlag.

Wilke, M., Leopold, D., and Logothetis, N. (2002). Flash suppression without interocular conflict. In *Society for Neuroscience Annual Meeting.* Orlando, Fla.: Society for Neuroscience.

Wolfe, J. (1984). Reversing ocular dominance and suppression in a single flash. *Vision Research, 24*, 471–478.

Zola-Morgan, S., and Squire, L. R. (1993). Neuroanatomy of memory. *Annual Review of Neuroscience, 16*, 547–563.

# 13 Binocular Rivalry and the Illusion of Monocular Vision

David A. Leopold, Alexander Maier, Melanie Wilke, and Nikos K. Logothetis

A primate's visual impression of the world is shaped by highly refined cortical mechanisms for registering and interpreting images cast on the retinas. The act of seeing is normally so efficient and effortless that one seldom considers the inherent difficulty in the process. The eyes and brain, presented with a two-dimensional image of light, dark, and color, must extract the structure and spatial relationships of objects from which illuminating light is reflected. In particular, the visual cortex is thought to employ diverse stages of processing that together integrate the detection of sensory motifs in a scene with mechanisms that actively interpret and understand the physical structures from which they arise. Interestingly, among these multiple levels of representation, some of the neural elements critical in securing robust perception are not themselves enlightened as to the ultimate percept.

## AMBIGUITY IN VISION

The problem of local ambiguity in vision is illustrated in figure 13.1, which demonstrates that even a well-posed visual problem is, at some level, composed of many smaller ambiguous ones. An apparently important task in perceptual organization[1] is the disambiguation of local information based upon global and configural properties of a scene, to generate unified perception of shapes and objects (Gregory, 1997; Koffka, 1935; Purves et al., 2001). Local analysis is implemented at many levels of visual processing. For example, a neuron in the primary visual cortex (V1) monitors only a small portion of the world (its receptive field), and responds only if a particular feature is present there. Such neural responses, when considered in isolation, are inherently ambiguous. For example, suboptimal stimulation of a typical V1 cell can be achieved by any number of combinations of

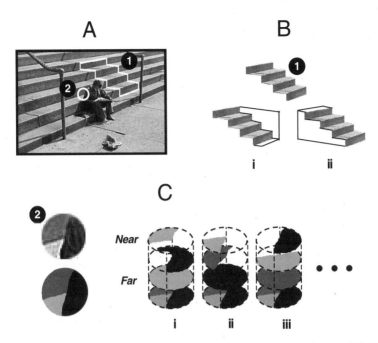

**Figure 13.1** Illustration of local ambiguity present in a natural scene. (*A*) Unambiguous photograph of a boy sitting on steps, with two local regions of the image denoted (1 and 2). (*B*) The extracted portion of the stairway (1), having lost its global context, is ambiguous. The brain alternately interprets this pattern in the configurations indicated by (i) and (ii). (*C*) Small portion of the scene (2), comparable to that monitored by a spatially localized receptive field. The three intersecting texture regions arise from a combination of local 3-D geometry, occlusion, and shading. However, in the absence of global information, the depth-ordering problem is entirely ambiguous. Three of many possible solutions are shown (i, ii and iii). Note that despite the abundance of local ambiguity, the global information ensures that this ambiguity does not reach perceptual awareness.

orientation, contrast, and spatial frequency. Second, even if the neuron's optimal feature is present in the receptive field, it might belong to any of an infinite number of global shapes and objects. The activation of such "feature detectors," while subject to moderate cognitive influences, is generally assumed to be an automatic consequence of the underlying connectivity, and their activity can be demonstrated even when an animal is under general anesthesia.

It is interesting to note that normally visual ambiguity is completely hidden from our perception, because global and redundant information generally ensures the uniqueness of a single, "correct," holistic impression of a scene. Nonetheless, it is relatively simple to create artificial stimuli that are ambiguous for all levels of visual processing and thus do not provide a unique interpretation see figure 13.1B). Confronted with such patterns, our visual impression does something highly uncharacteristic—it begins to waver. The result is a percept that is multistable in nature, adopting a certain configuration for a period, then often abruptly switching to an alternative interpretation. These perceptual alternations are thought to reflect a frequent reevaluation of activity in the visual cortex due to an inherently ambiguous or conflicting visual input. The class of multistable patterns is diverse, involving changes in visibility (Bonneh, Cooperman, and Sagi, 2001; Campbell and Howell, 1972; Levelt, 1965; Pritchard, 1961; Troxler, 1804), perceived depth (Necker, 1832; Rubin, 1921), or motion (Schiller, 1933; Wallach and O'Connell, 1953). While opinions regarding the basis of this phenomenon are varied, multistable stimuli have been valuable in the arsenal of tools employed by visual scientists to study interpretive elements of vision (Gregory, 1997; Koffka, 1935; Rock, 1984).

But how do visually responsive neurons in the early cortical areas fare when observing a multistable pattern, such as that shown in figure 13.1B? Are they active participants in the perceptual alternations, with their activity changes driving perception, or do they simply provide an impartial sensory signal upon which higher perceptual mechanisms can draw? A number of recent neurophysiological studies in monkeys using multistable stimuli suggest that the answer to this question may be quite complicated. While some neurons in the early cortical areas clearly modulate their responses according to perception, a larger fraction appears to respond purely on the basis of the physical structure of the stimulus, regardless of the perceptual state (Bradley, Chang, and Andersen, 1998; Dodd et al., 2001; Grunewald, Bradley, and Andersen, 2002; Leopold and Logothetis, 1996; Logothetis and Schall, 1989). In other studies examining the disambiguation of local features by applying different global contexts, neuron responses were similarly divided (Albright and Stoner, 2002; Heider, Meskenaite, and Peterhans, 2000; Lamme, Rodriguez-Rodriguez, and Spekreijse, 1999; Lee et al., 2002; Pack and Born, 2001; Rossi, Rittenhouse, and Paradiso, 1996; Sugita, 1999; Zhou, Friedman, and Von der Heydt, 2000). These and other experiments illustrate the complexity inherent in interpreting the perceptual relevance of signals in the sensory areas. Namely, in most cases of normal vision, activity in the visual cortex appears to consist of a mixture of local sensory processing, global contextual effects, and additional response modulation whose expression is not uniquely defined by the retinal input.

## BINOCULAR RIVALRY

In recent years, the bistable phenomenon of binocular rivalry has been studied extensively, using a variety of psychophysical and physiological techniques (Blake and Logothetis, 2002). As described in previous chapters, rivalry refers to the spontaneous alternation between periods of left- and right-eye dominance that emerges when conflicting stimuli are presented separately to the two eyes. At any point in time, a stimulus in one of the eyes is seen to dominate perception while that in the other eye is completely invisible. Yet this condition is only temporary, since after a few seconds the other eye becomes dominant, and visibility switches to the previously suppressed pattern. Perception during binocular rivalry is so "monocular" in nature that under appropriate conditions, it can be closely approximated by alternate closure of the two eyelids. Experiments testing the generality of rivalry suppression revealed that it was indiscriminate with regard to particular stimulus features, adding support to the notion that the entire eye's input is uniformly blocked (Blake, Westendorf, and Overton, 1980; Fox and Check, 1966a, 1968; Wales and Fox, 1970; but see Smith et al., 1982).

Yet while these observations support the notion of pure monocular vision during rivalry, other psychophysical experiments suggest that information from the perceptually suppressed eye penetrates deep into the cortical processing machinery. For example, in many cases, unperceived stimuli can generate adaptational aftereffects[2] that are of the same strength as continually visible stimuli (Blake and Fox, 1974; Lehmkuhle and Fox, 1975). Furthermore, interocular transfer[3] of such aftereffects is unattenuated during rivalry (Blake and Overton, 1979; O'Shea and Crassini, 1981), while the monocular component of such aftereffects can cause rivalry between monocular stimuli that are identical (Blake et al., 1998).

These results suggest that the mechanisms responsible for binocular rivalry lie at a relatively advanced stage of sensory processing, beyond both monocular and binocular mechanisms responsible for simple adaptational aftereffects. Thus psychophysical experiments have long called into question the intuitive notion that perception during rivalry stems from monocular processing. More recent studies have demonstrated that high-level organizational principles can override interocular alternation (Kovács et al., 1996; Logothetis, Leopold, and Sheinberg, 1996). Although such "stimulus rivalry" occurs only under a restricted set of conditions (Lee and Blake, 1999), it nonetheless presents additional difficulty for rivalry theories rooted in monocular suppression.

David A. Leopold and colleagues

Neurophysiological investigation of the mechanisms of rivalry has suggested that the activity of many neurons, particularly those at the earliest stages of processing, is entirely unaffected by the perceptual state. For example, in the lateral geniculate nucleus (LGN), where monocular signals are segregated, extracellular recordings failed to demonstrate any perception-related modulation during rivalry (Lehky and Maunsell, 1996; Sengpiel, Blakemore, and Harrad, 1995). A similar indifference was displayed by monocular neurons in the primary visual cortex of monkeys reporting their spontaneous perceptual changes (Leopold and Logothetis, 1996). In that study, the activity of a minimal fraction of binocular neurons in areas V1 and V2 correlated directly with the monkey's changing interpretation of the rivalry stimulus. Ascension in the cortical hierarchy revealed an ever-increasing fraction of neurons whose responses were in agreement with perception (Leopold and Logothetis, 1996; Logothetis and Schall, 1989; Sheinberg and Logothetis, 1997; for a review, see Leopold and Logothetis, 1999).

Interestingly, perception-modulated neurons were often neatly interwoven with those whose responses were dictated only by the sensory stimulus. These results suggest that binocular rivalry is not the consequence of a highly specialized mechanism imposed upon incoming monocular information (but see Polonsky et al., 2000; Tong and Engel, 2001). Interestingly, subsequent neurophysiological studies using bistable (structure-from-motion) 3-D object rotation have revealed very similar results (Bradley, Chang, and Andersen, 1998; Dodd et al., 2001; Grunewald, Bradley, and Andersen, 2002). Thus binocular rivalry appears to be related to other multistable phenomena (see chapter 8 in this volume) that have long been thought to employ principles of perceptual organization derived from natural vision.

We have previously reviewed the many parallels between binocular rivalry and other multistable stimuli, with particular attention paid to the nature of the alternation process (Leopold and Logothetis, 1999). In the next sections, we ignore for a moment those aspects of rivalry related to alternation, and focus instead on the mechanisms responsible, at any point in time, for the perceptual dominance of one stimulus over another. Specifically, we ask whether this subjective condition is dictated by, or at least reflected in, the activity of neurons in the early cortical visual areas. We address this question using an offshoot of binocular rivalry termed flash suppression (see also chapters 11 and 12 in this volume), which allows one to deterministically bestow perception during rivalry with a particular state of dominance (Wolfe, 1984).

Flash suppression refers to the sudden and persisting perceptual dominance achieved when two rivalrous patterns are presented asynchronously to the two eyes (figure 13.2). Under these conditions, the latter pattern dominates perceptually over the first, as long as they differ sufficiently in their structure (Wolfe, 1984). This paradigm, which affords the experimenter excellent control over the subject's perceptual state, is of great value in neurophysiological experiments, and was previously used to study perception-related single-cell responses in cats (Sengpiel, Blakemore, and Harrad, 1995; see also chapter 11 in this volume), monkeys (Sheinberg and

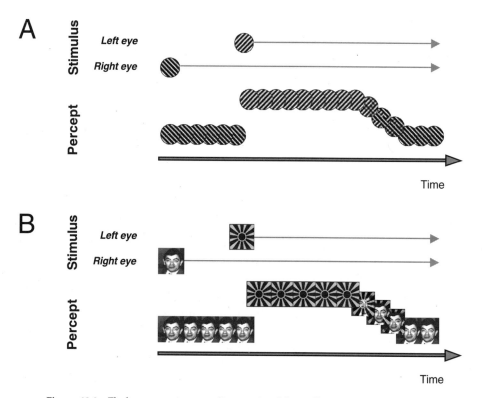

**Figure 13.2** Flash suppression paradigms using (*A*) small grating patterns and (*B*) large complex patterns and natural images. In all cases, monocular stimuli were presented for at least 500 msec before the addition of the rivalrous stimulus in the other eye. This asynchronous presentation reliably results in the immediate and persistent perception of the second stimulus, accompanied by complete suppression of the first.

Logothetis, 1997; Leopold, 1997), and, most recently, humans (Kreiman, Fried, and Koch, 2002; see also chapter 12 in this volume). For two identical rivalry presentations (except for the immediate history), flash suppression thus allows the experimenter to impose two very different perceptual states.

## Methods

To examine the expression of the alternate perceptual states during rivalry, we recorded activity in the visual cortex of three monkeys—A (90013), B (90004), and C (K97)—as they experienced flash suppression. The animals were required to fixate a small spot during two testing conditions. In the first, the position and extent of receptive fields were mapped. In the second, two conflicting stimuli were presented asynchronously to the two eyes, resulting in flash suppression. Monkey C was additionally required to report his percept following the flash. For monkeys A and B, stimuli consisted of small ($\approx 1°$) orthogonal grating patterns at the center of gaze (figure 13.2A), which are known to elicit excellent flash suppression in humans. Single units were isolated in the foveal representations of V1, V2, and V4, and recorded one at a time. The gratings were optimized in their orientation and spatial frequency to maximally stimulate each neuron's receptive field. Stimuli were presented separately to each eye by means of a polarization shutter system (see Leopold and Logothetis, 1996).

For monkey C, flash suppression was induced between diverse patterns, such as the image of a face and a geometrical pattern (figure 13.2B). The stimuli were large ($\approx 6°$), and optimized not according to the specific neural preferences but, rather, to perceptual criteria. Stimuli were presented separately to the two eyes by means of a mirror stereoscope. Extracellular single- and multiple-unit signals were conducted, using multiple electrodes distributed anterior to and posterior to the lunate sulcus. For most recording sites, the receptive fields' centers were located between $0°$ and $3°$ of the fixation spot.

## Single-Unit Responses During Flash Suppression

The responses of single neurons during flash suppression are shown for several visual areas in figure 13.3. Data from monkeys A and B are combined in the first three quadrants, corresponding to responses in V1, V2, and V4. The last quadrant presents data redrawn from Sheinberg and Logothetis (1997), showing equivalent data from IT. In each quadrant, the

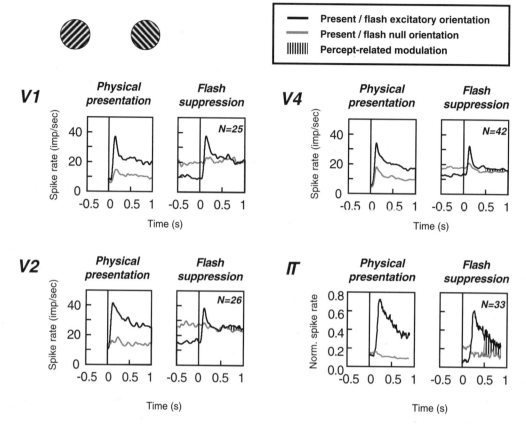

**Figure 13.3** Single–unit responses during physical presentation and flash suppression in several cortical visual areas. Excitatory and nonexcitatory patterns consisted of the preferred orientation and null (orthogonal) orientations in areas V1, V2, and V4, and of images or complex patterns in IT. Prior to testing, the excitatory and nonexcitatory stimuli were tailored to the preferences of each neuron. Physical presentations consisted of monoptic (or dioptic) placement of the stimulus in the neuron's receptive field for at least 1 sec. During flash suppression, the two patterns were shown dichoptically and asynchronously, with a 500 msec interval, resulting in perception of the second pattern. The hatched regions illustrate the difference in neural activity corresponding to the very different perceptual states. Note that this activity difference is markedly higher in the inferotemporal cortex (IT) than in the earlier visual areas (V1, V2, V4). (IT data adapted from Sheinberg and Logothetis, 1997.)

left panel shows mean responses over all neurons to the presentation of neurons' preferred (black line) versus null (gray line) orientations. Stimuli used for the inferotemporal cortex in the bottom right quadrant did not consist of oriented grating patterns, but of images and patterns similar to those shown in figure 13.2B. The right panels compare the flash suppression responses when the preferred (black line) and null stimuli (gray line) became dominant.

Perceptually, the conditions portrayed in the left and right panels, corresponding to the nonrivalry and rivalry conditions, respectively, are nearly identical, a fact that might lead one to speculate that the underlying neural activity is similar in the two cases. Nonetheless, figure 13.3 shows that the cells in the early cortical areas responded very differently during nonrivalry and rivalry, and generally showed less discrimination between the two orientations during perceptual, as compared to physical, stimulus changes. This was particularly true for cortical areas V1, V2, and V4, where perception-related modulation following flash suppression was modest compared to the preferred and null stimuli presented alone. Following initial transients (whose relevance to the perceptual state is difficult to assess, and which are put aside in the present analysis in favor of more sustained responses reflecting the prolonged perceptual state), activity in V1 was nearly indistinguishable for the two perceptual conditions during flash suppression. Areas V2 and V4 demonstrated a small but significant persisting difference between preferred and null dominance (hatched areas).

Thus, although the percepts experienced during the physical presentation and flash suppression conditions are highly similar, the unseen suppressed stimulus has a marked influence on the firing of neurons in the visual cortex. Responses in the inferotemporal cortex during flash suppression bore a much stronger resemblance to those seen during physical presentation of effective and ineffective stimuli (bottom right panel of figure 13.3) (Sheinberg and Logothetis, 1997). In contrast to the earlier areas, neural responses in IT reflected perception during flash suppression in a manner predicted by the neural selectivity.

While we have previously speculated that such differences among areas during free-running rivalry reveals their respective roles in natural vision, direct comparison is difficult because of the dissimilar nature of the stimuli used in flash suppression. Although binocular rivalry, including flash suppression, is highly robust to different stimulus types, it might be possible that the expression of perceptual dominance throughout the visual cortex depends on the types of stimuli used. For example, natural or complex patterns might produce fundamentally different global activity patterns, which could contribute to the differences observed. To test the effects of stimulus type directly, we next recorded from the early visual areas, using stimuli that were similar in nature to those used in the previous inferotemporal study.

## Flash Suppression with Natural Stimuli

Data were collected from the early visual areas in monkey C during flash suppression, using a variety of patterns of the type shown in figure 13.2B. The stimuli were optimized according to perceptual criteria, to provide uniform and reliable flash suppression. In addition to monitoring single–unit activity, we collected multiunit activity (MUA), corresponding here to the absolute value of the band-pass-filtered raw signal (500 Hz–3 kHz). Average MUA data for all recording sites in areas V1, V2, and V4 are shown in figure 13.4 during physical reversal between the two stimuli (left panels) and flash suppression (right panels). As with the data reported above, these two conditions were perceptually highly similar. For each recording site, the two competing stimuli were divided into effective and ineffective, based upon responses during physical reversal only (i.e., without regard to responses during flash suppression). Physical presentation of the effective stimulus (black lines) thus always resulted in higher activity than the ineffective stimulus (gray lines).

The corresponding patterns of responses during flash suppression were, as before, substantially different. In area V1, for example, there was no significant activity difference during perceptual dominance of the effective versus ineffective stimuli, as long as both were simultaneously present. This is consistent with the single–unit data presented above. In contrast, area V2, and particularly area V4, displayed an increased activity difference related to the perceptual state (hatched areas). Thus, consistent with flash suppression with gratings above, as well as with our earlier binocular rivalry results (Leopold and Logothetis, 1996), neural activity related to perception increased at higher stages of cortical processing.

## Discussion

The single–unit and multiunit results, taken together, demonstrate that the neural expression of a given perceptual state following flash suppression is distinctly different from that observed in the absence of interocular competition. In other words, in accordance with the psychophysical results described above, the unperceived, "suppressed" pattern continues to have a large impact on neurons throughout early striate and extrastriate cortical processing stages. Given the similarity in the single–unit and multiunit data, as well as in flash suppression between pairs of simple and

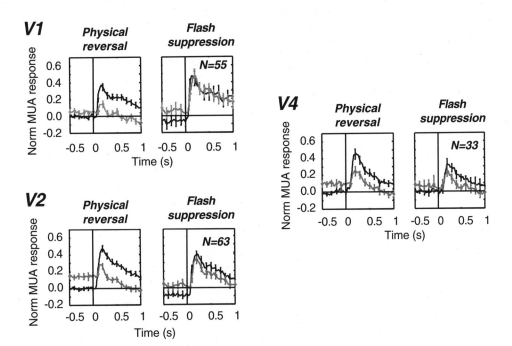

**Figure 13.4** Multiunit responses collected in areas V1, V2, and V4 during physical reversal and flash suppression of complex patterns. In this case, complex stimuli were selected based on perceptual criteria, and sorted into effective and ineffective based upon the responses during the physical reversal trials. During physical alternation trials (left panels), one pattern was shown monocularly for at least 1.0 sec (0.5 sec is shown to the left of the vertical line), and then replaced by the other pattern in either the same or the opposite eye (at time t = 0 sec). In the flash suppression trials, the second pattern was always shown to the opposite eye after at least 0.5 sec, while the first pattern remained. This manipulation resulted in a percept that was very similar to the physical reversal condition, although both stimuli were simultaneously present after the flash. The mean responses at each recording site were normalized by the nonrivalry, preferred responses. The baseline before presentation of the preferred stimulus (when the nonpreferred was present) was first subtracted in all conditions, and this trace was divided by the magnitude of the preferred response. The error bars represent the standard error of the mean among sites normalized in this way.

pairs of complex stimuli, what might account for the stark differences between early and late areas of visual processing?

The answer may lie in a fundamental difference in the roles of the various areas regarding the disambiguation of local stimulus information. Neurons responding to local visual primitives in the primary visual cortex necessarily pass ambiguous information on to higher processing stages. While their responses may be subject to modification by lateral interactions within the same area (Kapadia, Westheimer, and Gilbert, 2000; Stettler et al., 2002) and by feedback from higher visual areas (Angelucci et al., 2002; Hupé et al., 1998; Lamme and Roelfsema, 2000), these influences are limited. The increased perception-related responses in the extrastriate areas may signify their increasingly interpretive role in vision.

This finding parallels those of several other recent studies demonstrating that activity in area V2 more closely matches the perception of a locally ambiguous region than of primary visual cortex (Bakin, Nakayama, and Gilbert, 2000; Heider, Meskenaite, and Peterhans, 2000; Zhou, Friedman, and Von der Heydt, 2000). In the inferotemporal cortex, neural responses may play a distinctly different role in perception. Since inferotemporal neurons sit beyond cortical stages where ambiguous features are represented explicitly, their activation may reflect a visual problem for which a solution has already been found. This is one explanation that could account for the high fraction of neurons which modulate with perception in the inferotemporal cortex during binocular rivalry (Sheinberg and Logothetis, 1997).

While this is likely to be an oversimplified view of a process in which there is great interaction between diverse brain areas, it is possible to consider that the responses of IT neurons already represent a "commitment" on the part of the visual system, and are therefore much more closely linked with perception than responses in other areas which, by nature, remain ambiguous. But it is important to emphasize that even if IT were the first stage of cortical processing in which neural responses consistently match the perceived stimulus, it would not be implicated as being the site of binocular rivalry. On the contrary, the results presented here, taken in the context of other neurophysiological and psychophysical results, suggest that binocular rivalry does not have a single site in which it is implemented, but instead reflects competitive and interactive processes distributed over many levels of visual processing (Blake and Logothetis, 2002; Logothetis, 1998). In the next section, we consider how, given this distribution of neural activity in the cortex during rivalry, perception takes the form that it does.

# THE NATURE OF BINOCULAR RIVALRY

The flash suppression results shown here, taken together with several other psychophysical and physiological studies, suggest that most binocular neurons in the striate and early extrastriate areas continuously receive input from both eyes during binocular rivalry. But why, then, do we have the subjective impression that we only see one eye's stimulus at a time? What, then, is responsible for this monocular perception? If, as we have previously speculated, perception during rivalry is a product of central competitive mechanisms, why does it default to a form that could, in theory, be implemented in a much simpler way? Here we explore these points by drawing upon examples of interocular conflict present in natural vision. We first show that during normal binocular vision, the brain is frequently forced to resolve interocular conflict arising from diverse factors, and that it generally does so by defaulting locally to a monocular view. We then propose that perception during binocular rivalry is governed by similar principles, dictated by perceptual constraints and implemented well beyond the site of binocular combination in primary visual cortex.

## Interocular Conflict in Natural Vision

Primates, with their frontally mounted eyes separated by several centimeters, necessarily process two slightly different monocular views of the three-dimensional world. Discrepancies in the two eyes' images can arise from numerous factors, some of which are illustrated in figure 13.5 (see plate 4), which shows monocular and binocular regions of a human's horizontal plane of view. Note that each monocular field, for example, has a sharp discontinuity at its medial border representing the edge of the nose. With the eyes aimed straight ahead, these discontinuities define the horizontal borders of the binocular visual field, which subtends roughly 114°, and produce two monocular flanks extending an additional 37° in each direction (figure 13.5A) (Howard and Rogers, 2002). Despite the abrupt transition from monocular to binocular, there is no perceptual discontinuity at the edges of the binocular zone. This cannot be accounted for solely by the eccentric position of the border, since visual experience is similar even when the center of gaze is shifted directly into an unpaired monocular zone (figure 13.5B).

In this condition, the contralateral eye is aimed at the nose and cannot see the target. While introspection can bring us to notice the faint outline of our nose, we are generally unaware that our vision is monocular, a fact

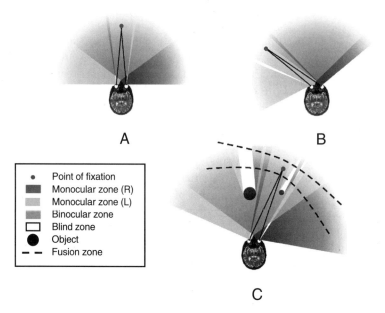

A

B

C

Point of fixation
Monocular zone (R)
Monocular zone (L)
Binocular zone
Blind zone
Object
Fusion zone

**Figure 13.5** Monocular and binocular regions of the visual field are mixed during natural vision. (*A*) During normal viewing of an object, a portion of each eye's view is blocked by the nose. For straight-ahead viewing, this results in a binocular field of roughly 114° visual angle centered on the object of interest. In addition to the unpaired temporal crescents, each eye's blind spot adds a monocular region nearer to the center of gaze. (*B*) A gaze shift (version) results in a smaller binocular visual field due to enhanced obstruction from the nose. Shown here is a large version in which the center of gaze is itself monocular. (*C*) Cluttered scenes lead to a highly inhomogeneous field of monocular, binocular, and blind zones, even in Panum's fusional area (dashed lines). See plate 4 for color version.

that can be easily verified by closing the contralateral eye. Other monocular regions in the visual field correspond to the blind spot representations on the horizontal meridian, arising from the receptor-free optic disk on each retina. These monocular zones are depicted by the thin blue and yellow streaks protruding at 12–15° from the gaze center in figure 13.5A. As with the monocular flanks, there are virtually no perceptual consequences to these unpaired zones during binocular vision, since we simply see that region of the world through the eye that is able. Finally, and perhaps most important, the presence of nearby objects in the real world differentially occludes the eyes, and thereby casts different images on the retinas.

Figure 13.5C demonstrates that in addition to the factors mentioned above, the presence of objects in a scene leads to large, unpaired monocular

David A. Leopold and colleagues

zones, which are also largely unnoticed. Thus, in considering the information originating within regions of space corresponding to Panum's fusional zone[4] (processing outside of Panum's area, while also potentially of great interest, is not discussed here), our natural vision often contains a complex constellation of monocular, binocular, and blind regions. Experiments have demonstrated that in binocular vision without interocular conflict, singleness of vision is due to the fusion of images from both eyes rather than suppression of one (Blake and Camisa, 1978; Fox and Check, 1966b). But how are the unpaired monocular zones treated? Clearly they cannot be fused, since they have no counterpart in the other eye. This commonly encountered situation in cyclopean vision[5] may be a fundamental problem of perceptual organization, in which the brain hides the complexity of the underlying binocular problem in favor of seeing continuous objects and surfaces.

Many observations have underscored the need for the intervention of higher-order perceptual principles to contend with interocular conflict, in particular the unpaired monocular zones that occur during binocular object vision. Leonardo da Vinci, for example, was aware of their existence, and was continually frustrated that they, along with the alternate perspectives afforded by the two eyes, prevented him from directly translating a binocularly viewed scene onto a flat canvas (Howard and Rogers, 2002; Ono, Wade, and Lillakas, 2002). Recently, models of stereoscopic vision have incorporated these zones as a means to disambiguate three-dimensional structure (Anderson and Nakayama, 1994; Gillam and Borsting, 1988; Nakayama and Shimojo, 1990). Interestingly, Shimojo and Nakayama demonstrated that during stereoscopic viewing, monocular zones which are "ecologically valid" (i.e., those which correspond to the geometry of natural vision) escape binocular rivalry entirely (Shimojo and Nakayama, 1990), and that points lying in these zones are assigned depth based upon global occlusion constraints rather than on local binocular matching (Shimojo and Nakayama, 1994). Thus, these and other experiments have revealed a strong link between fundamental mechanisms of binocular vision and other aspects of perceptual organization concerned with object and surface properties.

How, then, might the visual cortex draw upon this patchwork of monocular and binocular zones to synthesize a continuous and accurate percept? The need for an eye-of-origin signal has prompted speculation that such real–world constraints of binocular vision are implemented early in the visual system, where information from the two eyes is still largely segregated (Shimojo and Nakayama, 1990, 1994). At higher processing stages, binocular neurons would be unable to discriminate between right-eye and left-eye stimulation, and thereby could not judge whether a visual feature should be dominant or suppressed.

Similar arguments have been put forth for other aspects of stereoscopic vision as well, including the detection of binocular disparity. Since the seminal work of Julesz (1960), binocular disparity has been recognized as a sufficient cue for the perception of depth. Following the discovery of disparity-tuned neurons in the primary visual cortex (Barlow, Blakemore, and Pettigrew, 1967), and the subsequent demonstration that edges defined by disparity alone could activate orientation-selective neurons (Poggio et al., 1985), the convergence of monocular signals in the primary visual cortex has been thought to be an important contributor to the mechanisms underlying our stereopsis (for a review, see Cumming and DeAngelis, 2001).

Yet it is important to emphasize that even for aspects of perception that depend upon detecting large or small interocular discrepancies, there is no a priori reason to believe that problems of binocular vision must be resolved at the earliest stages of binocular combination. First, while humans' poor performance on utrocular discrimination[6] suggests that eye-of-origin information is inaccessible to perception, experiments in monkeys have revealed that many neurons carry eye-specific information well beyond the primary visual cortex. Although the vast majority of neurons in extrastriate cortex are binocular, meaning that they do not respond exclusively to stimuli placed in one eye or the other, a fraction of neurons in most areas tested display biases in their ocular preferences (Burkhalter and Van Essen, 1986; Maunsell and Van Essen, 1983; Uka et al., 2000). Even more pervasive in extrastriate areas is selectivity for interocular disparity, which is commonly found in the extrastriate areas (Burkhalter and Van Essen, 1986; Felleman and Van Essen, 1987; Hinkle and Connor, 2002; Janssen, Vogels, and Orban, 2000; Maunsell and Van Essen, 1983; Taira et al., 2000; Uka et al., 2000).

The role of ocular biases in interpreting the structure of objects and scenes is unknown, although recent evidence obtained with cortical microstimulation provides compelling evidence that extrastriate disparity responses are directly linked to the perception of stereoscopic depth (DeAngelis and Newsome, 1999). Most important, regardless of where interocular conflict is detected, its resolution must be smoothly integrated with diverse information arising from many other aspects of vision, including global cues applied in the reconstruction of three-dimensional structure (Cavanagh, 1987). A number of studies, including those mentioned above, suggest that neural activity bears increasing resemblance to perception as one moves beyond primary visual cortex. Recent physiological recordings assessing neural responses to absolute versus relative disparity[7] suggest that this principle is true even for stereopsis itself (Cumming and Parker, 1999; Thomas, Cumming, and Parker, 2002). In that study, many neurons in cortical area V2, but not in primary visual cortex, responded according to the relative disparity in a binocular pattern, capturing the aspect of stereopsis for which humans are most sensitive. This finding parallels several other recent studies demonstrating that activity in area V2 more closely matches stereoscopic perception and figure-ground depth ordering than that in primary visual cortex (Bakin, Nakayama, and Gilbert, 2000; Heider, Meskenaite, and Peterhans, 2000; Zhou, Friedman, and Von der Heydt, 2000).

Thus, close examination of natural binocular vision reveals an abundance of interocular mismatches. Small horizontal disparities, which are registered in the activity of neurons throughout the visual cortex, are generally exploited to provide information about three-dimensional structure. Resolution of larger interocular conflicts, whose explicit representation in extrastriate areas is less clear, generally takes the form of exclusive monocular dominance, although this is largely hidden from our perception. In all cases, interocular conflict arising in natural vision is coordinated with interpretive elements of vision to generate a unified and robust percept. In the final section, we return to binocular rivalry, and explore the possibility that its monocular percept is due to similar high-level organizational principles that guide the resolution of interocular conflict during normal vision.

## Binocular Rivalry and Perceptual Organization

When patterns in the two eyes are beyond reconciliation, binocular rivalry arises and perception becomes monocular. But given the evidence presented earlier, what is the neural basis of this monocular vision? Above we discussed evidence that interocular conflict is a common feature of natural vision, whose "monocular" resolution is smoothly integrated with other aspects of perceptual organization. Here we propose that vision during binocular rivalry derives from similar processes, and that its suppression, while powerful in shaping our percept, is in many respects only apparent.

One characteristic of rivalry consistent with this hypothesis is the surprisingly small magnitude of changes in sensitivity during suppression. Experiments measuring the effect of rivalry on perceptual thresholds have generally found that the sensitivity of the suppressed eye is impaired by only 0.3–0.5 log unit (Blake and Camisa, 1978; Blake and Logothetis, 2002; Fukuda, 1981; Norman, Norman, and Bilotta, 2000; Wales and Fox, 1970). This dissociation—strong perceptual suppression despite weak impairment of probe detection—is consistent with monocular perception being implemented at a central stage of processing. This point is further underscored by similar results obtained from other experiments, unrelated to binocular vision, in which basic visual sensitivity is shown to vary according to subjective figure/ground organization. In the "context superiority effect," test probes are more difficult to detect when a region is perceived as background than when it is perceived as figure (Weitzman, 1963; Wong and Weisstein, 1982). Most important, the sensitivity changes measured in such experiments are very similar to those measured during dominance and suppression phases of binocular rivalry, where the visibility of the stimulus is continually changing.

These experiments, taken together, suggest that the small changes observed in test probe detectability occurring in the suppressed eye during rivalry reflect a decrease in the perceptual prominence of its context (i.e., the suppressed stimulus) rather than a general disruption of monocular information. Such context effects are thought to be important in influencing not only the sensitivity but also the balance of dominance and suppression during multistable perception (Alais and Blake, 1999; Peterson and Gibson, 1993; Yu and Blake, 1992). An additional example of the similarity between rivalry and figure/ground reversals is shown in figure 13.6, which compares different effects of manipulating stimulus salience in binocular rivalry and a classic ambiguous figure (Rubin, 1921). Note that in the rivalry condition, the mean duration of rivalry dominance is determined by the contrast of the suppressed, rather than the visible, stimulus (Levelt, 1965), indicating that the brain can extract even quantitative information from an unperceived pattern. Even in the pathological condition of strabismic suppression, in which misalignment of the eyes results in a percept that is always monocular, evidence suggests that suppression is superficial. While distinct from rivalry, strabismic suppression affects test probe sensitivity by roughly the same small magnitude (Smith et al., 1985). Furthermore, strabismic suppression, like binocular rivalry, is similarly incapable of preventing the formation of adaptational aftereffects (Blake and Lehmkuhle, 1976).

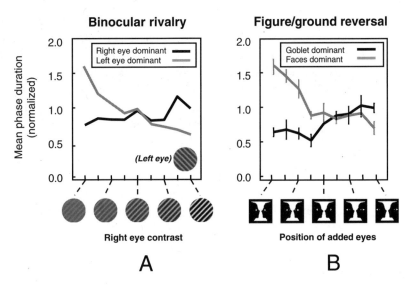

**Figure 13.6** Parametrically changing one stimulus during multistable perception can alter the balance of dominance and suppression. (*A*) For binocular rivalry, this is traditionally demonstrated by changing the contrast of a pattern in one eye while leaving that in the other eye constant. These data, from one subject, are typical, and demonstrate that the mean dominance of the unchanged stimulus is primarily affected. (*B*) The alternation dynamics can also be influenced by stimulus manipulations in other forms of multistable perception. Here, changing the position of two eyes added to Rubin's faces/vase pattern systematically changes the mean dominance time (N = 5).

These results, taken together, demonstrate that state-dependent changes in sensitivity are not unique to binocular rivalry, but appear to represent a more general mechanism related to perceptual organization. Nor is perceptual suppression dependent upon interocular conflict, since many phenomena exist in which complete visual suppression, often resembling binocular rivalry, exist in the absence of interocular conflict (Andrews and Purves, 1997; Bonneh, Cooperman, and Sagi, 2001; Campbell and Howell, 1972; Magnussen et al., 2001; Pritchard, 1961; Troxler, 1804).

One final troubling point for most theories of binocular rivalry, including those implicating high-level mechanisms, is the fractionation of the rivalry percept. Particularly for large patterns containing a high density of visual structure, perception does not consist of uniform alternation between the two monocular targets, but instead develops into a dynamic spatial mosaic of left- and right-eye dominance. This piecemeal percept illustrates that at some level, the resolution of interocular conflict during rivalry must take place on a spatially localized level. Experiments using high spatial frequency grating patterns as rivalry targets have suggested that the fundamental size for a zone of unitary perception during this piecemeal rivalry is linked to representations in the primary visual cortex. In particular, the spatial scale of fractionation varies with eccentricity in a manner consistent with the human magnification factor[8] in primary visual cortex (Blake, O'Shea, and Mueller, 1992).

Furthermore, a recent elegant study has quantified the dynamic properties of "waves" of perceptual dominance during rivalry, and suggested that they propagate with a constant speed over the cortical sheet, independent of eccentricity (Wilson, Blake, and Lee, 2001). This last result, providing strong evidence that some aspects of binocular rivalry resolution must refer back to representations in the topographic cortical areas, in addition offers a novel and useful paradigm to study the electrophysiological basis of piecemeal percepts during rivalry. While the suggestion that piecemeal rivalry reflects a perceptual investment in the early visual areas is difficult to refute, it is possible that other, higher-level factors might also contribute. For example, during normal vision, in contrast to rivalry or strabismus, zones of interocular conflict arising from binocular geometry are generally restricted in their spatial extent, particularly near the center of gaze. Vergence eye movements ensure that a properly fixated object and its immediate surroundings will lie within Panum's fusional area, whereas objects at larger eccentricities tend to contribute larger zones of monocularity or interocular conflict.

While these observations do not explain the generation of piecemeal rivalry, they offer some expectation that the brain might tend toward disbelief of a global monocular solution. Organizational mechanisms might thus fractionate the percept based on several factors, including the approximate size of monocular zones common in normal vision. It may be revealing that under some conditions, such fractionation can indeed work in a cooperative manner (e.g., Alais and Blake, 1999) with other elements of perceptual organization to form a unified percept. This is illustrated, for example, by old and new experiments in which principles of interocular grouping draw cooperatively from portions of the two eyes at once, in accordance with basic Gestalt principles (Diaz-Caneja, 1928; Kovács et al., 1996; Kulikowski, 1992; Leopold, 1997). Thus, mixed percepts in rivalry suggest that perception is at least constrained by feature representations in the early cortical areas, but that these constraints are subject to modification by global information. Recent results have argued that basic sensory representations might similarly constrain higher-order aspects of perception during binocular rivalry (Suzuki and Grabowecky, 2002).

## SUMMARY

The evidence presented in this chapter argues that the dominance and suppression during binocular rivalry stem from central, interpretive neural processes that have access to both eyes' views. Most psychophysical and nearly all electrophysiological experiments (but not all neuroimaging experiments) are in agreement that an unperceived stimulus penetrates well beyond the site of binocular combination, and thereby makes a significant mark on cortical neurons at many processing stages. In considering why central mechanisms might choose to entirely discard one eye's image from perception, we argue that interocular conflict is a common feature of natural binocular vision, and that in most cases it is settled by adopting one eye's information. From these points, we conclude that our percept during rivalry derives from principles of normal binocular vision. Given the processing of both eyes' patterns, but the visibility of only one pattern, we suggest that monocular perception during rivalry is in its very nature illusory. It is a thinly cast veil over a binocular sampling of the world, perhaps serving to protect our ultimate percept from the chaotic mixing of incompatible images.

## NOTES

1. *Perceptual organization* is a concept introduced by Gestalt psychologists (Wertheimer, 1923) to describe the active, interpretive elements of vision, such as grouping, motion correspondence, and figure/ground organization. Neural mechanisms underlying perceptual organization pose a great challenge for modern brain scientists, as they are thought to involve integrated processing among diverse brain areas.

2. *Adaptational aftereffects* are perceptual distortions following prolonged viewing of visual patterns. Adaptation, sometimes referred to as the "psychophysicist's electrode" is thought to isolate and temporarily diminish the contribution of specific subpopulation of neurons normally contributing to perception. While their physiological basis remains poorly understood, most are known to have a cortical origin.

3. *Interocular transfer* (IOT) refers to the presence of an aftereffect measured in an eye contralateral to that in which monocular adaptation was performed. In the motion aftereffect, for example, IOT accounts for roughly half the full aftereffect magnitude (Mather et al., 1998). The magnitude of IOT has often been used to gauge the relative contribution of monocular vs. binocular neurons.

4. During binocular vision, a point in three-dimensional space may or may not fall on corresponding regions of the two retinae. The set of all points for which this is the case is defined as the *horopter*, which is a function of eye position and, in particular, vergence. For a given fixation point, there exists a region of 3-D space surrounding the horopter in which binocular fusion is possible. This is commonly referred to as Panum's fusional area after the nineteenth-century German scientist (Panum, 1858), although its existence has been described since the time of Alhazen in the eleventh century (Howard and Rogers, 2002). Information impinging the retina from objects outside this region produces retinal projections that cannot be binocularly combined.

5. *Cyclopean vision* refers to the fact that our binocular view in the world subjectively appears to emerge from a single eye located halfway between the actual eyes (Howard and Rogers, 2002; Julesz, 1971).

6. *Utrocular discrimination* refers to a subject's identification of the eye through which a target pattern is shown. In general, humans are extremely poor or incapable of performing such a discrimination (von Helmholtz, 1925).

7. *Absolute disparity* refers to the horizontal difference in the location of a point striking each retina with respect to the two foveae. *Relative disparity* refers to the distance between absolute disparities of two features in three-dimensional space. Unlike absolute disparity, perception of relative disparity is robust to uniform distance changes and vergence movements, and is therefore thought to serve as the basis for human stereo judgments (Thomas et al., 2002).

8. The cortical *magnification factor* refers to the transformation by which visual space is mapped onto the visual cortex. In the primary visual cortex, there is a large overrepresentation of the central portion of visual field.

## REFERENCES

Alais, D., and Blake, R. (1999). Grouping visual features during binocular rivalry. *Vision Research, 39*, 4341–4353.

Albright, T. D., and Stoner, G. R. (2002). Contextual influences on visual processing. *Annual Review of Neuroscience, 25*, 339–379.

Anderson, B. L., and Nakayama, K. (1994). Towards a general theory of stereopsis: Binocular matching, occluding contours, and fusion. *Psychological Review, 101*, 414–445.

Andrews, T. J., and Purves, D. (1997). Similarities in normal and binocularly rivalrous viewing. *Proceedings of the National Academy of Sciences of the United States of America, 94*, 9905–9908.

Angelucci, A., Levitt, J. B., Walton, E. J. S., Hupé, J. M., Bullier, J., and Lund, J. S. (2002). Circuits for local and global signal integration in primary visual cortex. *Journal of Neuroscience, 22*, 8633–8646.

Bakin, J. S., Nakayama, K., and Gilbert, C. D. (2000). Visual responses in monkey areas V1 and V2 to three-dimensional surface configurations. *Journal of Neuroscience, 20*, 8188–8198.

Barlow, H. B., Blakemore, C., and Pettigrew, J. D. (1967). The neural mechanism of binocular depth discrimination. *Journal of Physiology, 193*, 327–342.

Blake, R., and Camisa, J. (1978). Is binocular vision always monocular? *Science*, 200, 1497–1499.

Blake, R., and Fox, R. (1974). Adaptation to invisible gratings and the site of binocular rivalry suppression. *Nature*, 249, 488–490.

Blake, R., and Lehmkuhle, S. W. (1976). On the site of strabismic suppression. *Investigative Ophthalmology*, 15, 660–663.

Blake, R., and Logothetis, N. K. (2002). Visual competition. *Nature Reviews: Neuroscience*, 3, 13–21.

Blake, R., O'Shea, R. P., and Mueller, T. J. (1992). Spatial zones of binocular rivalry in central and peripheral vision. *Visual Neuroscience*, 8, 469–478.

Blake, R., and Overton, R. (1979). The site of binocular rivalry suppression. *Perception*, 8, 143–152.

Blake, R., Westendorf, D. H., and Overton, R. (1980). What is suppressed during binocular rivalry? *Perception*, 9, 223–231.

Blake, R., Yu, K., Lokey, M., and Norman, H. (1998). Binocular rivalry and motion perception. *Journal of Cognitive Neuroscience*, 10, 46–60.

Bonneh, Y. S., Cooperman, A., and Sagi, D. (2001). Motion-induced blindness in normal observers. *Nature*, 411, 798–801.

Bradley, D. C., Chang, G. C., and Andersen, R. A. (1998). Encoding of three-dimensional structure-from-motion by primate area MT neurons. *Nature*, 392, 714–717.

Burkhalter, A., and Van Essen, D. C. (1986). Processing of color, form and disparity information in visual areas VP and V2 of ventral extrastriate cortex in the macaque monkey. *Journal of Neuroscience*, 6, 2327–2351.

Campbell, F. W., and Howell, E. R. (1972). Monocular alternation: A method for the investigation of pattern vision. *Journal of Physiology*, 225, 19P–21P.

Cavanagh, P. (1987). Reconstructing the third dimension: Interactions between color, texture, motion, binocular disparity and shape. *Computer Vision, Graphics, and Image Processing*, 37, 171–195.

Cumming, B. G., and DeAngelis, G. C. (2001). The physiology of stereopsis. *Annual Review of Neurosciences*, 24, 203–238.

Cumming, B. G., and Parker, A. J. (1999). Binocular neurons in V1 of awake monkeys are selective for absolute, not relative, disparity. *Journal of Neuroscience*, 19, 5602–5618.

DeAngelis, G. C., and Newsome, W. T. (1999). Organization of disparity-selective neurons in macaque area MT. *Journal of Neuroscience*, 19, 1398–1415.

Diaz-Caneja, E. (1928). Sur l'alternance binoculaire. *Annales d'Oculistique*, 165 (october), 721–731.

Dodd, J. V., Krug, K., Cumming, B. G., and Parker, A. J. (2001). Perceptually bistable three-dimensional figures evoke high choice probabilities in cortical area MT. *Journal of Neuroscience*, 21, 4809–4821.

Felleman, D. J., and Van Essen, D. C. (1987). Receptive field properties of neurons in area V3 of macaque monkey extrastriate cortex. *Journal of Neurophysiology, 57,* 889–920.

Fox, R., and Check, R. (1966a). Forced-choice form recognition during binocular rivalry. *Psychonomic Science, 6,* 471–472.

Fox, R., and Check, R. (1966b). Binocular fusion: A test of the suppression theory. *Perception and Psychophysics, 2,* 331–334.

Fox, R., and Check, R. (1968). Detection of motion during binocular rivalry suppression. *Journal of Experimental Psychology, 78,* 388–395.

Fukuda, H. (1981). Magnitude of suppression of binocular rivalry within the invisible pattern. *Perceptual and Motor Skills, 53,* 371–375.

Gillam, B., and Borsting, E. (1988). The role of monocular regions in stereoscopic displays. *Perception, 17,* 603–608.

Gregory, R. (1997). *Eye and Brain: The Psychology of Seeing.* 5th ed. Princeton, N.J.: Princeton University Press.

Grunewald, A., Bradley, D. C., and Andersen, R. A. (2002). Neural correlates of structure-from-motion perception in macaque V1 and MT. *Journal of Neuroscience, 22,* 6195–6207.

Heider, B., Meskenaite, V., and Peterhans, E. (2000). Anatomy and physiology of a neural mechanism defining depth order and contrast polarity at illusory contours. *European Journal of Neuroscience, 12,* 4117–4130.

Helmholtz, H. von. (1925). *Treatise on Physiological Optics,* New York: Dover. J. P. C. Southall, trans.

Hinkle, D. A., and Connor, C. E. (2002). Three-dimensional orientation tuning in macaque area V4. *Nature Neuroscience, 5,* 665–670.

Howard, I. P., and Rogers, B. J. (2002). *Seeing in Depth.* Thornhill, Ontario, Canada: I. Porteus.

Hupé, J. M., James, A. C., Payne, B. R., Lomber, S. G., Girard, P., and Bullier, J. (1998). Cortical feedback improves discrimination between figure and background by V1, V2 and V3 neurons. *Nature, 394,* 784–787.

Janssen, P., Vogels, R., and Orban, G. A. (2000). Three-dimensional shape coding in inferior temporal cortex. *Neuron, 27,* 385–397.

Julesz, B. (1960). Binocular depth perception of computer generated patterns. *Bell System Technical Journal, 39,* 1125–1162.

Julesz, B. (1971). *Foundations of Cyclopean Perception.* Chicago: University of Chicago Press.

Kapadia, M. K., Westheimer, G., and Gilbert, C. D. (2000). Spatial distribution of contextual interactions in primary visual cortex and in visual perception. *Journal of Neurophysiology, 84,* 2048–2062.

Koffka, K. (1935). *Principles of Gestalt Psychology.* New York: Harcourt, Brace and World.

Kovács, I., Papathomas, T. V., Yang, M., and Fehér, A. (1996). When the brain changes its mind: Interocular grouping during binocular rivalry. *Proceedings of the National Academy of Sciences of the United States of America, 93,* 15508–15511.

David A. Leopold and colleagues

Kreiman, G., Fried, I., and Koch, C. (2002). Single-neuron correlates of subjective vision in the human medial temporal lobe. *Proceedings of the National Academy of Sciences of the United States of America*, 99, 8378–8383.

Kulikowski, J. J. (1992). Binocular chromatic rivalry and single vision. *Ophthalmic and Physiological Optics*, 12, 168–170.

Lamme, V. A., Rodriguez-Rodriguez, V., and Spekreijse, H. (1999). Separate processing dynamics for texture elements, boundaries and surfaces in primary visual cortex of the macaque monkey. *Cerebral Cortex*, 9, 406–413.

Lamme, V. A., and Roelfsema, P. R. (2000). The distinct modes of vision offered by feedforward and recurrent processing. *Trends in Neurosciences*, 23, 571–579.

Lee, S. H., and Blake, R. (1999). Rival ideas about binocular rivalry. *Vision Research*, 39, 1447–1454.

Lee, T. S., Yang, C. F., Romero, R. D., and Mumford, D. (2002). Neural activity in early visual cortex reflects behavioral experience and higher-order perceptual saliency. *Nature Neuroscience*, 5, 589–597.

Lehky, S. R., and Maunsell, J. H. R. (1996). No binocular rivalry in the LGN of alert macaque monkeys. *Vision Research*, 36, 1225–1234.

Lehmkuhle, S. W., and Fox, R. (1975). Effect of binocular rivalry suppression on the motion aftereffect. *Vision Research*, 15, 855–859.

Leopold, D. A. (1997). Brain mechanisms of visual awareness: Using perceptual ambiguity to investigate the neural basis of image segmentation and grouping. Ph.D. dissertation, Baylor College of Medicine.

Leopold, D. A., and Logothetis, N. K. (1996). Activity changes in early visual cortex reflect monkeys' percepts during binocular rivalry. *Nature*, 379, 549–553.

Leopold, D. A., and Logothetis, N. K. (1999). Multistable phenomena: Changing views in perception. *Trends in Cognitive Sciences*, 3, 254–264.

Levelt, W. J. M. (1965). *On Binocular Rivalry*. Soesterberg, The Netherlands: Institute for Perception RVO-TNO.

Logothetis, N. K. (1998). Single units and conscious vision. *Philosophical Transactions of the Royal Society of London*, B353, 1801–1818.

Logothetis, N. K., Leopold, D. A., and Sheinberg, D. L. (1996). What is rivalling during binocular rivalry? *Nature*, 380, 621–624.

Logothetis, N. K., and Schall, J. D. (1989). Neuronal correlates of subjective visual perception. *Science*, 245, 761–763.

Magnussen, S., Spillman, L., Stuerzel, F., and Werner, J. S. (2001). Filling-in of the foveal blue scotoma. *Vision Research*, 41, 2961–2967.

Mather, G., Verstraten, F. A., and Anstis, S. (1998). *The Motion Aftereffect: A Modern Perspective.* Cambridge, Mass.: MIT Press.

Maunsell, J. H., and Van Essen, D. C. (1983). Functional properties of neurons in middle temporal visual area of the macaque monkey. II. Binocular interactions and sensitivity to binocular disparity. *Journal of Neurophysiology*, 49, 1148–1167.

Nakayama, K., and Shimojo, S. (1990). Da Vinci stereopsis: Depth and subjective occluding contours from unpaired image points. *Vision Research*, 30, 1811–1825.

Necker, L. A. (1832). Observations on some remarkable optical phaenomena seen in Switzerland; and on an optical phenomenon which occurs on viewing a figure of a crystal or geometrical solid. *London and Edinburgh Philosophical Magazine and Journal of Science*, 1, 329–337.

Norman, H. F., Norman, J. F., and Bilotta, J. (2000). The temporal course of suppression during binocular rivalry. *Perception*, 29, 831–841.

Ono, H., Wade, N. J., and Lillakas, L. (2002). The pursuit of Leonardo's constraint. *Perception*, 31, 83–102.

O'Shea, R. P., and Crassini, B. (1981). Interocular transfer of the motion after-effect is not reduced by binocular rivalry. *Vision Research*, 21, 801–804.

Pack, C. C., and Born, R. T. (2001). Temporal dynamics of a neural solution to the aperture problem in visual area MT of macaque brain. *Nature*, 409, 1040–1042.

Panum, P. L. (1858). *Physiologische Untersuchungen über das Sehen mit Zwei Augen*. Kiel, Germany: Schwerssche Buchhandlung.

Peterson, M. A., and Gibson, B. S. (1993). Shape recognition inputs to figure/ground organization in three-dimensional grounds. *Cognitive Psychology*, 25, 383–429.

Poggio, G., Motter, B., Squatrito, S., and Trotter, Y. (1985). Responses of neurons in visual cortex (V1 and V2) of the alert macaque to dynamic random dot stereograms. *Vision Research*, 25, 397–406.

Polonsky, A., Blake, R., Braun, J., and Heeger, D. J. (2000). Neuronal activity in human primary visual cortex correlates with perception during binocular rivalry. *Nature Neuroscience*, 3, 1153–1159.

Pritchard, R. M. (1961). Stabilized images on the retina. *Scientific American*, 204, 72–78.

Purves, D., Lotto, R. B., Williams, S. M., Nundy, S., and Yang, Z. (2001). Why we see things the way we do: Evidence for a wholly empirical strategy of vision. *Philosophical Transactions of the Royal Society of London*, B356, 285–297.

Rock, I. (1984). *Perception*. New York: Scientific American Library.

Rossi, A. F., Rittenhouse, C. D., and Paradiso, M. A. (1996). The representation of brightness in primary visual cortex. *Science*, 273, 1104–1107.

Rubin, E. (1921). Visuell wahrgenommene figuren. Translated in *Figure and Ground*, Steven Yantis, ed., 225–229. Philadelphia: Psychology Press/Taylor & Francis.

Schiller, P. V. (1933). Stroboskopische alternativversuche. *Psychologische Forschung*, 17, 179–214.

Sengpiel, F., Blakemore, C., and Harrad, R. (1995). Interocular suppression in the primary visual cortex: A possible neural basis of binocular rivalry. *Vision Research*, 35, 179–195.

Sheinberg, D. L., and Logothetis, N. K. (1997). The role of temporal cortical areas in perceptual organization. *Proceedings of the National Academy of Sciences of the United States of America*, 94, 3408–3413.

Shimojo, S., and Nakayama, K. (1990). Real world occlusion constraints and binocular rivalry. *Vision Research*, 30, 69–80.

Shimojo, S., and Nakayama, K. (1994). Interocularly unpaired zones escape local binocular matching. *Vision Research*, 34, 1875–1881.

Smith, E. L., Levi, D. M., Harwerth, R. S., and White, J. M. (1982). Color vision is altered during the suppression phase of binocular rivalry. *Science*, 218, 802–804.

Smith, E. L., Levi, D. M., Manny, R. E., Harwerth, R. S., and White, J. M. (1985). The relationship between binocular rivalry and strabismic suppression. *Investigative Ophthalmology and Visual Science*, 26, 80–87.

Stettler, D. D., Das, A., Bennett, J., and Gilbert, C. D. (2002). Lateral connectivity and contextual interactions in macaque primary visual cortex. *Neuron*, 36, 739–750.

Sugita, Y. (1999). Grouping of image fragments in primary visual cortex. *Nature*, 401, 269–272.

Suzuki, S., and Grabowecky, M. (2002). Evidence for perceptual "trapping" and adaptation in multistable binocular rivalry. *Neuron*, 36, 143–157.

Taira, M., Tsutsui, K., Jiang, M., Yara, K., and Sakata, H. (2000). Parietal neurons represent surface orientation from the gradient of binocular disparity. *Journal of Neurophysiology*, 83, 3140–3146.

Thomas, O. M., Cumming, B. G., and Parker, A. J. (2002). A specialization for relative disparity in V2. *Nature Neuroscience*, 5, 472–478.

Tong, F., and Engel, S. A. (2001). Interocular rivalry revealed in the human cortical blind-spot representation. *Nature*, 411, 195–199.

Troxler, D. (1804). *Ueber das Verschwinden Gegebener Gegenstaende Innerhalb Unseres Gesichtskreises*. Jena: Fromman.

Uka, T., Tanaka, H., Yoshiyama, K., Kato, M., and Fujita, I. (2000). Disparity selectivity of neurons in monkey inferior temporal cortex. *Journal of Neurophysiology*, 84, 120–132.

Wales, R., and Fox, R. (1970). Increment detection thresholds during binocular rivalry suppression. *Perception and Psychophysics*, 8, 90–94.

Wallach, H., and O'Connell, D. N. (1953). The kinetic depth effect. *Journal of Experimental Psychology*, 45, 205–217.

Weitzman, B. A. (1963). A threshold difference produced by a figure-ground dichotomy. *Journal of Experimental Psychology*, 66, 201–205.

Wertheimer, M. (1923). Untersuchung zur lehre von der gestalt II. *Psychologische Forschung*, 4, 301–350.

Wilson, H. R., Blake, R., and Lee, S. H. (2001). Dynamics of travelling light waves in visual perception. *Nature*, 412, 907–910.

Wolfe, J. M. (1984). Reversing ocular dominance and suppression in a single flash. *Vision Research*, 24, 471–478.

Wong, E., and Weisstein, N. (1982). A new perceptual context superiority effect: Line segments are more visible against a figure than against a ground. *Science*, 218, 587–588.

Yu, K., and Blake, R. (1992). Do recognizable figures enjoy an advantage in binocular rivalry? *Journal of Experimental Psychology: Human Perception and Performance*, 18, 1158–1173.

Zhou, H., Friedman, H. S., and Von der Heydt, R. (2000). Coding of border ownership in monkey visual cortex. *Journal of Neuroscience*, 20, 6594–6611.

# 14 The Functional Role of Oscillatory Neuronal Synchronization for Perceptual Organization and Selection

Pascal Fries, Miguel Castelo-Branco, Andreas K. Engel, and Wolf Singer

This chapter deals with the role of oscillatory neuronal synchronization for perceptual organization and selection. The first part focuses on stimulus selection during interocular rivalry and the role of neuronal gamma-frequency synchronization for the corresponding neuronal group selection. The second part deals with perceptual organization during the viewing of ambiguous plaid stimuli and the role of neuronal synchronization for the flexible grouping of neurons.

## OSCILLATORY NEURONAL SYNCHRONIZATION AS A CORRELATE OF PERCEPTUAL SELECTION DURING INTEROCULAR RIVALRY

### Firing Rates Correlate with Perception in Late but Not Early Visual Areas

Interocular rivalry is one of the most clear-cut cases of stimulus selection. Each eye is presented with its own stimulus, but only one of those two stimuli is perceived. Studies in awake and behaving monkeys have demonstrated that neurons in the inferotemporal (IT) cortex respond as if there were only the perceived stimulus (Sheinberg and Logothetis, 1997; see also chapter 13 in this volume). A given IT neuron might respond strongly, for example, to a face stimulus but only weakly to a sunburst picture. If those two stimuli are then used in a rivalry situation, the neuron will display its usual strong response to the face when the face is actually perceived, but only the weak response evoked by the sunburst when the sunburst is perceived.

Thus firing rates of the IT neurons reflect the actual perceptual selection. However, the mechanisms underlying the generation of those firing rate effects are still unclear. Neurons in IT cortex receive their main input from neurons in areas TEO and V4, and those areas in turn receive their input from V2 and V1. Recordings in V4 revealed that only about half the neurons modulate their firing rates according to the perceptual selection of the monkey (Leopold and Logothetis, 1996). Surprisingly, only about half of those modulating neurons show a positive correlation between their firing-rate modulation and the perceptual selection. Firing rates in the other half are negatively correlated with perception (i.e., neurons respond during rivalry as if only the *non*perceived stimulus were present). Finally, in area V1, only a minority of neurons show firing rate modulations with perceptual alternations, and again those can be of either sign (Leopold and Logothetis, 1996).

How, then, do neurons in V1 and V4 that represent the perceived stimulus control IT neurons despite the fact that they do not change their firing rates in a consistent way? One possibility is that the population of V1 and V4 neurons representing the perceived stimulus increases its impact through enhanced synchronization (Salinas and Sejnowski, 2001). Precise synchronization has been shown, both in vitro and in vivo, to enhance the impact of a given number of input spikes (Alonso, Usrey, and Reid, 1996; Azouz and Gray, 2000; Salinas and Sejnowski, 2000).

**The Strabismic Animal as a Model for Stimulus Selection**

We tested the hypothesis that perceptual selection is achieved through synchronization in primary visual cortex of awake, behaving strabismic cats. Strabismus essentially establishes permanent interocular rivalry. As during nonstrabismic rivalry, the input to the two eyes cannot be fused and the input from one of the two eyes is selected for perception. The strabismic cat model offers several advantages:

1. Most cells in early visual cortex are monocular (Hubel and Wiesel, 1965), permitting unambiguous association with the respective eye's stimulus.

2. Strabismic subjects always experience interocular rivalry (rivalry between the eyes) and not figural rivalry (rivalry between two stimuli, parts of which can be distributed in different eyes). They experience rivalry even when both retinas receive congruent stimulation (Holopigian, Blake, and Greenwald, 1988).

3. In strabismic subjects, one eye often develops perceptual dominance (Enoksson, 1968; Von Noorden, 1990). The dominant eye stimulus benefits from a permanent competitive advantage and suppresses the

nondominant eye stimulus. This can be exploited in the present context. Eye dominance can be determined once and then used to predict the outcome of stimulus competition when stimulus selection is not directly assessed (Fries et al., 1997; Fries, Schröder, et al., 2001; Fries et al., 2002).

For these reasons, we examined neuronal correlates of stimulus selection in adult cats that had been made strabismic at 3 weeks of age. We first dichoptically presented gratings moving in opposite directions in the two eyes of the cats (temporonasally for each eye). During 60-second periods of such stimulation, the cats typically developed optokinetic nystagmus (OKN). During rivalry, OKN direction is strongly and reliably correlated with the perceived stimulus (Fox, Todd, and Bettinger, 1975; Logothetis and Schall, 1990). Monocular stimulation always resulted in OKN driven by that stimulus, while dichoptic stimulation with equal contrast for both eyes typically resulted in almost permanent selection of the dominant eye. After determining for each animal which eye was dominant, we implanted the primary visual cortex with up to 34 electrodes. Since the electrodes were implanted on the basis of gross cortical anatomy but without knowledge of the stimulus and ocular selectivities at each site, the first recordings were used to assess each site's preferences for eye and orientation.

As expected in strabismic animals, most sites were monocularly driven by only one of the two eyes (Hubel and Wiesel, 1965). For subsequent recording sessions, we selected groups of eight electrodes (the number of available amplifiers) that preferred stimulation of the same eye and that could be coactivated by a grating of one orientation. To test the effects of perceptual selection during rivalry, we used two stimuli. One was in the preferred eye and of the preferred orientation for the recorded neurons, and was called the "activating stimulus." The other was in the nonpreferred eye and orthogonal to the activating stimulus, and was called the "nonactivating stimulus." Those stimuli were then presented monocularly or dichoptically in randomly interleaved trials while neuronal activity was recorded. The movement direction of the gratings was reversed every 1.5 sec, which was sufficient to avoid eye movements entirely (Fries et al., 2002). The activating and the nonactivating stimuli were turned on either simultaneously or with a relative temporal offset of 3 sec (corresponding to one cycle of the movement direction).

This design allowed us to analyze the effect of stimulus selection or suppression in several different ways. The different paradigms and the results obtained with them are described in the following sections.

## Neurons activated by dominant eye

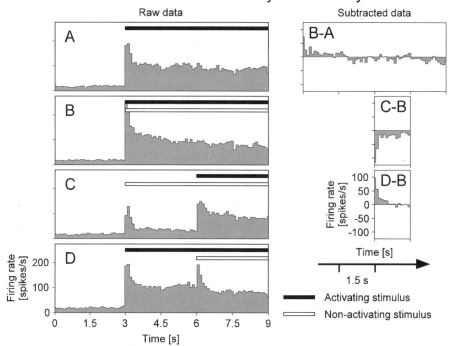

## Neurons activated by non-dominant eye

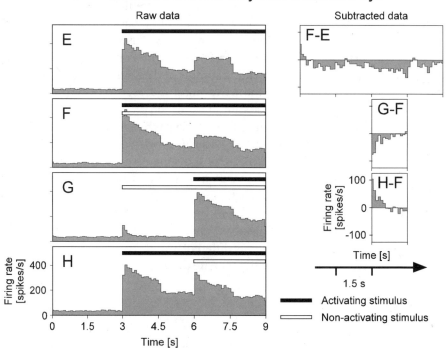

## Selection of an Activating Stimulus in the Dominant Eye

We recorded from neurons activated by the dominant eye and compared monocular stimulation of the dominant eye with dichoptic stimulation. Under both conditions, the stimulus in the dominant eye was the activating stimulus and the one that was perceived. Only when a competing, nonactivating stimulus was presented to the nondominant eye was there active selection of the activating stimulus in the dominant eye. Otherwise, the latter stimulus was the only one present. In figure 14.1, panels A and B show firing rates of primary visual cortex neurons obtained with this paradigm. Panel A shows the firing rate at a recording site in primary visual cortex when an optimally oriented grating stimulus is presented to the dominant eye. The response is strong and sustained throughout the stimulation period. Panel C (3–6 sec) shows the response of the same site when the nondominant eye is presented with an orthogonal but otherwise identical stimulus. There is only a short response to stimulus onset and only a slight elevation of the sustained firing rate. Panel B shows the response when both stimuli are presented simultaneously. During this rivalry condition, the stimulus in the dominant eye, which is the main activating stimulus, has to be selected actively. Despite active stimulus selection, the firing rate stays unchanged relative to monocular stimulation of the dominant eye.

Figure 14.2, panels A and B, shows an analysis of oscillatory neuronal synchronization in the same data set. Panel A shows spike-triggered averages (STAs) of local field potentials (LFPs) for the monocular (gray) and the rivalry (black) conditions. STAs were computed by averaging local field potential traces at ±128 msec around the time of occurrence of spikes. Spikes and LFPs were taken from two electrodes separated by several millimeters but both activated by the stimulus in the dominant eye. The negative LFP deflection peaking just before the spike (time 0) indicates synchronization between neuronal activities at both sites, because LFP negativities reflect neuronal activation. The strong oscillatory modulation of the STAs indicates that synchronization occurs between oscillating neuronal activities. When the activating stimulus is selected during rivalry, oscillatory neuronal synchronization is strongly enhanced. The frequency and strength of oscillatory neuronal synchronization can best be studied

◀ **Figure 14.1**  Examples of firing rate histograms under monocular and rivalry stimulation conditions. Further explanation is in the text.

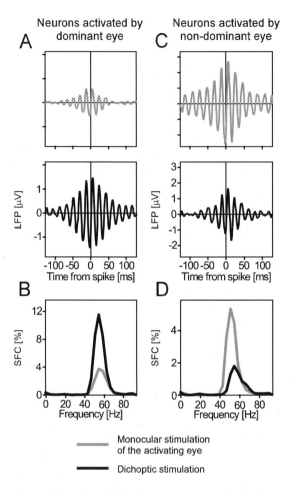

**Figure 14.2** (*A*) and (*B*) show an example of stimulus-selection-related enhancement of gamma-frequency synchronization among neurons activated by the dominant eye. (*C*) and (*D*) show an example of stimulus-suppression-related reduction in gamma-frequency synchronization among neurons activated by the nondominant eye.

by calculating spike-field coherence (SFC) spectra, as shown in panel B. The SFC spectra are the power spectra of the STAs normalized to the average power of the LFP traces used to compile the STAs. SFCs thus reflect synchronization between spikes and LFPs independent of eventual changes in firing rate or spectral content of the LFP. The SFCs show a pronounced peak between 40 and 70 Hz (in the gamma-frequency range, which is strongly enhanced by active stimulus selection).

## Suppression of an Activating Stimulus in the Nondominant Eye

We also recorded from neurons activated by the nondominant eye and compared monocular stimulation of that eye with dichoptic stimulation. In this comparison, for both conditions, the stimulus in the nondominant eye was the activating stimulus. This activating stimulus was perceived under monocular stimulation but was perceptually suppressed when there was a competing nonactivating stimulus in the dominant eye. Figure 14.1, panels E and F, shows the respective firing rates of a site in primary visual cortex. Panel E shows stimulation of the nondominant eye with the optimally oriented grating, leading to a very strong response. The response indicates a slight direction selectivity of the recording site, because movement direction reversals occuring every 1.5 sec modulate the firing rate. Monocular stimulation of the dominant eye with an orthogonal grating, as shown in panel G (3–6 sec), is ineffective in activating this site. When both stimuli are combined to instigate rivalry, the activating stimulus in the nondominant eye is perceptually suppressed. Nevertheless, as shown in panel F, firing rates remain virtually unchanged. In contrast, oscillatory neuronal synchronization is strongly affected. Figure 14.2, panels C and D, shows the STAs and SFCs for the same data set from neurons activated by the nondominant eye. Panel D shows that perceptual suppression of the activating stimulus during rivalry leads to a profound reduction in gamma-frequency synchronization.

While these results establish that gamma-frequency synchronization is a correlate of the selection of an activating stimulus presented to the dominant eye of a strabismic animal, it might be argued that this is a special case and that the situation might be different when selection is due to factors other than strabismic eye dominance. For this reason, we manipulated the relative dominance of the two stimuli by manipulating their relative contrasts or onset timings.

## Selection of a Newly Appearing Stimulus

When a stimulus is introduced into one eye against a stimulus that has already been presented to the other eye for some seconds, the newly appearing stimulus is reliably perceptually selected. This is known as flash suppression (Wolfe, 1984; Sheinberg and Logothetis, 1997; see chapters 11 and 12 in this volume). Thus, we could analyze the first 1.5-sec period after the introduction of an activating stimulus against a nonactivating stimulus that had already been presented to the other eye for 3 sec. This was compared against the first 1.5 sec after simultaneous presentation of activating and nonactivating stimuli in normal rivalry trials. Since this paradigm is explicitly independent of stimulus selection due to strabismic eye dominance, data from neurons activated by either eye can be treated alike. For neurons activated by the dominant eye, figure 14.1, panels B and C, shows the respective firing rates. For neurons activated by the nondominant eye, firing rates are shown in figure 14.1, panels F and G. Overall, the selection of the newly appearing activating stimulus resulted in a slight reduction of firing rates relative to the condition with simultaneous stimulus onsets. By contrast, neuronal gamma-frequency synchronization was enhanced when the activating stimulus was selected. This is demonstrated in figure 14.3, panels A and B.

**Suppression by a Newly Appearing Stimulus**

When a stimulus is introduced to one eye against a preexisting stimulus in the other eye, and therefore selected, the previous stimulus is suppressed. Thus, we can analyze perceptual suppression of an activating stimulus by a temporally delayed nonactivating stimulus and compare the results against normal rivalry trials with simultaneous stimulus onset. Firing rates for those conditions are shown in figures 14.1B and 14.1D for neurons activated by the dominant eye and in figure 14.1F and 14.1H for neurons activated by the nondominant eye. The suppression of an activating stimulus due to the introduction of a novel, nonactivating stimulus led to a slight increase in firing rates. By contrast, gamma-frequency synchronization was reduced when the activating stimulus was suppressed (figures 14.3C and 14.3D).

An earlier study on interocular competition used a very similar stimulation paradigm (Sengpiel and Blakemore, 1994; and see chapter 11 in this volume), but observed firing rate reductions. The animals in Sengpiel's study were anesthetized and paralyzed, and not examined behaviorally before the experiments. We repeated our measurements under general anesthesia in two of our animals with implanted electrodes, and recorded from the same electrodes as in the awake condition. The effects were very similar to those described by Sengpiel, suggesting anesthesia as the main reason for the discrepancy.

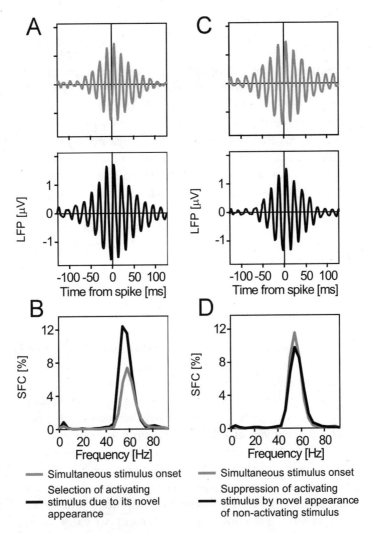

**Figure 14.3** (A) and (B) show an example of enhanced gamma-frequency synchronization among neurons activated by a stimulus that is selected because it has just appeared. (C) and (D) show an example of reduced gamma-frequency synchronization among neurons activated by a stimulus that is suppressed because a nonactivating stimulus has just appeared in the other eye.

The Role of Oscillatory Neuronal Synchronization

## Selection of a High-Contrast Stimulus in the Nondominant Eye

Another powerful parameter to manipulate the relative dominance of a stimulus is its luminance contrast. The luminance contrast of a stimulus is positively correlated with the total duration of time the stimulus is perceptually selected. By placing a high-contrast stimulus into the non-dominant eye and a low-contrast stimulus into the dominant eye, we could effectively render the dominant eye nondominant and vice versa (Fries, Schröder, et al., 2001). We then could repeat the procedures used to study selection and suppression due to strabismic eye dominance, but now with the selection of the high-contrast stimulus rather than the dominant-eye stimulus. The results from those experiments confirm the results from the other paradigms (Fries et al., 2002), showing that gamma-frequency synchronization is enhanced among the neurons activated by the selected stimulus.

## Neuronal Gamma-Frequency Synchronization as a Fundamental Mechanism of Neuronal Group Selection

Taken together, the results suggest that a group of neurons might be selected by synchronizing their respective responses in the gamma-frequency range. Precisely synchronized output of the selected neurons will arrive simultaneously at subsequent processing stages and will therefore have a stronger impact on coincidence-sensitive neurons at the next stage.

This mechanism of selecting a neuronal group seems to be a general mechanism that is not restricted to the case of interocular rivalry. In a related set of experiments, the relation between attentional stimulus selection and neuronal gamma-frequency synchronization was tested (Fries, Reynolds, et al., 2001). Attentional selection exhibits many similarities with stimulus selection during interocular rivalry because it allocates most processing resources to the selected stimulus while other stimuli are ignored or suppressed. Interestingly, neuronal gamma-frequency synchronization is enhanced when one attends to the activating stimulus compared to ignoring it. Thus, modulating gamma-frequency synchronization might be a fundamental mechanism for fast and flexible modulation of the impact of a neuronal group, and thereby for the selection or exclusion of the group.

The finding that neuronal synchronization correlates with stimulus selection during rivalry might be interpreted as a consequence of stronger binding among features of the selected stimulus. To further test this hypothesis, we turned to another bistable phenomenon that has already been described in some detail (see chapter 8 in this volume), the phenomenon of bistable plaid motion perception.

## NEURONAL SYNCHRONIZATION AS A CORRELATE OF PERCEPTUAL SELECTION DURING MOTION RIVALRY

Plaid stimuli provide a tool for investigating neural mechanisms underlying surface segmentation (figure 14.4A). The stimuli are composed of superimposed gratings that move in different directions. Because of the aperture problem, purely local signals lack the information required to disambiguate the motion of the whole grating, and therefore the veridical motion of plaid patterns is perceived as ambiguous (Adelson and Movshon, 1982). This ambiguity can be solved only through processes that group the responses to the same object and integrate across the local motion cues. In the case of plaids, competition processes bias perception toward either component-motion (two transparent surfaces sliding on top of one another) or pattern-motion conditions (two surfaces fused into a single surface).

Bistable plaids are thus ideal for studying the putative mechanisms underlying the binding and perceptual grouping of local features. We tested the hypothesis that perceptual selection between competing pattern- and component-motion conditions could be achieved through synchronization in cat motion-sensitive areas.

Movshon et al. (1985) defined a "conjunction detector" that serves to recombine local vectors through an "intersection of constraints" rule (Fennema and Thompson, 1979). They identified similarity criteria, such as contrast, velocity, and spatial frequency, that could serve as cues for the perceptual binding of surface contours. These rules are quite reminiscent of Gestalt binding criteria, and were extended to the color domain by Krauskopf and Farell (1990) and to the flicker domain by Alais, Blake, and Lee (1998).

When deploying bistable plaids in physiological studies, one must decide whether to use an awake, behaving animal or an anesthetized animal. The awake animal can report perceived direction of motion, but eye movements can complicate neural responses. Extraneous eye movements are less of a problem in anesthetized animals, but it is necessary to use nonambiguous stimuli. The dominant percept (component motion or pattern motion) can be predetermined by exploiting the relation between physical and perceptual rules of transparency (Stoner, Albright, and

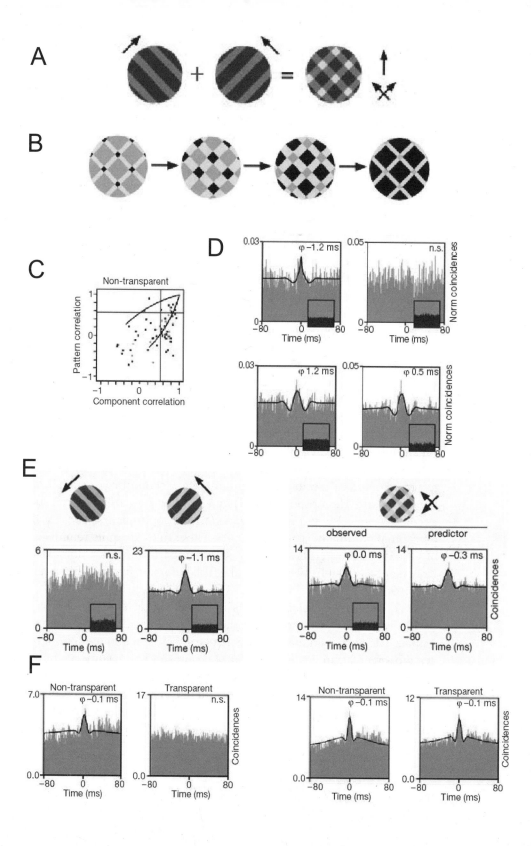

Ramachandran, 1990; Castelo-Branco et al., 2000). In the animal experiments reported below, we manipulated the physical properties of stimuli according to these rules, so that they were perceived as either transparent or nontransparent.

## Neurophysiological Models of Plaid Perception

We have specifically addressed the prediction that neurons responding to contours of the same surface should synchronize more often than neurons responding to contours of different surfaces. Whether both members of a cell pair will respond to the same given surface will depend on transparency conditions, and on how the preferred directions of the cells match the direction of plaid components. The likelihood that the pair is activated by the same surface depends in addition on the RF properties of the cell pairs. If they have overlapping RFs or prefer the same direction of motion or are aligned collinearly, it is very likely that they will always code for the same surface.

To begin, it is worth reviewing some alternative neural models of plaid perception. Movshon et al. (1985) proposed a serial two-stage model for

◀ **Figure 14.4** (*A*) Plaid stimuli, composed of superimposed gratings, elicit two alternative perceptual interpretations. Arrows indicate direction of perceived movements: two global surface vectors for component motion, and one global surface vector for pattern motion. (*B*) A progressive change in duty cycle (by increasing the width of thin bars) induces a change from nontransparent to transparent motion because of a flip in foreground versus background perceptual assignment of grating intersections. (*C*) Scatter plots identifying cells as component-selective (abscissa) or pattern-selective (ordinate) obtained from responses to nontransparent plaids. Continuous lines indicate significance of classification. Cells in upper left and lower right are classified as pattern-selective and component-selective, respectively. Cells outside these regions or inside the curved area are unclassified. For details on methods to compute this classification, see Castelo-Branco et al., 2000. (*D*) Synchronization between neurons with different direction preferences recorded from A18. Top, correlograms of responses evoked by a nontransparent (left) and a transparent (right) plaid moving in a direction intermediate to the cells' preferences. Bottom, correlograms of responses to two other types of nontransparent plaids, defined by distinct local contrasts. (*E*) Component-motion-induced synchrony for PMLS neurons with collinearly oriented overlapping RFs that prefer the same direction of motion. Observed synchrony corresponds to the linear predictor, which estimates synchrony as predicted from summed coincidences obtained from responses to gratings presented in isolation (from Castelo-Branco et al., 2000). (*F*) Dependence of synchrony on the direction of plaid motion and transparency conditions (duty cycle paradigm) for two cell pairs in A18 with discordant (left) and concordant (right) RF configuration. Cross-correlograms were obtained for responses to nontransparent and transparent plaids moving in a direction intermediate between the cells' preferences.

plaid perception in order to explain the computation of pattern motion from local components. This model allowed for the classification of visual neurons into pattern and component motion-sensitive classes. The model is, however, incomplete because it does not incorporate the integration/segregation rules that are necessary to perceptually segregate surfaces at different depth levels.

Another argument against a simple serial model comes from observations in a patient with posterior cortical atrophy (Victor and Conte, 1994) whose perception of motion of a single grating was more severely impaired than perception of plaid motion. The authors took this finding as evidence against a simple feedforward model. This suggests the existence of feature-tracking mechanisms other than those activated by oriented bars (Alais et al., 1996).

A similar argument is suggested by the finding that thresholds for the discrimination of speed or direction are often found to be quite different for single gratings and plaids (Welch, 1989; Victor and Conte, 1994). Since responses of MT neurons are substantially nonlinear, it becomes questionable whether traditional linear partial-correlation models are sufficient to explain neuronal responses. In fact there has been an intensive search for alternative models. Skottun (1999) has, for example, shown that a simple multiplicative rule among the outputs of conventional orientation-selective V1 neurons is sufficient to generate pattern-motion responses in MT neurons.

We have therefore tested whether a model based on synchrony could provide some further insight into the neural basis of plaid perception. A notion that is pivotal in our hypothesis is that pattern- and component-motion conditions are the result of competition between alternative states of coherence.

## Problems with the Definition of Coherence

In the case of random dot kinematograms (RDK), the level of coherence is specified according to the percentage of dots moving in the same direction. Superimposing two dot patterns that are 100% coherent and drifting in different directions produces a stimulus that is perfectly coherent but bidirectional, with a slight depth separation perceived between each dot pattern. This suggests that it may be misleading to label transparent plaid motion as noncoherent. Perception of two gratings moving transparently in fact implies that local responses have been integrated into two assemblies that support the perception of two independent but coherent surfaces. By contrast, a truly noncoherent plaid would imply that one perceives individual, local contours moving in a given direction, not a global surface textured by those contours. As will become evident in the next subsection, this distinction is crucial for any interpretation of neuronal mechanisms involved in surface segmentation and binding.

**Studies of Plaid Perception in Humans and Animals**

We have investigated whether flexible binding of local elements into one or more global surfaces might be implemented by dynamic synchronization or desynchronization of neuronal responses in areas 18 and PMLS of the anesthetized cat (Castelo-Branco et al., 2000). Stimulus transparency was manipulated in two different ways. In the first approach, component gratings were superimposed (figure 14.4A) and the luminance of the gratings' intersections was manipulated to generate either transparent or nontransparent plaids. In the second approach (figure 14.4B), we induced the transition between pattern and component motion, within the same trial, by gradually changing the relative width (duty cycle) of the bars of the gratings. This gradual change in duty cycle is associated with a sudden change of the figure–ground assignment (larger intersections are perceived as background and vice versa). It is the association of nontransparent intersections with the background (figure 14.4B) that induces a concomitant shift between pattern- and component-motion conditions. This procedure is convenient because it allows one to study synchrony within a single trial without major changes in the stimuli's Fourier components, thereby minimizing the likelihood of contrast-induced artifacts.

**Firing Rates Do Not Distinguish Between Pattern- and Component-Motion Conditions in Early Visual Areas**

We have used the method described by Movshon et al. (1985) to determine whether a rate-based linear classifier (figure 14.4C) could separate visual area 18 (A18) and the posteromedial lateral suprasylvian area (PMLS) neurons according to their responses to transparent and nontransparent stimuli. In general, cells are classified as component-selective if the directional tuning curve obtained with plaids correlates with the tuning predicted from summation of the responses to the respective component gratings. Otherwise, cells either are classified as pattern-selective (if the tuning curves obtained with plaids are significantly correlated with those obtained by stimulation with a single grating) or remain unclassified. One would predict that for nontransparent stimuli, more cells should classify as pattern-selective than for transparent stimuli. We found, however, that even for pattern-motion conditions, there was a very clear bias toward cells classified as component-selective (figure 14.4C). This suggests that at least in early visual areas, rate modulations do not correlate with stimulus selection.

### Synchronization as a Mechanism That Tags Responses to the Same Surface

We have hypothesized that neurons should synchronize if they respond to contours of the same surface, irrespective of whether responses are evoked by the pattern-motion or the component-motion condition. Synchronization should occur more often in the pattern-motion than in the component-motion condition for those neuron pairs whose members respond to different surfaces in the component-motion conditions. This is the case, for example, when the units in a cell pair each have a different directional preference that matches the direction of motion of one of the two component gratings. If they are activated by an appropriately oriented plaid stimulus, they should synchronize in the pattern-motion, but not in the component-motion, condition. An example of such a constellation is shown for an A18–PMLS pair in figure 14.4D. The cross-correlograms in the two bottom and left top panels show a significant synchronization peak. The respective responses were elicited by three different versions of nontransparent stimuli that differed in local contrast but moved in a direction intermediate to the ones preferred by the respective cells. In contrast, responses did not synchronize when they were evoked by a transparent stimulus (top right).

As mentioned above, synchronization probability should depend not only on transparency conditions but also on the configuration of the respective RFs. Accordingly, we have found that transparency-dependent changes in synchrony were more likely to occur for pairs whose RFs differed not only with respect to direction preference but also with respect to overlap and collinearity ($p \ll 0.01$, ANOVA).

We have often observed oscillatory synchrony in responses to single gratings moving in directions intermediate to those preferred by the respective cell groups, which is in agreement with the data reported above on binocular rivalry (see also Castelo-Branco, Neuenschwander, and Singer, 1998). However, an oscillatory patterning of responses was less frequent for moving plaids, even though synchrony was preserved. At present it is unclear why oscillations are more pronounced with single gratings than with the more complex plaid stimuli.

### Neuronal Synchrony Is Preserved Under Component-Motion Conditions If Neurons Respond to the Same Transparent Surface

As discussed above, transparent plaids can be considered as two coherent stimuli. In this condition, two assemblies of motion-selective cells, each responding to one of the two surfaces, should emerge.

According to our hypothesis, what determines whether cells respond or do not respond to the same surface is their RF configuration. If cells have a collinear arrangement of their RFs and prefer similar directions of motion, then they should exhibit synchrony for a grating moving in that direction, and synchrony should be maintained even when another transparent grating is superimposed.

Using a linear predictor, one can test to what extent the responses to the respective gratings predict the responses to the plaid. This is illustrated in figure 14.4E for a cell pair whose responses are not expected to desynchronize under component-motion conditions. PMLS neurons with collinearly aligned overlapping RFs that prefer the same direction of motion show the same amount of synchrony to the plaid as is predicted from the summed synchronicity in the responses to the individual gratings presented alone.

Thiele and Stoner (2003) analyzed plaid responses in awake monkeys performing passive fixation. The general result was that if data from pairs of cells are pooled, no clear relation exists between neuronal synchrony and the transparency condition. These results need not contradict our findings and conclusions, because experimental conditions and the tested hypothesis were very different. In the cited study, responses were compared only between transparent and nontransparent conditions, and the authors assumed that transparent plaids are totally noncoherent.

A further complicating factor in Thiele and Stoner's (2003) study is that selective attention probably played an important role. In the case of the depth-ordered (with a bright foreground grating) stimulus, the animal followed this foreground grating in at least 97% of the trials (and neglected the dark background grating). Thus, the animal signaled to perceive a single coherent surface moving in a single direction. By contrast, for the "coherent" nontransparent plaid, only 66% of the eye movements were in pattern direction, suggesting that the animal perceived this stimulus as less coherent. If this was the perception of the animal, Thiele and Stoner's data actually support our results because synchrony was higher with depth-ordered plaids than with pattern motion.

## Examining Changes in Plaid Evoked Neuronal Responses Within a Trial

The duty cycle paradigm described in figure 14.4B introduces changes in transparency conditions by manipulating physical parameters other than local luminance or contrast. Furthermore, the change occurs gradually over a trial, which allows one to study dynamic changes in synchrony in a more realistic manner.

The two right panels of figure 14.4F show that synchrony is present for a pair of units in area A18, under both transparent and nontransparent conditions. Both units had similar direction preferences and collinearly aligned overlapping RFs. They were therefore likely always to respond to the same surface.

The two panels on the left show, for two A18 pairs with differing directional tuning, that synchrony was present only for nontransparent conditions. Time-resolved analysis of changes in synchrony revealed a significant drop to nonsignificant levels under transparent conditions.

We believe that the duty cycle paradigm is of special interest in the context of behavioral animal studies, since it allows for the generation of predictable perceptual changes over time, and hence for a tight correlation between perception and neural activity patterns.

## An fMRI Study on the Perception of Bistable Plaids

It would be very interesting to directly correlate neuronal activity to behavioral reports of changing plaid perception while physical stimulation remains constant. Accordingly, we applied the fMRI technique to identify the neural correlates of plaid perception. In particular, we were interested in investigating whether changes in activity patterns in specific cortical areas could be correlated with simple model assumptions on activity shifts within a motion coherence map. Ambiguous plaid stimuli elicit bistable perceptual transitions between integration (one-surface, pattern-motion) and segmentation (two-surfaces, component-motion) processes.

One interpretation of this perceptual switch is based on the notion of activity shifts within a motion coherence map. The assumption is that there exists a map for global motion in hMT+/V5, which is similar to the one hypothesized for monkey MT (DeAngelis and Newsome, 1999). Each part of the map contains populations of neurons preferring the same direction of global motion, and in some cases also a preferred stimulus depth. This organization is thought to resemble the columnar organization of other visual areas. When one perceives component motion with bistable plaids, then two moving surfaces should be simultaneously represented in the motion coherence map. This would predict the existence of two active direction-selective clusters of neurons in hMT+/V5. Pattern-motion perception should then be associated with only one active neural population that represents the global motion of the perceived single surface. Perception of two surfaces should then result in more hMT+/V5 activity than perception of one surface, because in the latter case two populations of neurons are active instead of one.

Our recent fMRI data on plaid perception (Castelo-Branco et al., 2002) show that there is indeed a positive gradient of activity levels in hMT+/V5 depending on the number of surfaces perceived by the subjects ($P < 0.0001$ for component vs. pattern in left and right hMT+/V5, and $P < 0.01$ for left V3/V3A, ANOVA). These results were first obtained for unambiguous stimuli but then generalized to ambiguous bistable conditions.

The neuronal network activated by perceptual switches of either ambiguous or unambiguous plaids included hMT+/V5 as a pivotal area (figure 14.5A; plate 5). This area showed increased activity when subjects perceived two surfaces instead of one (figure 14.5B), which is consistent with two assemblies being active in the former case instead of just one. We found a very robust convergence of results obtained with a general linear model and a data-driven approach (independent-component analysis, which has the advantage of not imposing any a priori model on the data).

Interestingly, the higher activity observed for component-motion conditions was modulated by selective attention. Specifically, if the subjects had to attend continuously to a plaid feature (angle task, during which subjects had to compare plaid angle and fixation cross angles), then there was a significant difference between activity elicited by component and pattern motion in hMT+/V5 (figure 14.5C). If attention was not focused on plaids (color task, during which subjects compared the color of the fixation cross with the color of the aperture line), this difference vanished.

In summary, our fMRI results suggest that perceptual switches generate differential activation of hMT+/V5, and that those switches are associated with a rearrangement of the activity of cell ensembles in a motion coherence map within this area.

A

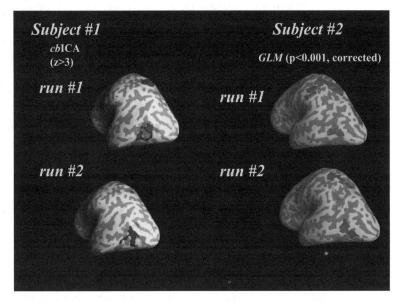

B

C

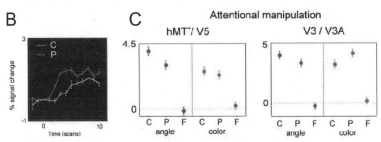

**Figure 14.5** (A) The sensorimotor network activated by perceptual switches of ambiguous plaids includes hMT+/V5 and the hand motor area (perceptual reports were indicated by finger button presses). This network is revealed both by GLM (general linear model) and cortex-based ICA (independent component analysis). Note the similar dynamics across subjects and across runs, regardless of whether GLM or ICA analysis was applied. (B) Motion responses in hMT+/V5 to an ambiguous stimulus as compared to a common rest baseline (nonrest baselines suffer from possible buildup of adaptation phenomena, as well as from the occurrence of irregular perceptual switches). The response associated with perception of component motion is significantly higher than the response associated with the perception of pattern motion ($p < 0.0001$, paired t-test) (adapted from Castelo-Branco et al., 2002). (C) Average group activity in hMT+/V5 and V3/V3A in an experiment that included different tasks manipulating attention (color and angle tasks). In the angle task, which requires subjects to pay equal attention to both pattern and component conditions, the response to component motion in hMT+/V5 was significantly higher than the response to pattern motion (ANOVA and post hoc tests, $p = 0.02$, for comparison between component and pattern motion response). C, component stimulus; P, pattern stimulus; F, fixation. See plate 5 for color version.

## CONCLUSIONS

Taken together, our human and animal data show that the neuronal processes underlying bistable percepts of global surfaces probably involve dynamic reconfiguration of cell assemblies. The reported neurophysiological results suggest that segmentation and binding of local motion cues into surfaces occur through synchronization of the responses of neurons to contours associated with the same surface. Active desynchronization may occur when neurons start responding to contours of different surfaces. Our fMRI study suggested that activity changes in hMT+/V5 reflect perceptual switches involving differential binding of stimulus components moving in different directions. Future studies should clarify the role of selective attention and adaptation mechanisms in modulating such processes.

## REFERENCES

Adelson, E. H., and Movshon, J. A. (1982). Phenomenal coherence of moving visual patterns. *Nature, 300,* 523–525.

Alais, D., Blake, R., and Lee, S. H. (1998). Visual features that vary together over time group together over space. *Nature Neuroscience, 1,* 160–164.

Alais, D., Van der Smagt, M. J., et al. (1996). Monocular mechanisms determine plaid motion coherence. *Vision Neuroscience, 13,* 615–626.

Alonso, J. M., Usrey, W. M., and Reid, R. C. (1996). Precisely correlated firing in cells of the lateral geniculate nucleus. *Nature, 383,* 815–819.

Azouz, R., and Gray, C. M. (2000). Dynamic spike threshold reveals a mechanism for synaptic coincidence detection in cortical neurons in vivo. *Proceedings of the National Academy of Sciences of the United States of America, 97,* 8110–8115.

Castelo-Branco, M., Formisano, E., et al. (2002). Activity patterns in human motion-sensitive areas depend on the interpretation of global motion. *Proceedings of the National Academy of Sciences of the United States of America, 99,* 13914–13919.

Castelo-Branco, M., Goebel, R., Neuenschwander, S., and Singer, W. (2000). Neural synchrony correlates with surface segregation rules. *Nature, 405,* 685–689.

Castelo-Branco, M., Neuenschwander, S., and Singer, W. (1998). Synchronization of visual responses between the cortex, lateral geniculate nucleus, and retina in the anesthetized cat. *Journal of Neuroscience, 18,* 6395–6410.

DeAngelis, G. C., and Newsome, W. T. (1999). Organization of disparity-selective neurons in macaque area MT. *Journal of Neuroscience, 19,* 1398–1415.

De Oliveira, S. C., Thiele, A., and Hoffmann, K. P. (1997). Synchronization of neuronal activity during stimulus expectation in a direction discrimination task. *Journal of Neuroscience, 17,* 9248–9260.

Enoksson, P. (1968). Studies in optokinetic binocular rivalry with a new device. *Acta Ophthalmologica* (Copenhagen), 46, 71–74.

Fennema, C. L., and Thompson, W. B. (1979). Velocity determination in scenes containing several moving objects. *Computer Graphics and Image Processing*, 9, 301–315.

Fox, R., Todd, S., and Bettinger, L. A. (1975). Optokinetic nystagmus as an objective indicator of binocular rivalry. *Vision Research*, 15, 849–853.

Fries, P., Reynolds, J. H., Rorie, A. E., and Desimone, R. (2001). Modulation of oscillatory neuronal synchronization by selective visual attention. *Science*, 291, 1560–1563.

Fries, P., Roelfsema, P. R., Engel, A. K., König, P., and Singer, W. (1997). Synchronization of oscillatory responses in visual cortex correlates with perception in interocular rivalry. *Proceedings of the National Academy of Sciences of the United States of America*, 94, 12699–12704.

Fries, P., Schröder, J. H., Roelfsema, P. R., Singer, W., and Engel, A. K. (2002). Oscillatory neuronal synchronization in primary visual cortex as a correlate of stimulus selection. *Journal of Neuroscience*, 22, 3739–3754.

Fries, P., Schröder, J., Singer, W., and Engel, A. K. (2001). Conditions of perceptual selection and suppression during interocular rivalry in strabismic and normal cats. *Vision Research*, 41, 771–783.

Holopigian, K., Blake, R., and Greenwald, M. J. (1988). Clinical suppression and amblyopia. *Investigative Ophthalmology and Visual Science*, 29, 444–451.

Hubel, D. H., and Wiesel, T. N. (1965). Binocular interaction in striate cortex of kittens reared with artificial squint. *Journal of Neurophysiology*, 28, 1041–1059.

Krauskopf, J., and Farell, B. (1990). Influence of colour on the perception of coherent motion. *Nature*, 348, 328–331.

Leopold, D. A., and Logothetis, N. K. (1996). Activity changes in early visual cortex reflect monkeys' percepts during binocular rivalry. *Nature*, 379, 549–553.

Logothetis, N. K., and Schall, J. D. (1990). Binocular motion rivalry in macaque monkeys: Eye dominance and tracking eye movements. *Vision Research*, 30, 1409–1419.

Movshon, J. A., Adelson, E. H., Gizzi, M. S., and Newsome, W. T. (1985). The analysis of moving visual patterns. In *Pattern Recognition Mechanisms*, C. Chagas, R. Gattass, and C. Gross, eds., 117–151. New York: Springer-Verlag.

Salinas, E., and Sejnowski, T. J. (2000). Impact of correlated synaptic input on output firing rate and variability in simple neuronal models. *Journal of Neuroscience*, 20, 6193–6209.

Salinas, E., and Sejnowski, T. J. (2001). Correlated neuronal activity and the flow of neural information. *Nature Reviews: Neuroscience*, 2, 539–550.

Sengpiel, F., and Blakemore, C. (1994). Interocular control of neuronal responsiveness in cat visual cortex. *Nature*, 368, 847–850.

Sheinberg, D. L., and Logothetis, N. K. (1997). The role of temporal cortical areas in perceptual organization. *Proceedings of the National Academy of Sciences of the United States of America*, 94, 3408–3413.

Skottun, B. C. (1999). Neuronal responses to plaids. *Vision Research, 39*, 2151–2156.

Stoner, G. R., Albright, T. D., and Ramachandran, V. S. (1990). Transparency and coherence in human motion perception. *Nature, 344*, 153–155.

Thiele, A., and Stoner, G. (2003). Synchrony does not underlie motion coherence in area MT. *Nature, 421*, 366–370.

Victor, J. D., and Conte, M. M. (1994). Investigation of a patient with severely impaired direction discrimination: Evidence against the intersection-of-constraints model. *Vision Research, 34*, 267–277.

Von Noorden, G. K. (1990). *Binocular Vision and Ocular Motility: Theory and Management of Strabismus*. St. Louis: Mosby.

Welch, L. (1989). The perception of moving plaids reveals two motion-processing stages. *Nature, 337*, 734–736.

Wolfe, J. M. (1984). Reversing ocular dominance and suppression in a single flash. *Vision Research, 24*, 471–478.

# 15  Perceptual Rivalry as an Ultradian Oscillation

## J. D. Pettigrew and O. L. Carter

Perceptual rivalry alternations are switches in perception that occur despite a constant, if ambiguous, sensory input. While being clearly and predictably influenced by the "external" rivalry-inducing stimulus (Levelt, 1965; Mueller and Blake, 1989), these internally driven changes in perceptual state also exhibit rhythmic properties (Carter and Pettigrew, 2003). It is this endogenously driven, externally influenceable nature of perceptual rivalry that has motivated the following comparison with the self-sustaining circadian oscillations of biological systems, despite the significant differences in periodicity.

Research into binocular rivalry and related bistable phenomena has largely focused on the mechanisms of suppression and awareness, with less consideration being directed toward the nature of the "switch" that drives the alternations in visual awareness. While the timing of the switches has been the subject of a number of studies (Borsellino et al., 1972; Walker, 1975; Lehky, 1995), the switches themselves are generally considered to be a consequence of a reciprocal inhibition between competing neural populations (Blake, 1989; Wilson, Blake, and Lee, 2001), with even the term "rivalry" implying direct competition. However, the observation that one can extend or truncate either suppression or dominance phase durations independently, through appropriate manipulation of the stimulus (Levelt, 1965; Sobel and Blake, 2002), raises questions about the envisaged nature of such "reciprocal" interactions.

Presented here is the thesis that binocular rivalry reflects the workings of an ultradian oscillator (an endogenously driven biological rhythm with a period of less than 24 hr). A key implication of this proposal is that the perceptual switches characteristic of rivalry are themselves generated by an oscillatory mechanism external to the level of perceptual representation. Previously proposed by Pöppel (1994), this is not a novel concept, but one that is being presented here with renewed vigor. While this is not the generally accepted viewpoint, a number of lines of recent evidence support the idea that the perceptual alternations and the relevant reciprocal interactions are driven by such an oscillatory mechanism (Pettigrew, 2001). Furthermore, since binocular rivalry is becoming increasingly linked to other forms of bistable and multistable visual phenomena (Carter and Pettigrew, 2003; Hupé and Rubin, 2003; see chapter 8 in this volume), and binocular rivalry is itself now being viewed as a process involving multiple brain regions (Blake and Logothetis, 2002), this proposal of a common oscillator for all forms of perceptual rivalry would seem well suited to unify and explain the present conglomeration of experimental results.

The thesis that perceptual rivalry alternations represent a form of ultradian oscillation was partly inspired by interactions at Caltech in the 1970s between one of the authors and Richard Feynman. Feynman conjectured, along with his friend David McDermott, that the brain might have a master oscillator, like the "clock" in a modern computer, which was responsible for coordinating all its rhythmic operations (e.g., Feynman, 1999). One corollary of Feynman's conjecture is that timing should be linked at different levels of scale. In line with this, our suggestion is that perceptual rivalries exhibit ultradian rhythms that can be linked to circadian rhythms, despite their different periodicities.

The notion of perceptual rivalry as an ultradian biological oscillation is not widely accepted (see Pöppel, 1994), but many of the difficulties in accepting this idea are similar to the objections that were raised originally with regard to circadian oscillations. In this chapter we will discuss evidence from several sources supporting the idea that the periods of perceptual rivalry rhythms reflect an underlying biological oscillator. Among these are the following:

1. Rivalry alternations look more regular and more like "free-running" biological oscillations when care is taken to minimize the potential "jitter" caused by *Zeitgebers* (literally, "time givers"; the term *Zeitgebers* will be used, in line with the biological rhythms literature, to refer to phase-shifting stimuli).

2. Despite considerable intraindividual stability, the rhythms of perceptual rivalries exhibit wide interindividual variation (over a more than tenfold range), similar to observed variations in circadian rhythms (Kerkhof, 1985).

3. The phase of a rivalry rhythm can be advanced or retarded in a manner analogous to the effects on circadian rhythms of *Zeitgebers*, such as light.

4. Twin studies show that rivalry rhythms have high heritability but must involve a very large number of genes.

5. The seconds-long cycles of perceptual rivalry rhythms appear to be driven by subcortical interhemispheric oscillators (for review, see Pettigrew, 2001) such as the suprachiasmatic nucleus, the daylong circadian oscillator that was also recently shown to be an interhemispheric oscillator (De la Iglesia et al., 2000).

## FEATURES OF CIRCADIAN RHYTHMS

The following discussion will pursue the relationship between circadian and perceptual rivalry oscillations by detailing the principal features of circadian rhythms mentioned above and examining the extent to which they can be applied to the ultradian rhythms of perceptual rivalry.

### The "Free-Running" Rivalry Period

Many consider it unlikely that relatively irregular rivalry rhythms have an affinity with circadian rhythms when the latter repeat themselves so regularly. In the absence of any *Zeitgebers*, free-running circadian rhythms have a regularity of minutes in 24 hr (< 0.1%). The problem here may be that the changes in the visual system induced by rivalry stimuli have a dual role as both input and output in perceptual rivalry studies. This is in stark contrast to characteristics of circadian rhythms, such as core body temperature (Refinetti and Menaker, 1992) and melatonin levels (Lewy et al., 1980), that can easily be measured in the absence of light cues. The action of this changing visual input may be to constantly reset the rivalry rhythm despite the fact that the ambiguous stimulus itself is held constant (elaborated below in the section on *Zeitgebers*). Such an influence of external factors, however, should not be considered as evidence against the role of an intrinsic oscillator. For example, a jet-setter constantly changing time zones will show an irregularity of circadian period that is not a true reflection of the highly reproducible circadian rhythm obtained when the influence of *Zeitgebers* is removed. If rivalry depends on the visual system for both input and output, it is impossible to consider the perceptual rhythms in isolation from the phase-shifting *Zeitgebers* in a manner equivalent to the light-controlled environments used to study circadian rhythms.

A crucial point here is that the same *Zeitgeber* has a completely different magnitude of effect, according to its timing, relative to the phase of rhythm. For example, there is a much greater effect of light at times when light is normally absent. If this also applies to rivalry, we would expect visual stimulation to act as a *Zeitgeber* that would vary in its effect according to the rhythm's phase, even though the stimulation was being held constant. A number of observations support this thesis of an underlying oscillator for perceptual rivalry whose stochastic qualities are a consequence of phase-dependent *Zeitgeber*-like interactions with the visual input.

First, if individual rivalry rhythms are measured under controlled conditions that recognize the possibility of phase-shifting inputs such as alterations in stimulus intensity, and great care is taken to reproduce the stimulus conditions exactly (with respect to image size, contrast, luminance, and even the testing procedure and location), test–retest reliability is 85% for the binocular rivalry rate of an individual (see figure 15.1) (Pettigrew and Miller, 1998). This level of reliability is impressively high for a psychometric measure, and it is also true for the rate of alternation of Bonneh's motion-induced blindness (MIB) (Bonneh, Cooperman, and Sagi, 2001), a perceptual oscillation shown to share remarkable temporal similarities with binocular rivalry (Carter, 2001; for an example of MIB, see www.weizmann.ac.il/~masagi/MIB/mib.html).

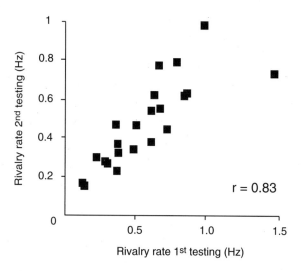

**Figure 15.1** Stability in time of perceptual rivalry rate when stimulus conditions are held constant. Selected data on binocular rivalry rate from 22 individuals, all measured over a period of years, using the same testing apparatus and in the same testing room (Pettigrew and Miller, 1998). Note the remarkable stability of rivalry rate in each individual, despite the interindividual variation.

J. D. Pettigrew and O. L. Carter

These two phenomena were thought to be distantly related only because each involves "suppression" of a stimulus that is continuously present. Our study suggests, however, that they may be united more fundamentally by a common oscillatory mechanism (Carter and Pettigrew, 2003). The proposal that a common oscillator may underlie all forms of perceptual rivalry has been further reinforced by the demonstration that plaid stimuli, a third kind of rivalry involving ambiguous motion, shares a number of temporal characteristics with binocular rivalry (Hupé and Rubin, 2002, 2003; see chapter 8 in this volume).

Second, extremely regular rivalry rhythms can be revealed by specific manipulations that appear to change the way in which visual input influences the oscillator. Perhaps the most extraordinary effect of this kind is the increased regularity of rivalry alternations that can be seen in the "rebound phase" after administration of hallucinogenic drugs such as LSD (Carter and Pettigrew, 2003) and psilocybin (Vollenweider, Hasler, Carter and Pettigrew, unpublished observations). This increased regularity, with multiple harmonically distributed modes, vividly suggests an underlying oscillator that the drug has revealed, conceivably, by reducing the impact of the "jitter" caused by visual input. This "harmonic oscillator" effect is seen in figure 15.2, where we show that it is exactly comparable in two different kinds of perceptual rivalry, Bonneh's MIB and binocular rivalry. Work is continuing to try to unravel the mechanism of this striking increase in the regularity of the rivalry rhythm in subjects under the influence of these drugs. In the meantime, whatever the mode of action, the fact that the same drug can reveal an underlying harmonic oscillator in two different kinds of perceptual rivalry provides support for the thesis that perceptual rivalry represents an ultradian oscillation.

### Interindividual Variability of Period

The circadian cycle typically runs over a period of 24 hr. However, in controlled environments—where the influence of *Zietgabers* is minimized, there is a considerable degree of interindividual variability in "free-running" circadian cycles (for review, see Kerkhof, 1985). The described range of circadian cycles is less than that described for rivalry cycles; however, the sample size is also smaller because measurement of this cycle is dependent on the subject spending many days within a light- and temperature-controlled environment. Nasal cycles in humans (another ultradian rhtythm that depends on the retrochiasmatic nucleus) vary from

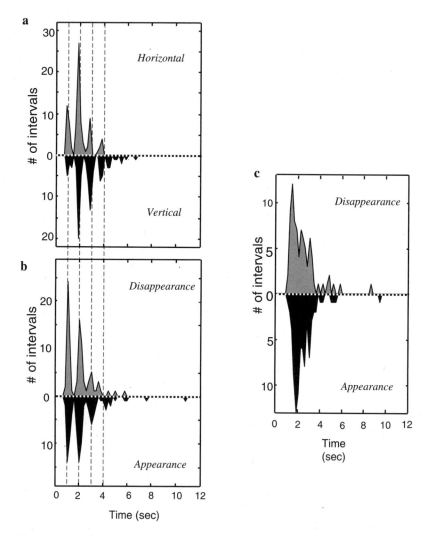

**Figure 15.2** A harmonic rivalry oscillator revealed by LSD. The existence of an underlying oscillator is strongly suggested by the greatly increased regularity in the phase durations and harmonic modes observed for a subject who had taken LSD 10 hr prior to being tested. The frequency histograms show (*a*) the distribution of dominance phase durations for periods lasting between 0 and 12 sec for binocular rivalry (gray = horizontal, black = vertical) and (*b*) for MIB (gray = appearance, black = disappearance); (*c*) shows the frequency histogram corresponding to phase durations reported for MIB by the same subject retested 2 mos later, when the subject was not under the influence of LSD (figure from Carter and Pettigrew 2003).

J. D. Pettigrew and O. L. Carter

20 min to 10 hours. This interindividual variability is similarly observed in the period of perceptual rivalry cycles, where there is an approximately tenfold variation between individuals (Pettigrew and Miller, 1998; also see figure 15.1). Furthermore, while both long-period and short-period circadian mutants are known, naturally occurring long-period mutants are more common. Similarly, the frequency distribution of individual rivalry periods is not normal but is skewed toward faster rhythms, with an extended tail toward slower periods.

It has been customary in the field, with a few exceptions (e.g., Leopold et al., 2002), to ignore these interindividual differences in rhythms through a process of "normalization" in which phase durations are represented, not in absolute terms but as a fraction of the mean phase duration. Even when data are normalized within observers, the results are rarely, if ever, considered in respect to interindividual variation.

### *Zeitgeber* Sensitivity Can Show Phase Dependence

The sensitivity of circadian rhythms to *Zeitgebers* is phase-dependent, with greater sensitivity observed at times when the relevant *Zeitgeber* stimulus is absent or low. This property is evident in the example of the circadian oscillator of the single-cell organism *Gonyaulax* (figure 15.3). The circadian cycle of this organism governs photosynthesis on the surface of the ocean during the day, and at night nitrogenous resources are harvested from the ocean depths (Roenneberg and Mittag, 1996). *Gonyaulax* has a precisely determined circadian cycle. If the *Gonyaulax* is deprived of nitrogen during the night, a late encounter with nitrogen will cause it to delay its ascent (Roenneberg and Rehman, 1996). In contrast to the earlier cycles, where continuously present nitrogen has no effect upon the circadian rhythm, this fourth cycle (shown in figure 15.3) is phase-delayed by the late encounter with nitrogen.

This example also illustrates the importance of oscillation in dealing with ambiguity. The late encounter of the nitrogenous resource does not result in a compromise in behavior, but in a phase delay of the switch from "stay" to "ascend." In respect to the human circadian cycle, similar phase-specific effects of light can be observed. Under constant "free-running" environmental conditions, light pulses presented against a background of constant darkness can cause shifts in the phase of these rhythms when presented during the animal's subjective night, but not during the subjective day (Minors, Waterhouse, and Wirz-Justice, 1991).

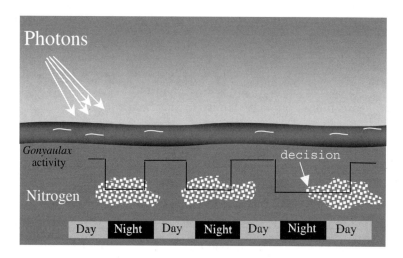

**Figure 15.3** Adaptability of the circadian oscillator of the single-cell organism *Gonyaulax*. During the day the circadian cycle of *Gonyaulax* governs photosynthesis on the surface of the ocean, and during the night nitrogenous resources are harvested from the ocean depths. Note that *Gonyaulax* has a precisely determined circadian cycle, as shown by the first three cycles of daytime surface activity and nocturnal descents. Of great interest to the present discussion about biological oscillators, both circadian and ultradian, is the "decision" faced by *Gonyaulax* in the third cycle illustrated, when no nitrogenous resources are encountered until dawn, the time for the organism to return to the surface. This "decision point" is marked by an arrow. Will *Gonyaulax* delay its ascent to take advantage of the resource, or should the precision of the circadian clock determine the outcome by forcing the organism to return to the surface? The phase shift in the clock that is illustrated here shows the adaptability of the circadian rhythm, even in this simple organism.

A set of experiments conducted by Leopold and colleagues (2002) showed the effectiveness of brief, intermittent stimulus exposure in increasing the duration of one phase of perceptual rivalry. In this study it was found that if a rivalrous stimulus (for example, a Necker cube or an ambiguously rotating sphere) was periodically removed for 5 sec, the individual's perceptual state could be maintained for prolonged periods, and in some cases perceptual alternations were prevented entirely. These results were reported to be evidence against an oscillator; however, reconsideration of the data shows otherwise. Specifically, a predictable relationship was found to exist between the individual's rivalry rate (during uninterrupted stimulus presentation) and the probability that the same individual will experience a perceptual alternation during intermittent exposure of the stimulus (figure 15.4). Under the intermittent condition (the stimulus with 5-sec blank periods), the individuals who showed the

J. D. Pettigrew and O. L. Carter

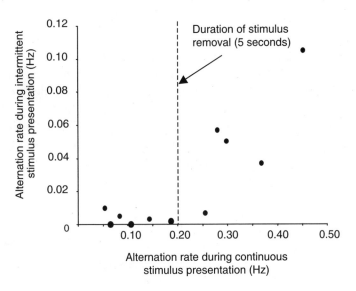

**Figure 15.4**  Replotted data from the "increased persistence" experiments of Leopold et al. (2002). For subjects who have fast rivalry switch rates (those on the right side of the dotted line), there is a linear relation between the rivalry rate under normal conditions and the rivalry rate during intermittent exposure. As indicated by the dotted line, this linear relationship intersects the x-axis at approximately 0.2 Hz (one switch per 5 sec). These results were claimed by the authors to be evidence against the involvement of an oscillator. However, when one considers the potential phase-shifting effects of intermittent stimulus exposure, the finding that perceptual "stabilization" (after removal of the stimulus for 5 sec) occurred predominantly in individuals who normally required a period of more than 5 sec to switch, is compatible with the current thesis that there is an underlying oscillator driving perceptual rivalry.

greatest degree of stabilization were those with an average phase duration of more than 5 sec (0.2 Hz). This finding is exactly what would be predicted if rivalry alternations were driven by an endogenous oscillator that can be "phase-shifted" by late-phase stimuli in the manner we are proposing.

### *Zeitgebers* Shift Phase of Perceptual Oscillation

Mammalian circadian rhythms are known to be driven by a network of endogenously oscillating neurons within the suprachiasmatic nucleus (Meijer and Rietveld, 1989). This bilateral nucleus is generally assumed to be synchronously active on both sides, but evidence shows that interhemispheric coordination of the paired nuclei can be asynchronous, or even 180° out of phase (De la Iglesia et al., 2000). The significance of interhemispheric circadian rhythms is yet to be fully elucidated, but this finding is consistent with the claim that binocular rivalry switching is associated with interhemispheric switching (Pettigrew, 2001).

As mentioned above, external cues such as light and temperature influence the durations of the respective phases of the circadian cycles, with exposure to bright light during the early day advancing the circadian rhythm and exposure to the same light stimulus in the evening delaying the rhythm (for review, see Van Esseveldt, Lehman, and Boer, 2000). In contrast to the detailed knowledge about the phase-shifting effects of *Zeitgebers* on the circadian cycle, information is still emerging about the influence of different stimuli on relative phases of binocular rivalry rhythms. For example, until recently it was generally accepted that manipulating the "strength" of one of the rivaling figures through increases in motion (Breese, 1909), contrast (Mueller and Blake, 1989), or spatial frequency (Fahle, 1982) will affect its overall predominance, not by prolonging its dominance phase but by reducing its suppression phase duration. (This is known as Levelt's second proposition; see Levelt, 1965, and chapters 8 and 17 of this volume.)

However, work by Sobel and Blake (2002) shows that the duration of dominance of one of the rivaling alternatives can also be increased directly by appropriate manipulations of the contextual salience of that phase (i.e., adding contextual cues can disproportionately enhance the global "significance" of one of the rivalry targets). The phase-shifting effects of *Zeitgebers* depend upon the phase in which they are applied. The new experiments showing these "anti-Levelt" effects provide evidence that rivalry is likewise phase-sensitive. This is particularly so if one considers MIB, where there is a simpler possible interpretation of phase than in binocular rivalry, where there is potential double confound (right eye "ON" is not, strictly speaking, synchronous with left eye "OFF," even if reciprocity is usually assumed). Plaid rivalry also reinforces the importance of pinning down phase, with the result that contextual effects can be more firmly attributed to one phase and the prediction that the effect might be reversed at the opposite phase. A detailed study of such context-specific reversals has been submitted for publication (Carter et al., submitted).

A possible unifying theme in the complicated interpretation of phase relations in biological rhythms is the idea that all may be interhemispheric rhythms, with each phase corresponding to the dominance of a different hemisphere. Since each hemisphere exhibits well-recognized asymmetries in function (Nicholls, 1996; Tzourio et al., 1998; Perry et al., 2001) and "cognitive styles" (Ramachandran, 1994), this phase-hemisphere correspondence could help elucidate phase changes. For example, in the case of

J. D. Pettigrew and O. L. Carter

Bonneh's MIB, the disappearance phase can be reliably linked to the activity of the left hemisphere by experiments using transcranial magnetic stimulation (TMS), and similar experiments link the appearance phase to activity of the right hemisphere (Pettigrew and Funk, 2001). This assignment is in line with the left hemisphere's "cognitive style" to ignore discrepancies (i.e., the stationary disks in the same depth plane and in complementary yellow color) with the main hypothesis (the moving 3-D cloud of blue dots). The return of the yellow disks, in contrast, is consonant with the right hemisphere's style to highlight discrepancies. In this case, the phase effects are particularly clear. Perhaps this approach will also illuminate the context versus stimulus strength problem of phase in other perceptual rivalries. In any case, if due regard is paid to the difficulty of identifying the phase of perceptual rivalry, it is clear that stimulus conditions can shift the phase of perceptual rivalry just as they can shift the phase of a circadian rhythm.

## High Heritability of Period—Multiple Genes

An increasing number of "circadian clock" genes have been discovered since the initial discovery of the *per* gene in *Drosophila* (Konopka and Benzer, 1971). While review of this literature is beyond the scope of this chapter (for review, see Helfrich-Förster, 1996), a number of features of circadian-rhythm genetics are relevant to the present comparison with rivalry rhythms. First, even though there is much to learn about how the many "clock genes" contribute to the generation of stable, $\sim$24 hr rhythms, there is overwhelming evidence that the circadian period is highly heritable. Studies of twins, still in progress, reveal that the period of the binocular rivalry rhythm is highly heritable, with monozygotic twins showing a high concordance (0.55). In contrast, fraternal twins have a low concordance for binocular rivalry period, close to zero. Modeling of these results is consistent with genetic determination of the rivalry rhythm involving a large number of genes. A larger sample size of twins will be needed to provide a more precise estimate of the number of genes that are likely to be involved, but the results so far support a high heritability and multigenic determination of rivalry rate, just as with circadian rate (Hansell et al., in preparation).

It has been suggested that rivalry alternation rate reflects neural adaptation under control of specific transmitter mechanisms, which would similarly be expected to have a strong genetic influence. In response to this claim we would like to put forward an interesting prediction: that perceptual rivalry rate will be buffered against changes in body temperature. Given that the rates of a number of physiological processes have been shown to be affected by temperature (Schoepfle and Erlanger, 1941; Hodgkin and Katz, 1949; Takeya, Hasuo, and Akasu, 2002), those who adhere to "habituation" as a mechanism of rivalry would have to admit the possibility that increased metabolism would affect its physiology and that a temperature change would alter the rate of rivalry alternations. In contrast, a functional prerequisite for circadian pacemakers is that the oscillator is temperature-compensated so that timekeeping will remain accurate over a range of physiological temperatures. Accordingly, the circadian rhythms have been found to show a remarkable ability to compensate for increases or decreases in temperature (Barrett and Takahashi, 1995; Huang, Curtin, and Rosbash, 1995; Ruby, Burns, and Heller, 1999).

## Genetic Coupling of Circadian to Ultradian Periods

A mysterious phenomenon links the genetics of both ultradian and circadian rhythms. A mutation that produces an increased period in a circadian rhythm (e.g., *per* long in *Drosophila*, ~30 hr) may produce a correspondingly increased ultradian rhythm in the same individual, such as the courtship rhythm in *Drosophila*, measured in seconds (Dowse and Ringo, 1987; Konopka, Kyriacou, and Hall, 1996). This phenomenon has been observed in a number of systems, including *C. elegans*, where the periods of three different rhythms at three different scales have been shown to be linked in this way. Similar observations are seen in human perceptual rivalry:

1. Individuals with a faster than usual rhythm, measured on one form of perceptual rivalry, also show a faster than usual rhythm on a different form of perceptual rivalry. This has been shown for binocular rivalry versus monocular rivalry and binocular rivalry versus Bonneh's MIB (Carter and Pettigrew, 2003).

2. Rivalry rhythms are linked to nasal cycle rhythms, with individuals exhibiting a fast or slow nasal cycle similarly experiencing rivalry alternations at a rate respectively faster or slower than the average (Pettigrew and Hekel, in preparation).

## DISCUSSION: FEYNMAN'S CONJECTURE

If the thesis that perceptual rivalries are ultradian oscillations is accepted for the moment, "how?" and "why?" questions arise immediately. Perhaps the most difficult aspect of the present thesis is the "how?" component of the connection between ultradian rhythms of different scales. Specifically, how is coupling achieved between rhythms that are as far apart as binocular rivalry (seconds) and nasal cycle (hours)? We draw the reader's attention to a phenomenon that supports Feynman's conjecture while providing an explanation for the coupling of biological rhythms at all temporal scales. This remarkable discovery involves a redox enzyme, expressed on cell surfaces, that has an ultradian rhythm of around 21 min. If the gene for the enzyme is manipulated to produce an altered ultradian rhythm, the cell's circadian rhythm is altered in direct proportion. For example, a new enzyme with a 30-min ultradian period results in a circadian period of 30 hr instead of 24 hr. This remarkable finding at the same time provides a biochemical mechanism for Feynman's conjecture and strong impetus for the present thesis linking the ultradian rhythms of rivalry to other biological rhythms (Morre et al., 2002).

To answer the "why?" question, we would like to return again to the unpublished conjecture by Richard Feynman. As mentioned previously, Feynman and McDermott proposed that the brain should have a master oscillator that would synchronize its activities in a manner comparable to the internal clock of a modern computer. In such a scheme one would expect lawful temporal relationships between rhythms of different scales, such as the coupling that we observe between different rivalry rhythms and between these rhythms and the much slower nasal cycle. This scheme also explains how the proposed existence of both high- and low-level forms of binocular rivalry (for review, see Blake and Logothetis, 2002) could be phenomenologically and temporally linked. While there is increasing evidence to support Feynman's conjecture, acceptance has been limited by the lack of any plausible underlying basis for coupling oscillators of different scale.

One might also ask why visual perception should be influenced by "clocks" at all. Such a question arises naturally if one adopts the common view of vision as a relatively passive hierarchical sensory process that was widely promulgated as a result of the success of the Nobel laureates Hubel and Wiesel. However, it is becoming increasingly clear that visual perception is necessarily bound to processes of visual decision-making, attention, and other high-level processes that might require precise timing information. Feynman himself seems to have recognized an inextricable link between perception and timing in his early experiments. He was particularly struck by the varying influence that verbal and visual information can have on an individual's internal clock (see Feynman, 1999, p. 218).

Recent work has shown a strong link between efference copy magnitude in an individual and that same individual's rivalry rate, two apparently distant phenomena that are linked obviously only by their mutual reliance on temporal information (Campbell et al., 2003). This precise, lawful relationship further strengthens the view that neural timing, as revealed by rivalry rhythm, is fundamentally determined.

In regard to the fundamental role of timing in perception, we draw attention to the work of Dale Purves on "inescapable ambiguity." Although ambiguity in visual perception is not a novel concept, his work emphasizes that ambiguity is often obligatory, and not a facultative issue that can ultimately be "solved" by, for example, bringing touch or other sensory information to bear upon the ambiguity. Faced with inescapable ambiguity, which is an inevitable property of the physical world, we propose that perception has evolved an oscillatory response. To help illustrate this role of perceptual oscillation in dealing with ambiguity, consider again the single-cell organism *Gonyaulax* that we show in figure 15.3. After a night at depth, on this particular dive *Gonyaulax* is completely deprived of the sparsely distributed nitrogenous substrates for which it descends each evening. What does *Gonyaulax* "decide" to do if it encounters a patch of nitrogen just as its biological clock indicates that it is time to ascend? As figure 15.3 shows, the single cell is capable of a very adaptive response, and delays its ascent to take advantage of the just-discovered resource.

It is easy to imagine a variety of scenarios where different concentrations of nitrogenous resources interact at different times during the night to provide a variety of "ambiguous" situations for which the outcome will be determined in a way that is difficult to determine in advance. The point is that the same sensory data concerning the nitrogenous resource will be "perceived" differently by *Gonyaulax* according to the phase of the circadian cycle, with a small signal triggering a phase delay if there has been a very low signal in the immediate past, while a large signal has no effect on behavior if it occurs following recent large signals.

Similarly, we propose that an ultradian oscillation has been incorporated into the decision-making of visual perception in recognition of the fact that ambiguity cannot be escaped, but must be accepted in the early stages of processing instead of being "solved" at some later stage. If there are at least two different interpretations of the same sense data, as Purves and colleagues have shown for lightness, brightness, color, motion, stereo depth, and geometrical relations (Purves et al., 2001), we suggest that the ground state should reflect this reality by oscillating between alternatives instead of assuming from the outset that there is a single "solution" that can be derived by the appropriate calculations. Andrews and Purves (1997) have speculated that binocular rivalry reflects a mechanism evolved to deal with conditions of perceptual uncertainty. We would like to go further and suggest that oscillations are an inextricable component of all forms of visual perception. We think that widening the debate in this way may help generate further interest and expand the relevance of perceptual rivalry beyond the visual sciences. Current investigations into the rivalry process are focused so intently on the neural correlates of visual suppression and awareness that there is a real danger of ignoring a more fundamental significance of the oscillatory aspect of the phenomena.

## REFERENCES

Andrews, T. J., and Purves, D. (1997). Similarities in normal and binocularly rivalrous viewing. *Proceedings of the National Academy of Sciences of the United States of America*, 94, 9905–9908.

Barrett, R. K., and Takahashi, J. S. (1995). Temperature compensation and temperature entrainment of the chick pineal cell circadian clock. *Journal of Neuroscience*, 15, 5681–5692.

Blake, R. (1989). A neural theory of binocular rivalry. *Psychological Review*, 96, 145–167.

Blake, R., and Logothetis, N. K. (2002). Visual competition. *Nature Reviews: Neuroscience*, 3, 13–21.

Bonneh, Y., Cooperman, A., and Sagi, D. (2001). Motion induced blindness in normal observers. *Nature*, 411, 798–801.

Borsellino, A., De Marco, A., Allazetta, A., Rinesi, S., and Bartolini, B. (1972). Reversal time distribution in the perception of visual ambiguous stimuli. *Kybernetik*, 10, 139–144.

Breese, B. (1909). Binocular rivalry. *Psychological Review*, 16, 410–415.

Campbell, T., Ericksson, G., Wallis, G., Liu G. B., and Pettigrew, J. D. (2003). Correlated individual variation of efference copy and perceptual rivalry timing. *Society for Neuroscience Abstract Program*, 550.

Carter, O. L. (2001). Alternations in visual perception: A measure of interhemispheric switching and bipolar disorder. Honors thesis, University of Queensland, Brisbane.

Carter, O. L., and Pettigrew, J. D. (2003). A common oscillator for perceptual rivalries? *Perception*, 32, 295–305.

Carter, O. L., Campbell, T., Wallis, G., Liu, G. B., and Pettigrew, J. D. (submitted). The contradictory effects of context on binocular rivalry.

De la Iglesia, H. O., Meyer, J., Carpino, A., Jr., and Schwartz, W. J. (2000). Antiphase oscillation of the left and right suprachiasmatic nuclei. *Science*, 290, 799–801.

Dowse, H. B., and Ringo, J. M. (1987). Further evidence that the circadian clock in *Drosophila* is a population of coupled ultradian oscillators. *Journal of Biological Rhythms*, 2, 65–76.

Fahle, M. (1982). Binocular rivalry: Suppression depends on orientation and spatial frequency. *Vision Research*, 22, 787–800.

Feynman, R. P. (1999). *The Pleasure of Finding Things Out: The Best Short Works of Richard P. Feyenman*. London: Penguin Books.

Hansell, N., Wright, M., Martin, N., Pettigrew, J. D., and Miller, S. (in preparation). Concordance for binocular rivalry rate in monozygotic and dizygotic twins.

Helfrich-Förster, C. (1996). *Drosophila* rhythms: From brain to behavior. *Seminars in Cell and Developmental Biology*, 7, 791–802.

Hodgkin, A. L., and Katz, B. (1949). The effect of temperature on the electrical activity of the giant axon of the squid. *Journal of Physiology*, 109, 240–249.

Huang, Z. J., Curtin, K. D., and Rosbash, M. (1995). PER protein interactions and temperature compensation of a circadian clock in *Drosophila*. *Science*, 267, 1169–1172.

Hupé, J.-M., and Rubin, N. (2002). Stimulus strength and dominance duration in perceptual bi-stability. Part II: From binocular rivalry to ambiguous motion displays. (Abstract). *Journal of Vision*, 2, 464a.

Hupé, J.-M., and Rubin, N. (2003). The dynamics of bi-stable alternation in ambiguous motion displays: A fresh look at plaids. *Vision Research*, 43, 531–548.

Kerkhof, G. A. (1985). Inter-individual differences in the human circadian system: A review. *Biological Psychology* 20, 83–112.

Konopka, R. J., and Benzer, S. (1971). Clock mutants of *Drosophila melanogaster*. *Proceedings of the National Academy of Sciences of the United States of America*, 68, 2112–2116.

Konopka, R. J., Kyriacou, C. P., and Hall, J. C. (1996). Mosaic analysis in the *Drosophila* CNS of circadian and courtship-song rhythms affected by a period clock mutation. *Journal of Neurogenetics*, 11, 117–139.

Lehky, S. R. (1995). Binocular rivalry is not chaotic. *Proceedings of the Royal Society of London*, B259, 71–76.

Leopold, D. A., Wilke, M., Maier, A., and Logothetis, N. K. (2002). Stable perception of visually ambiguous patterns. *Nature Neuroscience*, 5, 605–609.

Levelt, W. J. M. (1965). *On Binocular Rivalry*. Soesterberg, The Netherlands: Institute for Perception RVO-TNO.

Lewy, A. J., Wehr, T. A., Goodwin, F. K., Newsome, D. A., and Markey, S. P. (1980). Light suppresses melatonin secretion in humans. *Science*, 210, 1267–1269.

Meijer, J. H., and Rietveld, W. J. (1989). Neurophysiology of the suprachiasmatic circadian pacemaker in rodents. *Physiological Review*, 69, 671–707.

Minors, D. S., Waterhouse, J. M., and Wirz-Justice, A. (1991). A human phase-response curve to light. *Neuroscience Letters*, 133, 36–40.

Morre, D. J., Chueh, P. J., Pletcher, J., Tang, X., Wu, L. Y., and Morre, D. M. (2002). Biochemical basis for the biological clock. *Biochemistry*, 41, 11941–11945.

Mueller, T. J., and Blake, R. (1989). A fresh look at the temporal dynamics of binocular rivalry. *Biological Cybernetics*, 61, 223–232.

Nicholls, M. E. R. (1996). Temporal processing asymmetries between the cerebral hemispheres: Evidence and implications. *Laterality*, 1, 97–137.

Perry, R. J., Rosen, H. R., Kramer, J. H., Beer, J. S., Levenson, R. L., and Miller, B. L. (2001). Hemispheric dominance for emotions, empathy and social behaviour: Evidence from right and left handers with frontotemporal dementia. *Neurocase*, 7, 145–160.

Pettigrew, J. D. (2001). Searching for the switch: Neural bases for perceptual rivalry alternations. *Brain and Mind*, 2, 85–118.

Pettigrew, J. D., and Funk, A. P. (2001). Opposing effects on perceptual rivalry caused by right vs left TMS. *Society for Neuroscience Abstract Program*, 27, 10.10.

Pettigrew, J. D., and Hekel, A. P. (in preparation). Coupling of human rhythms and bipolar disorder.

Pettigrew, J. D., and Miller, S. M. (1998). A "sticky" interhemispheric switch in bipolar disorder? *Proceedings of the Royal Society of London*, B265, 2141–2148.

Pöppel, E. (1994). Temporal mechanisms in perception. *International Review of Neurobiology*, 37, 185–202.

Purves, D., Lotto, R. B., Williams, S. M., Nundy, S., and Yang, Z. (2001). Why we see things the way we do: Evidence for a wholly empirical strategy of vision. *Philosophical Transactions of the Royal Society of London*, B356, 285–297.

Ramachandran, V. S. (1994). Phantom limbs, neglect syndromes, repressed memories, and Freudian psychology. *International Review of Neurobiology*, 37, 291–333.

Refinetti, R., and Menaker, M. (1992). The circadian rhythm of body temperature. *Physiology and Behavior*, 51, 613–637.

Roenneberg, T., and Mittag, M. (1996). The circadian program of algae. *Seminars in Cell and Developmental Biology*, 7, 753–763.

Roenneberg, T., and Rehman, J. (1996). Nitrate, a nonphotic signal for the circadian system. *FASEB Journal*, 10, 1443–1447.

Ruby, N. F., Burns, D. E., and Heller, H. C. (1999). Circadian rhythms in the suprachiasmatic nucleus are temperature-compensated and phase-shifted by heat pulses in vitro. *Journal of Neuroscience*, 19, 8630–8636.

Schoepfle, G. M., and Erlanger, J. (1941). The action of temperature on the excitability, spike height and configuration, and the refractory period observed in the responses of single medullated nerve fibers. *American Journal of Physiology*, 134, 694–704.

Sobel, K. V., and Blake, R. (2002). How context influences predominance during binocular rivalry. *Perception*, 31, 813–824.

Takeya, M., Hasuo, H., and Akasu, T. (2002). Effects of temperature increase on the propagation of presynaptic action potentials in the pathway between the Schaffer collaterals and hippocampal CA1 neurons. *Neuroscience Research*, 42, 175–185.

Tzourio, N., Crivello, F., Mellet, E., Nkanga-Ngila, B., and Mazoyer, B. (1998). Functional anatomy of dominance for speech comprehension in left handers vs right handers. *Neuroimage*, 8, 1–16.

Van Esseveldt, K. E., Lehman, M. N., and Boer, G. J. (2000). The suprachiasmatic nucleus and the circadian timekeeping system revisited. *Brain Research Review, 33,* 34–77.

Walker, P. (1975). Stochastic properties of binocular rivalry alternations. *Perception and Psychophysics,* 18, 467–473.

Wearden, J. H., and Penton-Voak, I. S. (1995). Feeling the heat: Body temperature and the rate of subjective time, revisited. *Quarterly Journal of Experimental Psychology,* B48, 129–141.

Wilson, H. R., Blake, R., and Lee, S. H. (2001). Dynamics of travelling waves in visual perception. *Nature,* 412, 907–910.

# 16 Binocular Rivalry in the Divided Brain

## Robert P. O'Shea and Paul M. Corballis

### WHAT IS A DIVIDED BRAIN?

A person with a divided brain has had the corpus callosum, the large tract of fibers joining the two cerebral hemispheres, cut, usually to relieve epilepsy. This surgery does help control the epilepsy, but also has the fascinating side effect of revealing the lateralization of certain higher mental functions (Bogen and Gazzaniga, 1965; Gazzaniga, 1965; Gazzaniga, Bogen, and Sperry, 1962, 1965; Seymour, Reuter-Lorenz, and Gazzaniga, 1994). Specifically, the left hemisphere produces speech, understands speech, processes the right side of the sensory world, and controls the right side of the body. The right hemisphere understands spatial relations, understands some speech, processes the left side of the sensory world, and controls the left side of the body. Hereafter, we refer to people with such divided brains as split-brain observers.

In the intact brain, higher functions can be lateralized because the corpus callosum allows one hemisphere to access all of the sensorimotor world for that function. For example, spatial understanding can be lateralized to the right hemisphere because at that level of processing, the right hemisphere can represent the entire visual scene, both left and right of fixation.

### WHY IS IT INTERESTING TO STUDY BINOCULAR RIVALRY IN THE DIVIDED BRAIN?

It is interesting to study binocular rivalry in split-brain observers to determine whether rivalry is a higher, lateralized function. There are two theories holding that critical aspects of rivalry are lateralized, and one theory—ours—holding that the rivalry mechanism is essentially duplicated at a low level of each hemisphere.

According to Pettigrew and colleagues (Miller, 2001; Miller et al., 2000; Ngo et al., 2000; Pettigrew and Miller, 1998), rivalry is processed at a high level of the visual system, possibly in inferotemporal cortex. At this level, they say, each hemisphere adopts one of the rival stimuli, rivalry reflecting alternations in activation of left and right hemispheres controlled by subcortical oscillators. Pettigrew et al. have some challenging evidence for their theory (detailed in chapter 15 of this volume). For example, they have found that squirting cold water into the right ear (cold caloric stimulation), a procedure that increases blood flow to the left hemisphere, can arrest normal rivalry alternations, perception presumably settling on whichever rival stimulus the left hemisphere has adopted. They also have found that disrupting the left hemisphere with transcranial magnetic stimulation (TMS) can trigger a rivalry alternation on about 50% of trials (this would be when perception is supported by the left hemisphere) but makes no change on the remaining 50% of trials (when perception would be supported by the undisturbed right hemisphere). In addition, they have found that people with bipolar disorder, whom they argue have slower subcortical oscillators, have slower rivalry alternation rates than people without such a diagnosis.

According to Lumer, Friston, and Rees (1998), rivalry is controlled by a structure in the right frontoparietal cortex. They showed a red, moving grating to one eye and a green face to the other while they measured fMRI activity. Observers pressed keys to signal their experiences of rivalry. Later, Lumer et al. played each observer a nonrival display that was perceptually the same as he or she had reported for rivalry. Observers again pressed keys, and had their fMRI activity measured. The only difference was that in one case any changes in appearance occurred because of rivalry, and in the other case any changes occurred because of physical disappearance of one of the monocular stimuli. When Lumer et al. subtracted one fMRI record from the other, they found a region of strong activation in the right frontoparietal cortex.

From both theories, we predict that no rivalry will be reported when stimuli are confined to the left hemisphere of a split-brain observer. In Pettigrew et al.'s theory, a split-brain observer should report only the stimulus adopted by the left hemisphere. In Lumer et al.'s theory, a split-brain observer should report something unlike rivalry, because the left hemisphere is cut off from the switching mechanism in the right hemisphere.

Our theory, however, is that rivalry is processed at a low level of the visual system, possibly within cortical hypercolumns of the primary visual cortex, V1 (Blake, O'Shea, and Mueller, 1992; Mueller, 1990). At this

Robert P. O'Shea and Paul M. Corballis

level of the visual system, each hemisphere covers only its own half of the visual field. This means processing must be the same in the two hemispheres; otherwise, objects would appear to change as they moved from one side of the visual field to the other (which, as far as we know, has never been reported). If the rivalry mechanism is duplicated in each hemisphere, we predict similar rivalry from the left and right hemispheres of a split-brain observer.

## WHO ARE OUR SPLIT-BRAIN OBSERVERS?

Our split-brain observers are JW and VP (Gazzaniga et al., 1985). (We have done most work with JW.) JW is male, now 50 years old; VP is female, now 51 years old. They had callosotomies in 1979. They are right-handed. They have good visual acuity in each eye and can see the depth in random-dot stereograms. They are extremely experienced psychophysical observers.

## HOW DOES A SPLIT-BRAIN OBSERVER DESCRIBE RIVALRY?

We first tested our predictions by showing JW a pair of rival figures in a stereoscope (figure 16.1a). He described alternations between the stimuli, then said they looked like a black record with a white label alternating with a white record with a black label[1] (O'Shea and Corballis, 2001). Although we did not monitor JW's eye fixation in this experiment, this is such a beautifully poetic description that it could have come only from his left hemisphere. JW's right hemisphere is essentially mute.

Later, we conducted experiments in which we were able to monitor JW's fixation while presenting rival stimuli to the right or left field (to the left or right hemisphere, respectively). We also trained him and other observers, including VP, to report rivalry by pressing keys with the fingers of the right or left hand (controlled mainly by the left or right hemisphere, respectively). We asked observers to press one key whenever and for as long as they saw vertical with no trace of horizontal, and the other key whenever and for as long as they saw horizontal with no trace of vertical during 1-min trials. We first trained the observers to respond to pseudo rivalry changes (real changes to the stimuli that resembled rivalry alternations), and then tested rivalry. We monitored fixation with an eye tracker (SMI EyeView). We asked the observers to describe the stimuli after each trial.

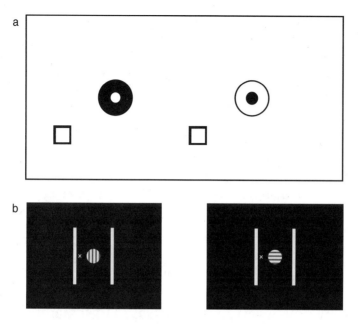

**Figure 16.1** (*a*) Reproduction of the stimuli we displayed in a Telebinocular stereoscope to JW. The black ring was presented to the left eye and the white ring, to the right eye. When JW fixated the square, these images would be processed only by his left hemisphere (admittedly we could not monitor JW's eye fixation in this experiment). JW reported normal rivalry (O'Shea and Corballis, 2001). (*b*) Reproduction of the monitor screens viewed by the left eye and right eye through a mirror stereoscope in O'Shea and Corballis's (2003a) experiments. Each screen was 17.85° × 13.52°. The white bars assisted binocular alignment. Observers fixated the ×, in this case placing the rival gratings in the right field for processing by the left hemisphere. JW reported normal rivalry with these stimuli.

After JW's first left-hemisphere rivalry trial, he said:

Strange. They change right in the middle of the screen. They change from up-and-down [vertical] to right-to-left [horizontal]. Sometimes I see one on one side and the other on the other [he demonstrated with his fingers, showing vertical on the left and horizontal on the right].

Later, in trials in which pseudo rivalry and real rivalry were interspersed, JW said of a left-hemisphere rivalry trial:

That's the one where there are two different ones the same time. Sometimes there would be [vertical] and [horizontal] together. Yuck! Sometimes I had one button halfway pressed while I decided what to do. Annoying because it changes so fast.

JW's reports leave us in no doubt that he experiences left-hemisphere rivalry in essentially the same way that intact-brain observers do. His

Robert P. O'Shea and Paul M. Corballis

reports testify to the chaotic nature of rivalry alternations, which we were unable to simulate with our pseudo rivalry displays. JW's reports are problematic for theories that place any critical aspect of rivalry in the right hemisphere, but are consistent with our theory that the rivalry mechanism is duplicated in the two hemispheres.

After JW's right-hemisphere trials, he gave much simpler descriptions. He would say things like "OK" or "Lots of changes that time." These reports also came from his left hemisphere, which had not seen the stimuli. We suspect that JW's left hemisphere was able to report on the number of changes because it either had felt the left hand pressing the keys (through ipsilateral afferents) or had heard the keys being pressed (through the right ear). To learn more of the right hemisphere's experiences of rivalry, we have to turn to key-press data.

## ARE THERE QUALITATIVE AND QUANTITATIVE DIFFERENCES OF RIVALRY FROM THE LEFT AND RIGHT HEMISPHERES?

To characterize rivalry fully, we analyzed four different aspects: exclusive visibility (the total time one response key or the other was pressed), rate (the number of key presses), period (the average time one response key or the other was pressed), and the distribution of durations of episodes of rivalry dominance. We have graphed the first three of these in figure 16.2.

As can be seen from figure 16.2, JW shows rivalry in both hemispheres that is similar to that of the intact-brain observer. (The intact-brain observer's results were similar to those of all the intact-brain observers we measured.) The only difference is that JW's periods from the left hemisphere are longer than those from the right. The other split-brain observer, VP, showed similar rivalry in the two hemispheres and longer periods from the left hemisphere (O'Shea and Corballis, 2001). This seems consistent with the response style of the two hemispheres: the right hemisphere is said to record every detail, whereas the left hemisphere is said to gloss over details (Ramachandran, 1994), perhaps ignoring brief departures from exclusive visibility. Our results do suggest that the qualitative experience of rivalry is the same in the two hemispheres.

In figure 16.3, we have plotted the distributions of durations of key presses from the left and right hemispheres of a split-brain observer and a representative intact-brain observer. These distributions have the classic gamma shape that is typical of rivalry (Blake, Fox, and McIntyre, 1971; Cogan, 1973; Fox and Herrmann, 1967; Lumer, Friston, and Rees, 1998).

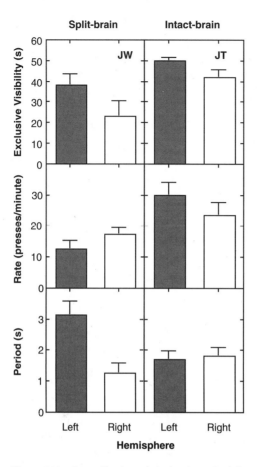

**Figure 16.2** Quantification of rivalry from the left and the right hemispheres of JW and of an intact-brain observer in response to the stimuli illustrated in figure 16.1b. Error bars are 1 standard error. JW's rivalry is similar to that of the intact-brain observer, although with longer periods from the left hemisphere (O'Shea and Corballis, 2003a).

Despite JW's longer durations from the left hemisphere, there are no marked differences in the shapes of the distributions between the hemispheres of either observer, or between the observers. This measure also suggests that the qualitative experience of rivalry is the same in the two hemispheres.

In split-brain observers we found qualitatively similar responses to rival stimuli, whether presented to the left or to the right hemisphere. This was true for orthogonal achromatic gratings of different sizes and

Robert P. O'Shea and Paul M. Corballis

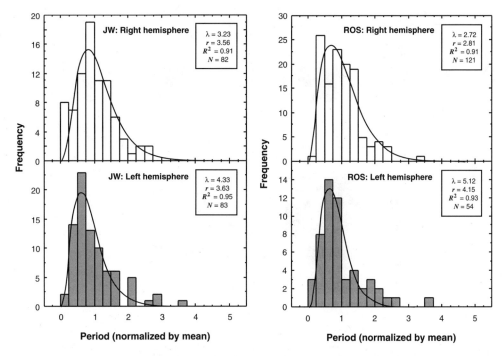

**Figure 16.3** Distributions of durations of episodes of rivalry dominance from the left and the right hemispheres of JW and of an intact-brain observer in response to the stimuli illustrated in figure 16.1b. All distributions are remarkably similar, showing the typical gamma shape, and are well-fitted by gamma distributions whose parameter values are shown in the top right-hand corner (O'Shea and Corballis, 2003a).

eccentricities, oppositely colored gratings and faces (figure 16.4a; plate 6) (O'Shea and Corballis, 2001), and coherence stimuli (Diaz-Caneja; see Alais et al., 2000; figure 16.4b, see O'Shea and Corballis, 2003b). Coherence stimuli are particularly important because rivalry is between complete gratings that are distributed across the two eyes, implicating interocular visual grouping. That is, we found similar interocular grouping in each of JW's hemispheres.

We also showed JW rival gratings on both sides of fixation and had him track rivalry on both sides simultaneously by pressing two keys with the left hand and two keys with the right hand. He was able to do this effortlessly, something that defeated all our intact-brain observers. His rivalry from the two hemispheres was essentially independent.

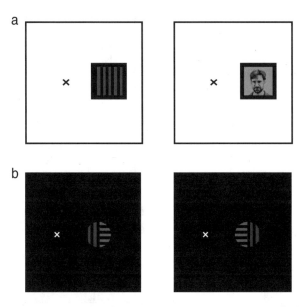

**Figure 16.4**   (*a*) Stimuli presented, one to each eye, to test whether rivalry between complex stimuli, similar to those used by Lumer, Friston, and Rees (1998), might yield differences between JW's hemispheres. No qualitative differences were found (O'Shea and Corballis, 2001). (*b*) Example of Diaz-Caneja-type rivalry stimuli. Occasionally, perception is of a red vertical grating alternating with a green horizontal grating, showing that visual grouping can operate across the eyes to yield coherence rivalry. JW reported similar coherence rivalry from his two hemispheres (similar to that of intact-brain observers) (O'Shea and Corballis, 2003b). See plate 6 for color version.

## DOES HAVING A CORPUS CALLOSUM MAKE ANY DIFFERENCE TO RIVALRY?

JW has an intact anterior commissure, so one might argue that the coordination of the two hemispheres required by Pettigrew et al. and Lumer et al. is accomplished via this pathway. This seems unlikely; in split-brain observers the only function ever demonstrated for the anterior commissure is exchange of olfactory information (Gazzaniga, 2000).

Nevertheless, to examine whether there were any interhemispheric effects on rivalry in our split-brain observer, we used a technique invented by Alais and Blake (1999). They presented pairs of gratings to one eye, and sets of random dots to the same locations in the other eye, for 60 sec. The gratings and dots engaged in rivalry. Alais and Blake asked their observers to press one key whenever one grating appeared (with no trace of

Robert P. O'Shea and Paul M. Corballis

dots), and another key whenever the other grating appeared (with no trace of dots). They computed joint predominance: the time both keys were pressed, divided by the total time either or both keys were pressed. This yielded a dimensionless number ranging from 0 (when neither key was pressed at the same time as the other) to 1 (when both keys were always pressed at the same time).

Using their technique, Alais and Blake manipulated the grouping characteristics of the gratings. That is, gratings could be collinear (so that the bars would join up if extended; good grouping), parallel (intermediate grouping), or orthogonal (minimal grouping). Also, the gratings could be confined within one visual half-field, and hence one hemisphere, or distributed between two half-fields, hence occupying two hemispheres. The essentials of their design are illustrated in figure 16.5.

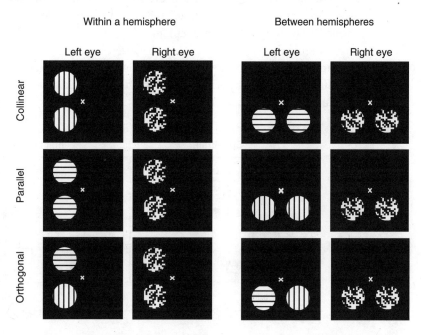

**Figure 16.5** Illustration of stimuli similar to those used by Alais and Blake (1999) and by us (O'Shea and Corballis, 2003b). The left panels show stimuli confined within a hemisphere, in this case the right (left field). Left-hemisphere stimuli also were tested. The right panels show stimuli distributed between the hemispheres. In this case, stimuli are displayed below the horizontal meridian; stimuli above the horizontal meridian also were tested. The top panels show gratings that are collinear. The middle panels show gratings that are parallel. The bottom panels show gratings that are orthogonal (HV). The other possible arrangement of orthogonal gratings (VH) also was tested.

Alais and Blake discovered that the joint predominance of the gratings was greater for collinear and parallel gratings than for orthogonal gratings, whether within or between hemispheres. They also calculated joint predominance expected from independent rivalry within each region. All conditions except for orthogonal gratings were significantly greater than this predicted level. Grouping effects on rivalry between hemispheres presumably depend on communication across the corpus callosum.

We conducted a similar experiment on JW and some intact-brain observers. For our experiment, we scaled up all dimensions of the stimuli to keep the pairs of rival stimuli off the area of nasotemporal overlap. We first trained our observers to respond to pseudo rivalry changes in the stimuli, and we monitored eye fixation. Our results were similar to Alais and Blake's for intact-brain observers (one shown on the right of figure 16.6).

Critically, JW's results (see the left panel of figure 16.6) also were similar when the stimuli were confined within one hemisphere. In these conditions, there were no differences in joint predominance from the left or right hemisphere. When the stimuli were distributed between the hemispheres, however, there were no significant grouping effects at all. Thus, we finally ran an experiment in which JW's lack of a corpus callosum made a difference to his rivalry.

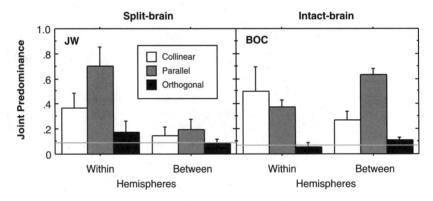

Figure 16.6 Joint predominance of JW and of an intact-brain observer in response to the stimuli illustrated in figure 16.5 (O'Shea and Corballis, 2003b). Error bars are 1 standard error. The gray line shows the level of joint predominance expected from independent rivalry in the two regions. JW shows the effect of visual grouping when the rival gratings were confined within one hemisphere, but no effects of visual grouping when the gratings fell in different hemispheres. The intact-brain observer's results are similar to those of Alais and Blake (1999), with grouping effects within and between hemispheres.

Robert P. O'Shea and Paul M. Corballis

JW's lack of any interhemispheric grouping of rivalry rules out any major contribution to rivalry of the anterior commissure, because otherwise Pettigrew et al. would have to hold it responsible for his normal visual-grouping effects with Diaz-Caneja stimuli (figure 16.4b) but not for between-hemisphere visual grouping effects (figure 16.6). It also demonstrates that JW has normal rivalry in each hemisphere, and that the effects of grouping are the same in each hemisphere. The effects of grouping probably arise from lateral interconnections between adjacent regions of the cortex analyzing adjacent regions of the visual field (e.g., Das and Gilbert, 1995; Gilbert, 1992). In intact-brain observers, these lateral connections must cross the corpus callosum to give grouping between the hemispheres. These connections are cut in JW's case.

To summarize this section, we find similar rivalry in each hemisphere of a split-brain observer, consistent with the rivalry mechanism being duplicated in each hemisphere. We doubt that such duplication has developed following the callosotomies of our split-brain observers. We think duplication represents the normal state of affairs in the intact brain, required because each hemisphere's rivalry mechanism covers only half of the visual field.

## HOW DO WE RECONCILE PETTIGREW ET AL.'S DATA WITH OURS?

We think there are alternative explanations of Pettigrew et al.'s results. For example, cold caloric stimulation and TMS may simply alter the rivalry mechanism within the hemisphere controlling responses to centrally presented rivalry stimuli. We note that Pettigrew et al. always presented the same rivalry stimulus to the same eye, thereby confounding stimulus with eye. It is possible that cold water in one ear or a magnetic pulse to that side of the head affects stimuli imaged in the eye on that side. Pettigrew et al.'s finding of slower alternations in people with bipolar disorder could be from the mood-stabilizing drugs used to control the disorder in the majority of Pettigrew and Miller's (1998) patients (see also Miller et al., 2003). Although the effects of these drugs on rivalry have never been specifically tested, other drugs, such as sedatives and alcohol, slow rivalry alternations (e.g., Platz, Uhr, and Miller, 1960; Ruttiger, 1963; Seedorff, 1956).

In any case, there is one major problem for Pettigrew et al.'s theory: rivalry composites. When rival stimuli cover large areas of the visual field, for much of a trial one sees small patches of one stimulus dynamically intermingled with small patches of the other. Only rarely do all the patches of one image coalesce to yield an episode of exclusive visibility. In

Pettigrew et al.'s terms, there must be many independent switches, one for each location in the visual field. The area over which rivalry dominance spreads, scales with spatial frequency in the same way as with fusion and stereopsis (O'Shea, Sims, and Govan, 1997), and binocular phenomena that Pettigrew may agree are processed in V1 (Barlow, Blakemore, and Pettigrew, 1967). In Pettigrew et al.'s terms, the independent switches must scale with spatial frequency. The area over which rivalry dominance spreads also matches that of receptive fields of V1 neurons at different eccentricities (Blake, O'Shea, and Mueller, 1992). In Pettigrew et al.'s terms, the independent switches must scale with eccentricity like V1 neurons, instead of neurons higher in the visual system, which have much larger receptive fields. The properties of the visual system revealed by rivalry composites require Pettigrew to duplicate many of the properties of V1 wherever the switches are located in the brain. It is more parsimonious to put the switches in V1. This is essentially our contention.

## HOW DO WE RECONCILE LUMER ET AL.'S DATA WITH OURS?

We think there are complex reasons for Lumer et al.'s finding rivalry-related fMRI activity in the frontoparietal cortex, regions supposed to be involved in allocating spatial attention. When we used Lumer et al.'s technique for producing pseudo rivalry, we noticed that the observer's task of pressing keys was much simpler than when the alternations were produced by rivalry. As JW's verbal reports attest, real rivalry is much more chaotic than pseudo rivalry; it is much more difficult to decide when to press keys. We are quite prepared to believe that the attention devoted to deciding when to press a key during rivalry involved the frontoparietal cortex.

It is also worth pointing out that Lumer et al.'s technique for producing pseudo rivalry actually involves rivalry. To produce an episode of pseudo rivalry dominance, say of red verticals, Lumer et al. increased the contrast of that stimulus to one eye while decreasing the contrast of the other stimulus to the other eye. During the changes, therefore, both stimuli were presented dichoptically, yielding the conditions for binocular rivalry. When the change was over, the red grating was presented to one eye and a gray field to the other, yet only the grating was perceived. Hering (1964) called this form of binocular rivalry contour dominance. It has now come to be called permanent suppression (e.g., Ooi and Loop, 1994). It is possible (although we think it unlikely) that the brain regions for conventional rivalry and permanent suppression differ at the level of the frontoparietal cortex.

In any case, in later research Lumer and Rees (1999) also found enhanced fMRI activity to rivalry in the left frontoparietal cortex, although this seemed weaker than in the right. According to the logic of Lumer et al., if each hemisphere has its own switching mechanism, we would predict no, or small, differences in rivalry in the isolated hemispheres—just what we found.

## CONCLUSIONS

Split-brain observers have essentially normal rivalry in each hemisphere; this is true even when the components of rival stimuli are distributed across the eyes (Diaz-Caneja stimuli) or across the visual field (Alais and Blake's stimuli).

In JW's case, there are no effects on rivalry of grouping between hemispheres, suggesting that grouping effects in intact-brain observers are mediated via the corpus callosum with little, if any, contribution from the anterior commissure.

Our results present difficulties for the theories of Pettigrew et al. and of Lumer, Friston, and Rees (1998) but are consistent with ours that the rivalry mechanism is duplicated in each hemisphere. Duplication is necessary at the level of the visual system at which each hemisphere processes only its own half of the visual field, namely, at low levels such as V1.

## ACKNOWLEDGMENTS

We are grateful to our split-brain observers, JW and VP, for their cheerful participation in our experiments; Mike Gazzaniga, for helpful discussion and encouragement; Malcolm Handley and Michael Bevin for programming; Barry Dingwall and Robin Gledhill for constructing the apparatus; Petya Radoeva, Ian Wilson, Mike McMath, Rebecca O'Connor, Judy Trevena, Amy Dillon, and Amar Dhand for assisting research; and Steven Miller for helpful comments. This research was partially funded by a Human Frontiers Science Program Grant (RG0161/1999-B) to PC, and Otago Research, Division of Sciences, Departmental, and NZ-US CSP (00-CSP-44) grants to ROS.

# NOTE

1. A *record* was a flat disk of vinyl into each side of which a spiral groove had been pressed. By rotating the disk on a record player, a needle picked up vibrations encoded in the path of the groove that were amplified as sounds, usually music. That is, a record was an analog sound recording device (similar to a CD) popular in JW's and ROS's youth.

# REFERENCES

Alais, D., and Blake, R. (1999). Grouping visual features during binocular rivalry. *Vision Research*, 39, 4341–4353.

Alais, D., O'Shea, R. P., Mesana-Alais, C., and Wilson, I. G. (2000). On binocular alternation. *Perception*, 29, 1437–1445.

Barlow, H. B., Blakemore, C., and Pettigrew, J. D. (1967). The neural mechanism of binocular depth discrimination. *Journal of Physiology*, 193, 327–342.

Blake, R., Fox, R., and McIntyre, C. (1971). Stochastic properties of stabilized-image binocular rivalry alternations. *Journal of Experimental Psychology*, 88, 327–332.

Blake, R., O'Shea, R. P., and Mueller, T. J. (1992). Spatial zones of binocular rivalry in central and peripheral vision. *Visual Neuroscience*, 8, 469–478.

Bogen, J. E., and Gazzaniga, M. S. (1965). Cerebral commissurotomy in man: Minor hemisphere dominance for certain visuospatial functions. *Journal of Neurosurgery*, 23, 394–399.

Cogan, R. (1973). Distribution of durations of perception in the binocular rivalry of contours. *Journal of General Psychology*, 89, 297–304.

Das, A., and Gilbert, C. D. (1995). Long-range horizontal connections and their role in cortical reorganization revealed by optical recording of cat primary visual cortex. *Nature*, 375, 780–784.

Fox, R., and Herrmann, J. (1967). Stochastic properties of binocular rivalry alternations. *Perception and Psychophysics*, 2, 432–436.

Gazzaniga, M. S. (1965). Psychological properties of the disconnected hemispheres in man. *Science*, 150, 372.

Gazzaniga, M. S. (2000). Cerebral specialization and interhemispheric communication: Does the corpus callosum enable the human condition? *Brain*, 123, 1293–1326.

Gazzaniga, M. S., Bogen, J. E., and Sperry, R. W. (1962). Some functional effects of sectioning the cerebral commissures in man. *Proceedings of the National Academy of Sciences of the United States of America*, 48, 1765–1769.

Gazzaniga, M. S., Bogen, J. E., and Sperry, R. W. (1965). Observations on visual perception after disconnection of the cerebral hemispheres in man. *Brain*, 88, 221–236.

Gazzaniga, M. S., Holzman, J. D., Deck, M. D. E., and Lee, B. C. P. (1985). MRI assessment of human callosal surgery with neuropsychological correlates. *Neurology*, 35, 682–685.

Gilbert, C. D. (1992). Horizontal integration and cortical dynamics. *Neuron*, 9, 1–13.

Hering, K. E. (1964). *Outlines of a Theory of the Light Sense*, L. M. Hurvich and D. Jameson, trans. Cambridge, Mass.: Harvard University Press. First published 1874.

Lumer, E. D., Friston, K. J., and Rees, G. (1998). Neural correlates of perceptual rivalry in the human brain. *Science*, 280, 1930–1934.

Lumer, E. D., and Rees, G. (1999). Covariation of activity in visual and prefrontal cortex associated with subjective visual perception. *Proceedings of the National Academy of Sciences of the United States of America*, 96, 1669–1673.

Miller, S. M. (2001). Binocular rivalry and the cerebral hemispheres: With a note on the correlates and constitution of visual consciousness. *Brain and Mind*, 2, 119–149.

Miller, S. M., Gynther, B. D., Heslop, K. R., Liu, G. B., Mitchell, P. B., Ngo, T. T., et al. (2003). Slow binocular rivalry in bipolar disorder. *Psychological Medicine*, 33, 683–692.

Miller, S. M., Liu, G. B., Ngo, T. T., Hooper, G., Riek, S., Carson, R. G., and Pettigrew, J. D. (2000). Interhemispheric switching mediates perceptual rivalry. *Current Biology*, 10, 383–392.

Mueller, T. J. (1990). A physiological model of binocular rivalry. *Visual Neuroscience*, 4, 63–73.

Ngo, T. T., Miller, S. M., Liu, G. B., and Pettigrew, J. D. (2000). Binocular rivalry and perceptual coherence. *Current Biology*, 10, R134–R136.

Ooi, T. L., and Loop, M. S. (1994). Visual suppression and its effect upon color and luminance sensitivity. *Vision Research*, 34, 2997–3003.

O'Shea, R. P., and Corballis, P. M. (2001). Binocular rivalry between complex stimuli in split-brain observers. *Brain and Mind*, 2, 151–160.

O'Shea, R. P., and Corballis, P. M. (2003a). Binocular rivalry in split-brain observers. *Journal of Vision*, 3, 610–615, http://journalofvision.org/3/10/3/.

O'Shea, R. P., and Corballis, P. M. (2003b). Visual grouping on binocular rivalry in a split-brain observer. Manuscript submitted for publication, University of Otago. Retrieved from http://psy.otago.ac.nz/r_oshea/coherence030703.pdf.

O'Shea, R. P., Sims, A. J. H., and Govan, D. G. (1997). The effect of spatial frequency and field size on the spread of exclusive visibility in binocular rivalry. *Vision Research*, 37, 175–183.

Pettigrew, J. D., and Miller, S. M. (1998). A "sticky" interhemispheric switch in bipolar disorder? *Proceedings of the Royal Society of London*, B265, 2141–2148.

Platz, A., Uhr, L., and Miller, J. G. (1960). A pilot experiment on the effects of meprobamate on stereoscopic retinal rivalry of complementary colors. *Perceptual and Motor Skills*, 10, 230.

Ramachandran, V. S. (1994). Phantom limbs, neglect syndromes, repressed memories, and Freudian psychology. *International Review of Neurobiology*, 37, 291–333.

Ruttiger, K. F. (1963). Individual differences in reaction to meprobamate: A study in visual perception. *Journal of Abnormal and Social Psychology*, 67, 37–43.

Seedorff, H. H. (1956). Effect of alcohol on the motor fusion reserves and stereopsis as well as on the tendency to nystagmus. *Acta Ophthalmologica* (Copenhagen), 34, 273–280.

Seymour, S. E., Reuter-Lorenz, P. A., and Gazzaniga, M. S. (1994). The disconnection syndrome: Basic findings reaffirmed. *Brain*, 117, 105–115.

# 17 Rivalry and Perceptual Oscillations: A Dynamical Synthesis

## Hugh R. Wilson

By their very nature, binocular rivalry and other perceptual oscillations represent a fascinating window onto the dynamics of competitive networks in the brain. The basic phenomenon of rivalry has been known at least since 1593, when Porta described the experience of viewing two separate book pages, one with each eye (cited by Wade, 1998). Extensive research, particularly since Levelt's (1965) study, has now given us a rather detailed characterization of many perceptual oscillations and their dependence on stimulus parameters. What is lacking is a comprehensive synthesis demonstrating how properties of perceptual oscillations arise as natural consequences of neural activity and network connectivity, although several significant strides have been made in this direction (e.g., Lehky, 1988; Blake, 1989; Laing and Chow, 2002).

In attempting to relate rivalry to networks in the brain, it is necessary to have some idea of the cortical locus at which rivalry activity is generated. One hypothesis is that rivalry emerges from competition between monocularly driven neurons in primary visual cortex (V1), and a second hypothesis is that rivalry represents competition between object representations in higher cortical areas (Blake and Logothetis, 2002). In support of the first hypothesis, one fMRI study has shown clear evidence for rivalry in V1 (Polonsky et al., 2000), and a second has shown that rivalry occurs within the V1 representation of the blind spot where input is exclusively monocular (Tong and Engel, 2001; see chapter 4 in this volume). However, another fMRI study can be interpreted as being consistent with rivalry between higher cortical representations of houses and faces (Tong et al., 1998), and some psychophysical work has also supported this higher cortical viewpoint (Kovács et al., 1996).

A critical experiment was performed by Logothetis, Leopold, and Sheinberg (1996) in an attempt to adjudicate between these two hypotheses.

They introduced temporal transients into the conventional rivalry paradigm by flickering orthogonal dichoptic gratings at 18.0 Hz and swapping the gratings between eyes at 1.5 Hz (i.e., every 333 msec). The striking result was that rivalry dominance intervals averaged about 2.3 sec, largely unchanged from the mean dominance interval for conventional static rivalry targets. Clearly, therefore, this dynamic flicker and swap (F&S) procedure produced a rivalry pattern that could not be explained by competition between monocularly driven neurons, since dominance durations spanned approximately seven interocular grating swaps. Rather, rivalry during F&S stimulation must reflect competition at a cortical level where monocular information has been combined binocularly. But does this mean that rivalry under all conditions reflects higher cortical interactions?

Following up on Logothetis, Leopold, and Sheinberg (1996), Lee and Blake (1999) conducted a detailed study of the temporal frequency conditions under which F&S rivalry produced prolonged dominance durations. They discovered that flicker near 18.0 Hz plus swapping at approximately 1.5 Hz was critical. To anyone familiar with nonlinear dynamics, such restriction to a narrow corner of stimulus parameter space is indicative of a switch or bifurcation in system response. Such a bifurcation is analogous to the transition in locomotory speed from a walk to a gallop in the neural control of gait. Given this allusion to a neural network that can change its response characteristics with oscillation frequency, perhaps the F&S procedure in rivalry triggers a dynamic transition in the underlying competitive cortical networks. Indeed, Wolfe (1996) suggested that the F&S procedure might somehow minimize normal monocular competition. Consistent with this, the nonlinear neural model presented here demonstrates that the F&S procedure can defeat or bypass an initial monocular rivalry stage and thereby reveal a higher stage of neural competition. This insight offers a dynamic resolution of the two rivalry hypotheses via synthesis into a hierarchy in which competition at multiple levels is necessary (see chapters 3, 4, 7, 11, and 13 in this volume).

**COMPETITIVE RIVALRY NETWORKS**

There is a nearly universal consensus that binocular rivalry and other perceptual oscillations result from inhibition between competing neural representations (see chapter 15 in this volume). Dynamics reveals that there are two requirements for a competitive network to generate oscillations (Wilson, 1999a). First, reciprocal inhibition between the competing representations must be sufficiently strong for one to suppress the other in a temporary "winner-take-all" manner. Second, the winner of the competition must fatigue or self-adapt to a point where it releases the suppressed representation from inhibition. To make these ideas concrete, let us consider the simplest possible neural model of rivalry in which two excitatory (E) neurons inhibit one another with strength **a.** (Explicit representation of inhibitory interneurons has been ignored as a mathematical convenience, which does not alter any of the arguments below.) In addition, each E neuron undergoes a slow self-adaptation governed by a variable $H$ (see figure 17.1A).

It is impossible to model any neural oscillation like rivalry without a nonlinearity in the system, and the simplest such nonlinearity is a threshold with a linear increase in firing rate above threshold with slope M. These concepts are embodied in the following equations:

$$\tau \frac{d E_L}{dt} = -E_L + M[L - a E_R - g H_L]_+$$

$$\tau_H \frac{d H_L}{dt} = -H_L + E_L$$

$$\tau \frac{d E_R}{dt} = -E_R + M[R - a E_L - g H_R]_+$$

$$\tau_H \frac{d H_R}{dt} = -H_R + E_R.$$

(17.1)

$L$ and $R$ denote left and right monocular inputs to $E_L$ and $E_R$, respectively. The expressions on the right within brackets incorporate the threshold

$$[X]_+ = \max(X, 0).$$

(17.2)

This is a threshold function such that a net negative argument $X$ shuts off firing and positive $X$ produces a linear firing rate above threshold. The heavy solid line in figure 17.2 shows that this function is a good approximation to the firing rate of a human neocortical neuron over a reasonable range (data from Avoli et al., 1994).

Self-adaptation in equation (17.1) is mediated by the $H$ variables, which necessarily have very slow time constants, so $\tau_H \gg t$. For excitatory neurons a typical value of t is 15 msec. This means that $\tau_H > 100$ msec, a figure that is far too long to describe any inhibitory neuron. However, excitatory neocortical neurons in humans and other mammals invariably have slow, hyperpolarizing membrane currents that are typically calcium

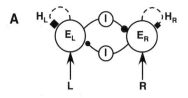

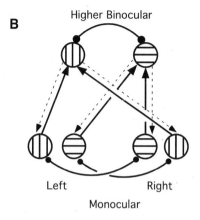

**Figure 17.1** Schematic of rivalry networks described by equation (17.1). (*A*) $E_L$ and $E_R$ are monocularly driven neurons with respective inputs L and R. Each inhibits the other via the I connections (separate inhibitory neurons are not explicitly represented in the model for mathematical convenience only). Slow hyperpolarizing membrane currents $H_L$ and $H_R$ reduce the spike rates of their respective nerons and are under neuromodulatory control (see text, "Conclusions and Conjectures"). (*B*) Two-level hierarchic model for rivalry competition. Left-eye-driven and right-eye-driven neurons comprise the lower, monocular level, with both vertical and horizontal orientation preferences (hatching) being represented. Interocular inhibitory competition occurs between orthogonal orientations at the monocular level, as represented by arcs ending in solid circles. Neurons at a higher binocular level sum excitatory inputs from monocular neurons with the same preferred orientations (heavy arrows). These higher-level binocular neurons also engage in strong inhibitory competition. Finally, the hierarchic model also incorporates weak recurrent excitation from the binocular neurons back to their monocular inputs (light, dashed arrows). All excitatory neurons have the hyperpolarizing H currents depicted in (*A*).

($Ca^{++}$)-mediated potassium ($K^+$) currents (Avoli et al., 1994; McCormick and Williamson, 1989; Connors and Gutnick, 1990). We have previously hypothesized that these currents drive perceptual reversals (Wilson, Krupa, and Wilkinson, 2000; Wilson, Blake, and Lee, 2001). In particular, human excitatory neurons are known to possess hyperpolarizing membrane currents with time constants averaging $\tau_H = 990$ msec (McCormick and Williamson, 1989). In the absence of any competitive interactions, this

Hugh R. Wilson

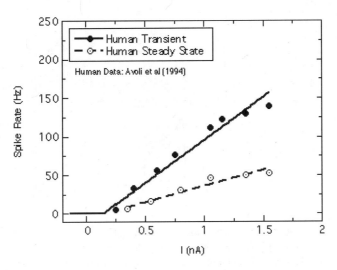

**Figure 17.2** Spike rates of a human excitatory neocortical neuron as a function of input current I (adapted from Avoli et al., 1994). Solid circles plot initial transient firing rates, and open circles plot sustained rates following spike-frequency adaptation. Solid and dashed lines illustrate that the simple threshold nonlinearity in equation (17.2) provides a good fit to the firing rate data.

slow hyperpolarizing current reduces the spike rate of a neuron by about a factor of 3 from its initial value. This is shown by the heavy dashed line fit of the model to cortical neuron data in figure 17.2. It is also important to note that these hyperpolarizing currents are under control of the modulatory neurotransmitters serotonin, dopamine, histamine, and acetylcholine (McCormick and Williamson, 1989). I shall return to this important fact later to explain individual variability in rivalry data.

Given the neural model in equations (17.1) and (17.2), it is a simple matter to derive necessary and sufficient conditions for rivalry alternations to occur. This is a standard form of nonlinear analysis based on the presence of separate fast and slow time scales governed by t and $\tau_H$, respectively (see Wilson 1999a). The results lead to two requirements:

$$a > \frac{1}{M}$$

$$g > a - \frac{1}{M}.$$

(17.3)

The first expression guarantees that the inhibitory gain **a** will be sufficiently strong so that each E neuron is able to suppress firing of the other, and the second inequality guarantees that self-adaptation by a dominant

Rivalry and Perceptual Oscillations

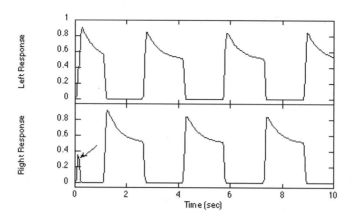

**Figure 17.3** Rivalry oscillation produced by equation (17.1) with parameters given in text. Upper and lower pannels are relative spike rates of $E_L$ and $E_R$, respectively. Although this model produces strictly deterministic limit cycle oscillations, analogous models describing individual action potentials generate a gamma distribution of dominance intervals via neural chaos (Laing and Chow, 2002; Wilson, 2003). Note that both competitive neurons are active during the first 150 msec (arrow), in agreement with psychophysical rivalry data (Wolfe, 1983).

E neuron will eventually weaken its response sufficiently to release the suppressed neuron from inhibition.

Simulation of equation (17.1) with parameters satisfying equation (17.2) ($M = 1.0, a = 1.7$, and $g = 1.0$) shows that alternate dominance intervals in response to orthogonal grating stimuli do indeed occur on a timescale comparable to binocular rivalry data (figure 17.3). Notice also that both E neurons fire simultaneously during the transient response at stimulus onset, which would correspond to the percept of a superimposed grating plaid. Only after about 150 msec does one neuron suppress the other, which agrees with psychophysical data (Wolfe, 1983). This is an unavoidable consequence of recurrent inhibition, which must always develop more slowly than the direct excitatory response to stimulation.

Although the alternation in figure 17.3 is a limit cycle oscillation (Wilson, 1999a), it is well known that empirical measurements of rivalry intervals generate a distribution of dominance intervals approximated by a gamma function (Fox and Herrmann, 1967; Borsellino et al., 1972). One possible way of producing gamma distributions from equation (17.1) is simply to add noise through a stochastic variable, as was shown by Lehky (1988). However, a more interesting possibility has arisen. Laing and Chow (2002) developed a model with the same competitive interactions as equation (17.1), except that they replaced $E_L$ and $E_R$ each by a large population of neurons described by Hodgkin–Huxley-type conduction dynamics. The resulting network generated dominance intervals approximating a gamma distribution via chaotic dynamics (Laing and Chow, 2002). Such chaos has been replicated using simplified equations describing human cortical neurons (Wilson, 1999b) in networks comprising as few as six spiking neurons (Wilson, 2003).

Indeed, chaos and gamma distributions may be an unavoidable ingredient in any neural network with strong reciprocal inhibition and self-adaptation. Although studies by Richards, Wilson, and Sommer (1994) and Lehky (1995) failed to find direct evidence of chaos in rivalry data, this is likely due to noisy data. This hypothesis is supported by the observation that removal of eye movement jitter using image stabilization still produces a gamma-function dominance distribution (Blake, Fox, and McIntyre, 1971). In sum, gamma distributions are easy to generate in networks such as equation (17.1) through addition of either noise or neural chaos among spiking neurons. Thus, it is legitimate to model key features of rivalry with periodic dynamics, with the understanding that gamma-function distributions can be easily and naturally generated if desired.

## LEVELT'S SECOND LAW

One defining feature of binocular rivalry is enshrined in Levelt's Second Law (Levelt, 1965). For patterns of variable contrast, a precise statement of this law is "Changes in the contrast of the lower contrast pattern primarily alter the mean dominance duration of the higher contrast pattern, dominance durations for the lower contrast pattern remaining largely unaffected." This behavior is manifested by the neural model in equation (17.1) and is illustrated in figure 17.4A. The solid line plots dominance durations for the neuron driven by a fixed, high-contrast stimulus for a range of contrasts of the weaker stimulus. While durations driven by the higher-contrast stimulus vary dramatically, those for the lower-contrast stimulus (dashed line) remain relatively unchanged. Figure 17.4B shows the oscillation produced by equation (17.1) when contrast of the weaker stimulus has been significantly reduced (arrow in figure 17.4A). Thus, the very simple model in equation (17.1) produces responses obeying Levelt's Second Law. Furthermore, spiking neuron equations producing chaos and gamma distributions also obey Levelt's Second Law (Laing and Chow, 2002).

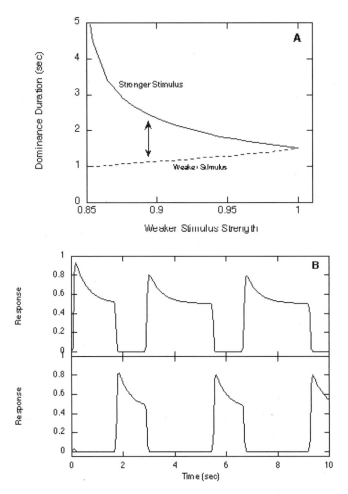

**Figure 17.4** Levelt's Second Law behavior resulting from the network in figure 17.1 and equation (17.1). (*A*) As the strength of the weaker stimulus is reduced from that of the stronger stimulus, stronger stimulus dominance intervals increase substantially (solid line), and weaker stimulus intervals decrease minimally (dashed line). (*B*) Neural activity in more strongly stimulated neuron (top panel) and weaker neuron (bottom pannel) for stimulus strengths shown by the double-headed arrow in (*A*). For comparison, figure 17.3 shows results when both neurons are equally stimulated with unity input.

## DOMINANCE WAVES IN RIVALRY

Anybody who has viewed large rivaling patterns knows that the patterns do not alternate as a whole. Rather, portions of one pattern will emerge locally and sweep across the field, suppressing the other monocular

Hugh R. Wilson

pattern in their wake. For years such spatial dynamics proved intractable experimentally, so researchers resorted to studying rivalry by using small stimulus patches that appear and vanish in a roughly unitary fashion. This simplification led to important discoveries, among them the observation that patch size for unitary pattern alternation increases with retinal eccentricity in accord with cortical magnification (Blake, O'Shea, and Mueller, 1992). This important insight implies that unitary rivalry reflects the local domain of neural inhibition.

To further understand rivalry, characterization of its spatial spread is necessary. A paradigm for studying the spread of monocular pattern dominance resulted from a serendipitous exposure to research in the field of $Ca^{++}$ waves in cardiac tissue. Nagai et al. (2000) employed an experimental paradigm in which $Ca^{++}$ waves were monitored while propagating around an annulus of cardiac tissue in a culture dish. This elegant paradigm forced two-dimensional waves to travel around what was effectively a one-dimensional race track annulus.

We adapted this approach to the study of dominance waves in rivalry (Wilson, Blake, and Lee, 2001). One such rivalry stimulus is depicted in figure 17.5A. The observer fixated the central fusion bull's-eye, and each trial began when the observer reported by button press that the high-contrast spiral annulus was completely dominant. At that point a brief (200 msec) contrast pulse restricted to a small portion of the suppressed radial pattern caused it to become dominant locally, and this triggered a dominance wave that swept around the annulus until it reached the designated point at the bottom. Measurement of dominance-wave travel time revealed that it was a linear function of distance around the annulus (see figure 17.5B), thus indicating travel at a constant speed (Wilson, Blake, and Lee, 2001). Further measurements with annuli of different mean diameters revealed that dominance-wave speed was constant at approximately 2.24 cm/sec when mapped into V1 cortical coordinates as measured by Horton and Hoyt (1991). Additional measurements showed that dominance-wave speed doubled when the pattern driving the waves was concentric (see figure 17.5B) rather than radial (Wilson, Blake, and Lee, 2001). This is consistent with the operation of weak but long-range excitatory connections mediating collinear facilitation in V1 (Malach et al., 1993; Das and Gilbert, 1995; Somers et al., 1998).

Propagation of dominance waves has been explained quantitatively by a simple extension of the rivalry model developed above. The model comprises two spatially extended, circular rings of competing E neurons representing the stimulus annulus. The only remaining ingredient in the model

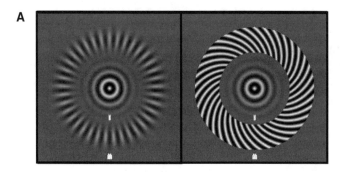

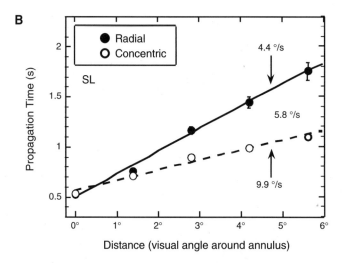

**Figure 17.5** Rivalry dominance waves. (*A*) One eye viewed a high-contrast spiral annulus that, due to Levelt's Second Law, dominated the lower-contrast radial annulus (Wilson, Blake, and Lee, 2001). Waves were then triggered in the low-contrast pattern at any of eight cardinal points, and the transit time to the marked point at the bottom was measured. Fixation was maintained on the fused central bull's-eyes. (*B*) Dominance-wave propagation data for one subject. Solid circles and line show propagation times as a function of distance around the radial annulus in (*A*) at a constant speed corresponding to 4.4° visual angle per sec. When waves were propagated around a concentric annulus (not shown), speed roughly doubled (open circles and dashed line). This speed increase is attributed to the effects of weak but long-range collinear facilitation.

is a spatial spread of the competitive inhibition. The spatial extent of this inhibitory spread was chosen to be 1.0 mm, the distance between adjacent ocular dominance columns in human V1 (Hitchcock and Hickey, 1980). This model produces traveling dominance waves with a speed of

Hugh R. Wilson

2.24 cm/sec (Wilson, Blake, and Lee, 2001), in agreement with psychophysics. The mechanism of wave propagation in the model is simple: when a neuron becomes dominant, its spatial spread of inhibition leads to disinhibition of its own monocular neighbors, so these waves propagate by disinhibition. Addition of longer-range collinear excitation in the model increases wave propagation speed to 4.4 cm/sec, thereby reproducing data obtained with concentric monocular stimuli (Wilson, Blake, and Lee, 2001). The one caveat is that collinear excitation must be weak to permit the network to continue producing oscillations, since even moderately strong collinear facilitation causes bifurcation to a winner-take-all network in which rivalry oscillations cannot occur (Wilson, 1999a).

## A COMPETITIVE RIVALRY HIERARCHY

Dominance waves in rivalry propagate at constant speed when mapped onto V1, and they exhibit collinear facilitation. Both of these observations support the hypothesis that these waves are a manifestation of interocular competition in V1. As discussed above, however, Logothetis, Leopold, and Sheinberg (1996) used their flicker and swap (F&S) procedure (18.0 Hz flicker with eye swapping at 1.5 Hz) and still obtained dominance intervals averaging about 2.3 sec, time for about seven swaps between eyes. This dramatic result clearly cannot be the result of competition between monocular neurons. Rather, binocular neurons must be the units competing in this case. To those conversant with nonlinear dynamics, these experiments strongly suggest that the F&S procedure causes a bifurcation of competitive network dynamics into a different regime (see Wilson, 1999a, for discussions of neuronal bifurcations).

I have incorporated these ideas into a hierarchical, two-stage competitive network that explains both traditional and F&S rivalry (Wilson, 2003). The architecture of this network is illustrated in figure 17.1B, where a monocular competitive network provides input to a higher level of competition between binocular neurons. The network also incorporates weak excitatory feedback from the binocular to the monocular level (dashed lines), although this is not necessary to its function. Both levels of the network can be described by equation (17.1) or by similar equations incorporating a Naka–Rushton nonlinearity (Wilson, 2003). Parameters are the same at both network levels, except that the inhibitory gain **a** must be stronger at the binocular level for reasons described below.

The network was first stimulated by a traditional rivalry pattern in which orthogonal monocular gratings were continuously presented. In this case the monocular level of the network generates the same rivalry oscillations as in figure 17.3; these oscillations in turn drive the binocular neurons, causing them to produce an identical oscillation (Wilson, 2003). Thus, the network accounts for normal rivalry as the result of monocular neural competition that is reflected at higher levels.

When the network is driven by F&S stimulation, a very different result ensues. As shown in figure 17.6, the F&S stimulus overcomes competition at the monocular level so that responses to both orthogonal gratings are continuously sent to the binocular level. Rivalry now occurs only at the binocular level, and dominance durations last through six to seven eye

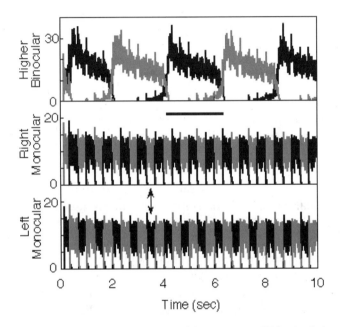

**Figure 17.6** Hierarchic rivalry model responses to F&S stimulation. Neurons preferring vertical orientations are plotted in black, and those preferring horizontal orientations are plotted in gray. The bottom two panels illustrate responses of the left and right monocular neurons, and the top panel plots responses of the higher-level binocular neurons. Note that the F&S stimulation paradigm defeats rivalry at the monocular stage so that both horizontal and vertical neural responses simultaneously pass through to the binocular level (indicated by vertical arrow). As described in the text and by Wilson (2003), rivalry now occurs at the binocular stage, and dominance durations are approximately 7.0 interocular switches in duration (horizontal solid line in middle panel). When traditional rivalry stimuli are used, however, the monocular network levels revert to the rivalry alternations depicted in figure 17.3, and these drive all activity at the binocular stage. Both levels of the hierarchy are necessary to account for both traditional and F&S rivalry.

Hugh R. Wilson

swaps, in complete agreement with psychophysics (Logothetis, Leopold, and Sheinberg, 1996). The temporal dynamics of the stimulus have eliminated competition at the monocular level, thereby revealing a higher level of binocular competition (Wilson, 2003).

This elimination of monocular competition at the first level may be understood from two related perspectives, one empirical and one dynamic. First, Wolfe (1983) has shown that rivalry does not develop within the first 150 msec following stimulus presentation, and neural models indicate that this is a consequence of recurrent inhibition that must lag behind its excitatory drive (see figure 17.3). During F&S stimulation, the stimulus is presented for only 27.8 msec at a time (half-cycle of 18.0 Hz). Furthermore, eye swapping every 333 msec guarantees that self-adaptation of E neurons via slow self-adaptation is minimal. Thus, on empirical grounds each 27.8 msec presentation of the stimuli is akin to the initial transient period of traditional rivalry, when superposition rather than alternation occurs (Wolfe, 1983). Logic then dictates that in the F&S procedure the rivalry oscillations must result from a higher competitive stage.

The second explanation for defeat of competition at the monocular stage is computational. Because the inhibitory neurons providing reciprocal inhibition are driven by the monocular excitatory neurons, ipso facto their responses must fall off more rapidly at higher temporal frequencies than their excitatory inputs. In consequence, the value of the inhibitory gain **a** in equation (17.1) will be reduced at high temporal frequencies, and at some frequency it will have been reduced sufficiently so that the first inequality in equation (17.3) fails. At this point $E_L = E_R$ becomes asymptotically stable, so oscillations at the first stage must vanish (see Wilson, 1999a). The empirical result that F&S stimulation does generate rivalry with dominance intervals extending over six to seven eye swaps (Logothetis, Leopold, and Sheinberg, 1996) then implicates a second, binocular stage of competition. This stage still receives 18.0 Hz modulated input from the first stage, however (indeed, flicker is perceptually apparent), so the second stage must have a stronger inhibitory gain **a;** otherwise, it, too, would succumb to the same fate as the first stage (Wilson, 2003). Simulations indicate that inhibition at the binocular stage must be roughly 1.6 times stronger than at the monocular stage for F&S rivalry to be obtained, and this inhibition is too strong to permit rivalry under traditional stimulus conditions, since the second inequality in equation (17.3) is violated.

To summarize, traditional rivalry is driven by monocular competition in the hierarchical model, and the binocular level merely oscillates in response to its monocular inputs, which is consistent with fMRI results obtained by Tong et al. (1998). With F&S rivalry stimuli, however, competition at the monocular stage is eliminated, and the stronger inhibition at the binocular stage is effectively reduced to the point where bifurcation to an oscillatory mode occurs. Thus, nonlinear modeling suggests that two hierarchical levels of neural competition are necessary to explain both traditional and F&S rivalry within a single coherent framework. This provides a synthesis of the opposing low-level and high-level views of rivalry.

Two further comments are in order. First, incorporation of weak excitatory feedback from the higher binocular to the lower monocular level (dashed arrows in figure 17.1B) has only a modest effect on rivalry: it can increase dominance durations by up to about 12%. Any stronger recurrent excitation causes a bifurcation from a regime supporting rivalry oscillations to a winner-take-all regime in which no oscillations are possible (Wilson, 2003). Thus, excitatory feedback within the hierarchy, while doubtless present anatomically, does not play an explanatory role in either traditional or F&S rivalry.

Second, one might question whether the simulation results presented here are an artifact resulting from the use of spike-rate equations in the dynamics. Can the same result be obtained in a neural network using spiking, Hodgkin–Huxley–type neurons? As discussed in greater detail elsewhere (Wilson, 2003), the answer is yes. To demonstrate this, a two-level hierarchic network with the same architecture as shown in figure 17.1B was simulated, using dynamic equations for the individual neurons (both excitatory and inhibitory) that provide an accurate description of action potential shapes and firing rates of human neocortical neurons (Wilson, 1999b). As mentioned above, this network produces alternations in response to traditional rivalry stimuli and generates a gamma distribution of dominance durations via neural chaos (see also Laing and Chow, 2002). When this network is driven by F&S stimuli, monocular neurons in the first level cease rivaling and fire simultaneously. The stronger inhibition in the higher binocular level now generates rivalry alternations that are again chaotic and produce a gamma distribution (Wilson, 2003). The dominance intervals again encompass six to seven eye swaps, so the hierarchic model architecture illustrated in figure 17.1B is robust with respect to both spike rate and action potential based descriptions of the constituent neurons.

Hugh R. Wilson

## CONCLUSIONS AND CONJECTURES

The neural model depicted in figure 17.1B demonstrates that both low-level monocular rivalry and higher-level binocular rivalry can coexist peacefully within a single competitive hierarchy. In attempting to relate the model to cortical physiology, one must confront the single-unit data reported by Leopold and Logothetis (1996). They recorded from various cortical areas while monkeys reported rivalry, and they found that 38% of V4 neurons and 43% of MT neurons alternated firing during rivalry, although only 18% of V1 neurons did so. Furthermore, almost all neurons displaying rivalry-linked activity received binocular inputs. However, this is compatible with the hierarchic model in figure 17.1B. First, the monocular neurons in this model need not be strictly monocular. Rather, it would suffice for them to belong to Hubel and Wiesel's (1968) ocular dominance classes 2, 3, 5, and 6. Each of these is dominated by input from one eye but also receives modest input from the other, and all of these would have been classified as binocular by Leopold and Logothetis (1996).

Second, the fact that a lower percentage of V1 neurons undergo rivalry alternations remains compatible with their being the driving force behind all traditional rivalry at higher cortical levels. For example, the higher binocular stage of the hierarchic rivalry network can receive constant inputs in addition to the rivaling monocular inputs, and still be driven by the lower-level rivalry inputs during traditional rivalry stimulation. In sum, primate rivalry physiology poses a number of interesting issues but certainly does not yet provide answers vis-à-vis human rivalry, so more primate work is clearly needed.

The physiological data of Leopold and Logothetis (1996) suggest that competitive interactions can occur in many cortical areas. The hierarchic rivalry model remains moot regarding the locus of higher binocular competition, which cannot be determined theoretically. Perhaps it is binocular neurons in V1, perhaps in V4, perhaps elsewhere. Indeed, we have obtained psychophysical evidence for competitive interactions in rivalry responses to Marroquin patterns (Marroquin, 1976) that likely occur in V4 (Wilson, Krupa, and Wilkinson, 2000; Wilkinson et al., 2001). Most probably there is a multilevel hierarchy of competitive inhibitory interactions within the cortical form vision system. It is significant that one computational model of pattern recognition postulates such multiple levels of inhibition as a key ingredient (Reisenhuber and Poggio, 1999). A multilevel generalization of the hierarchic rivalry model is obviously compatible with this.

Although this chapter has not focused on other forms of perceptual alternation, the basic theme embodied in equation (17.1) can explain many other perceptual phenomena. As one example, we have shown that the appearance and vanishing of illusory circles in the Marroquin (1976) illusion can be explained by a spatial extension of equation (17.1) in which a single two-dimensional sheet of E neurons competes via inhibition that is limited to a neighboring spatial region (Wilson, Krupa, and Wilkinson, 2000). Again the presence of slow hyperpolarizing potentials in the membranes of excitatory cortical neurons with time constants approaching 1.0 sec (McCormick and Williamson, 1989) is crucial to the generation of an oscillation. Given evidence that other forms of "object rivalry," such as the Necker cube and faces–vase alternations, are described by gamma functions similar to those of binocular rivalry (Borsellino et al., 1972), it is likely that these will also be subsumed under an elaborated rivalry hierarchy once more details of high-level form vision have been elucidated.

Finally, the hierarchic model can account for individual differences in mean rivalry dominance durations. It has been convincingly demonstrated that the slow hyperpolarizing membrane potentials in excitatory neurons, usually $Ca^{++}$-mediated $K^+$ potentials, are controlled by modulatory neurotransmitters: serotonin, histamine, dopamine, and acetylcholine (McCormick and Williamson, 1989). These modulatory transmitters alter the asymptotic level to which spike rates decline, which is represented by the parameter $g$ in equation (17.1) and plotted as a dashed line in figure 17.2. Rather small variations in the $g$ parameter can cause dramatic changes in mean dominance intervals. The simulation in figure 17.3 produced a dominance interval of 1.6 sec for $g = 1.0$. Modulatory neurotransmitters reduce $g$ (McCormick and Williamson, 1989), and simulations show that dominance intervals increase to 3.1 sec for $g = 0.75$; to 4.0 sec for $g = 0.72$; and to 6.6 sec for $g = 0.703$. Furthermore, the second inequality in equation (17.3) shows that a sufficient reduction in $g$ will destroy rivalry alternations via a bifurcation to a state where one monocular representation will win the competition forever. Thus, reductions in the slow $Ca^{++}$-mediated $K^+$ hyperpolarizing current ubiquitous in excitatory neocortical neurons can explain the reliable individual differences in mean dominance durations documented by others (see chapter 15 in this volume).

We have previously shown that changes in the strength of this same current can also explain individual differences in oscillations of perceptual circles in the Marroquin (1976) illusion (Wilson, Krupa, and Wilkinson, 2000). Since this current is under neuromodulatory control, it seems obvious that it evolved to be altered over time as a parametric control of local network properties. Therefore, minor variations in mean neuromodulatory level from person to person will naturally result in reliable differences in perceptual performance. A final important point to emphasize is that these slow $Ca^{++}$-mediated $K^{+}$ hyperpolarizing currents, with time constants averaging about 1.0 sec in humans (McCormick and Williamson, 1989), readily explain dominance durations for perceptual alternations, whereas recurrent self-inhibition cannot. Inhibitory feedback loops are simply too fast to produce dominance durations in the range of a few seconds.

In conclusion, rivalry alternations require at least a two-level competitive hierarchy to reconcile data on traditional interocular rivalry with the novel results discovered using F&S stimuli by Logothetis, Leopold, and Sheinberg (1996). The evidence that one level of neural competition can be eliminated by the F&S procedure suggests that analogous temporal transients might reveal competitive hierarchies in other sensory systems. Additional visual rivalry stages might also be revealed by using novel combinations of rivaling spatiotemporal patterns. Finally, psychophysical information concerning the cortical locus of higher rivalry stages might be obtained by measuring the size of unitary rivalry domains during F&S stimulation based on the approach of Blake, O'Shea, and Mueller (1992) for traditional rivalry. Thus, it now appears that we have a means of selectively tapping one of at least two competitive stages in vision.

## ACKNOWLEDGMENT

This research was supported in part by NSERC grant #OP227224.

## REFERENCES

Avoli, M., Hwa, G. G. C., Lacaille, J.-C., Olivier, A., and Villemure, J.-G. (1994). Electrophysiological and repetitive firing properties of neurons in the superficial/middle layers of the human neocortex maintained in vitro. *Experimental Brain Research,* 98, 135–144.

Blake, R. (1989). A neural theory of binocular rivalry. *Psychological Review,* 96, 145–167.

Blake, R. (2001). A primer on binocular rivalry, including current controversies. *Brain and Mind,* 2, 5–38.

Blake, R., Fox, R., and McIntyre, C. (1971). Stochastic properties of stabilized-image binocular rivalry alternations. *Journal of Experimental Psychology,* 88, 327–332.

Blake, R., and Logothetis, N. K. (2002). Visual competition. *Nature Reviews: Neuroscience,* 3, 13–21.

Blake, R., O'Shea, R. P., and Mueller, T. J. (1992). Spatial zones of binocular rivalry in central and peripheral vision. *Visual Neuroscience, 8*, 469–478.

Borsellino, A., De Marco, A., Allazetta, A., Rinesi, S., and Bartolini, B. (1972). Reversal time distribution in the perception of visual ambiguous stimuli. *Kybernetik, 10*, 139–144.

Connors, B. W., and Gutnick, M. J. (1990). Intrinsic firing patterns of diverse neocortical neurons. *Trends in Neurosciences, 13*, 99–104.

Das, A., and Gilbert, C. D. (1995). Long range cortical connections and their role in cortical reorganization revealed by optical recording of cat primary visual cortex. *Nature, 375*, 780–784.

Fox, R., and Herrmann, J. (1967). Stochastic properties of binocular rivalry alternations. *Perception and Psychophysics, 2*, 432–436.

Hitchcock, P. F., and Hickey, T. L. (1980). Ocular dominance columns: Evidence for their presence in humans. *Brain Research, 182*, 176–179.

Horton, J. C., and Hoyt, W. F. (1991). The representation of the visual field in human striate cortex: A revision of the classic Holmes map. *Archives of Ophthalmology, 109*, 816–824.

Hubel, D. H., and Wiesel, T. N. (1968). Receptive fields and functional architecture of monkey striate cortex. *Journal of Physiology, 195*, 215–243.

Kovács, I., Papathomas, T. V., Yang, M., and Fehér, A. (1996). When the brain changes its mind: Interocular grouping during binocular rivalry. *Proceedings of the National Academy of Sciences of the United States of America, 93*, 15508–15511.

Laing, C. R., and Chow, C. C. (2002). A spiking neuron model for binocular rivalry. *Journal of Computational Neuroscience, 12*, 39–53.

Lee, S. H., and Blake, R. (1999). Rival ideas about binocular rivalry. *Vision Research, 39*, 1447–1454.

Lehky, S. (1988). An astable multivibrator model of binocular rivalry. *Perception, 17*, 215–228.

Lehky, S. R. (1995). Binocular rivalry is not chaotic. *Proceedings of the Royal Society of London, B259*, 71–76.

Leopold, D. A., and Logothetis, N. K. (1996). Activity changes in early visual cortex reflect monkeys' percepts during binocular rivalry. *Nature, 379*, 549–553.

Levelt, W. J. M. (1965). *On Binocular Rivalry.* Soesterberg, The Netherlands: Institute of Perception RVO-TNO.

Logothetis, N. K., Leopold, D. A., and Sheinberg, D. L. (1996). What is rivalling during binocular rivalry? *Nature, 380*, 621–624.

Malach, R., Amir, Y., Harel, M., and Grinvald, A. (1993). Relationship between intrinsic connections and functional architecture revealed by optical imaging and in vivo targeted biocytin injections in primary striate cortex. *Proceedings of the National Academy of Sciences of the United States of America, 90*, 10469–10473.

Marroquin, J. L. (1976). Human visual perception of structure. Master's thesis, MIT.

McCormick, D. A., and Williamson, A. (1989). Convergence and divergence of neurotransmitter action in human cerebral cortex. *Proceedings of the National Academy of Sciences of the United States of America, 86*, 8098–8102.

Nagai, Y., González, H., Shrier, A., and Glass, L. (2000). Paroxysmal starting and stopping of circulating waves in excitable media. *Physical Review Letters,* 84, 4248–4251.

Polonsky, A., Blake, R., Braun, J., and Heeger, D. J. (2000). Neuronal activity in human primary visual cortex correlates with perception during binocular rivalry. *Nature Neuroscience,* 3, 1153–1159.

Reisenhuber, M., and Poggio, T. (1999). Hierarchical models of object recognition in cortex. *Nature Neuroscience,* 2, 1019–1025.

Richards, W., Wilson, H. R., and Sommer, M. A. (1994). Chaos in percepts? *Biological Cybernetics,* 70, 345–349.

Somers, D. C., Todorev, E. V., Siapas, A. G., Toth, L. J., Kim, D. S., and Sur, M. (1998). A local circuit approach to understanding integration of long range inputs in primary visual cortex. *Cerebral Cortex,* 8, 204–217.

Tong, F., and Engel, S. A. (2001). Interocular rivalry revealed in the human cortical blind-spot representation. *Nature,* 411, 195–199.

Tong, F., Nakayama, K., Vaughan, J. T., and Kanwisher, N. (1998). Binocular rivalry and visual awareness in human extrastriate cortex. *Neuron,* 21, 753–759.

Wade, N. J. (1998). *A Natural History of Vision.* Cambridge, Mass.: MIT Press.

Wilkinson, F., James, T. W., Wilson, H. R., Gati, J. S., Menon, R. S., and Goodale, M. A. (2000). An fMRI study of the selective activation of human extrastriate form vision areas by radial and concentric gratings. *Current Biology,* 10, 1455–1458.

Wilson, H. R. (1999a). Simplified dynamics of human and mammalian neocortical neurons. *Journal of Theoretical Biology,* 200, 375–388.

Wilson, H. R. (1999b). *Spikes, Decisions, and Actions: Dynamical Foundations of Neuroscience.* Oxford: Oxford University Press.

Wilson, H. R. (2003). Computational evidence for a rivalry hierarchy in vision. Submitted for publication.

Wilson, H. R., Blake, R., and Lee, S. H. (2001). Dynamics of travelling waves in visual perception. *Nature,* 412, 907–910.

Wilson, H. R., Krupa, B., and Wilkinson, F. (2000). Dynamics of perceptual oscillations in form vision. *Nature Neuroscience,* 3, 170–176.

Wolfe, J. M. (1983). Influence of spatial frequency, luminance, and duration on binocular rivalry and abnormal fusion of briefly presented dichoptic stimuli. *Perception,* 12, 447–456.

Wolfe, J. M. (1996). Resolving perceptual ambiguity. *Nature,* 380, 587–588.

# 18 A Neural Network Model of Top-Down Rivalry

## D. P. Crewther, R. Jones, J. Munro, T. Price, S. Pulis, and S. Crewther

Binocular rivalry is an involuntary alternation in perception. It occurs under conditions where sufficiently dissimilar stimuli are presented to the two eyes and has an experimental history extending for centuries, as summarized in chapter 1. From the late 1960s until the early 1990s, there was general acceptance that rivalry was the result of competition between the eyes, and more particularly between the monocular streams of information coming from the retinal output of the two eyes (summarized in Blake, 1989).

The neuroscience revolution of the 1980s and 1990s meant that new experimental techniques were applied to understanding the mechanism of binocular rivalry. The general finding from experiments in monkeys and humans on how objects are seen is that the complexity of neuronal processing increases along the pipeline of temporal cortical areas (reviewed in Logothetis, 1998a). This is exemplified by the activation of human fusiform cortex by face stimuli (Kanwisher, McDermott, and Chun, 1997; Puce et al., 1995) and other complex stimuli, such as scenes and places in the parahippocampal gyrus (Epstein and Kanwisher, 1998).

Under conditions of disparate inputs to the two eyes, the percentage of neurons responding in a fashion correlated with perceptual rivalry alternations also increases from area V1 to inferotemporal cortical regions (Leopold and Logothetis, 1996; Logothetis, 1998b; Logothetis, Leopold, and Sheinberg, 1996), with the event-related study of faces/place rivalry giving ample evidence in humans of high-level alternation of activation of brain regions in a way that reflects the perceptual categorization (between faces and houses) and resolution of rival percepts by this stage of processing (Tong et al., 1998). A separate challenge to the retinal rivalry theory has come from experiments demonstrating object completion or association of like attributes of objects between the retinal stimuli (interocular grouping) prior to the determination of rivalry (Kovács et al., 1996).

However, more recent studies using fMRI techniques have shown modifications in processing in the striate and early extrastriate cortex corresponding to perceptual switches that have been interpreted in terms of a relatively early site of the rival exchange mechanism (Lee and Blake, 2002; Polonsky et al., 2000; Tong and Engel, 2001).

## TWO COMPETING THEORIES

Several descriptors have been used for the rivaling theories: "early versus late," "low-level versus high-level," "sensory versus representational." All make reference to the first stage of processing in the brain, where fluctuations in activity correlate with perceptual switches. We would prefer to use the terminology "top-down versus bottom-up." By "bottom-up" is meant the process whereby at the earliest point of excitatory binocular interaction (i.e., striate cortex), disparate streams of information from the two eyes result in a suppression of one stream. In its strongest form, bottom-up rivalry implies that no information from the suppressed stream enters extrastriate cortex.

Top-down rivalry, on the other hand, implies the creation of high-level neural representations of the streams of information from the two eyes and a competition between these representations, with information on the outcome passed in a retrograde fashion. In its strongest form, such competition occurs between modules of neurons in inferotemporal cortex, the suggested site of categorical processing, as supported by several electrophysiological, MEG, and fMRI studies; these modules then inform the rest of the brain. The question of bottom-up or top-down is a vexed one because of the reentrant signaling that characterizes cortical connections (Bullier, 2001; Hupé et al., 2001; Lamme et al., 2000; Lamme, Van Dijk, and Spekreijse, 1992).

Thus it is possible that fluctuations occurring in striate cortex in synchrony with perceptual alternations may be top-down rivalry reporting back (retroinjecting) to striate cortex. Interpretation is made more difficult by the fact that binocular rivalry is a phenomenon with a characteristic perceptual exchange time on the order of seconds, while estimates from single-cell electrophysiology indicate that reentrant processing reaches striate cortex only about 120 msec after stimulation (Super, Spekreijse, and Lamme, 2001). To add to this, the first 150 msec or so of a binocular rivalry presentation usually result in false fusion (Wolfe, 1983).

Thus the percept is essentially evaluated in a steady-state fashion ("which of two stimuli are you currently seeing?"), a situation that is relatively hard to assess through event-related electrical potentials (though amenable to fMRI or steady-state MEG [Tononi et al., 1998] studies).

The notion that higher cortical areas feed information back to striate cortex and that this may affect the outcome of rivalrous stimulation is made clear by Kovács et al.'s (1996) observation that rivalry between complementary patchworks of intermingled stimuli results in the restoration of coherence in the images that rival. This could be viewed either as a rivalry imposed at a higher cortical level within binocular neurons or as an imposition or stamping of the higher-order temporal cortical regions back onto striate cortex.

Whichever way, we find it difficult to interpret these phenomena in terms of rivalry at an early level without access to global object information derived from higher cortical regions (conflicting views exist—compare Seghier et al., 2000; and Alais and Blake, 1999). The idea of an early imposition of rival choices with total suppression of the "loser" is further challenged by the observation that for moving gratings with rivaling orientations presented to the two eyes, information on the direction of motion of the suppressed image is available for the judgment of the overall motion (Andrews and Blakemore, 1999).

## NEURAL NETWORK MODELS

Computational modeling can help make underspecified abstract models more concrete. They allow an investigation of the impact of various parameters within a model and can provide predictions that can focus the direction of experimental investigation.

Several computational models of binocular rivalry have been published—from simple computational models mimicking the stochastic nature of rivalrous exchanges (Sugie, 1982), to reciprocal inhibition models that allow for presynaptic inhibition and a rivalry threshold for the temporal dynamics of binocular rivalry (Lehky, 1988; Mueller, 1990; Mueller and Blake, 1989). Lumer (1998) presented a model based on the synchronization of cell firings. The essential ingredient of the model is the principle that congruent and incongruent stimuli produce different effects on the relative timing of action potentials in primary visual cortex (V1).

The model by Dayan (1998) attempts to incorporate features of some of these "low-level models" while at the same time building on the influential work of Logothetis and colleagues implicating high-level mechanisms

(Leopold and Logothetis, 1996; Logothetis, Leopold, and Sheinberg, 1996; Logothetis and Schall, 1989), and forms the basis for our model. Dayan's model used competition between high-level neurons in the visual pathway that feed back to lower layers, thus recurrently affecting the responses in higher levels. His model comprised four layers, each representing an area further up the visual pathway. He termed these layers the retinal input layer, V1, early extrastriate cortex, and late extrastriate cortex. The cells in the higher levels of the hierarchy represent increasing levels of complexity, with the final layer containing a mere two cells acting as "categorical" cells (recognizing horizontal versus vertical elements). In order for the images presented to rival, Dayan also introduced a fatigue factor in V1 where excited cells would gradually reduce their activity over time.

Several features observed in experimental binocular rivalry are reproduced by Dayan's model, notably the lack of rivalry between low-strength inputs (Blake, 1977; Liu, Tyler, and Schor, 1992) and the dependence of suppression periods on the relative contrast of the stimuli (see also chapter 17 in this volume). Dayan noted that his model did not accurately describe the experimentally observed stability of monocular neurons during rivalry (Leopold and Logothetis, 1996). His model is also deterministic, ignoring the stochastic nature of suppression and dominance periods (which follow a gamma distribution). Also, there are no cells that respond when the images are presented binocularly and also fire when suppressed during rivaling. Neither are there cells that do not fire during binocular presentation but do fire during rivalry.

## AIMS

We wished to investigate the contrast dependence of a much more complex rivalry model. The number of input states and the number of categorical cells in the Dayan model were so restricted that statistical statements about the general behavior of the model under, say, contrast variation conditions would be hard to draw.

Furthermore, it was proposed to set up a model to meet the principles as set out by Levelt (1966):

• The percentage of total dominance of an image will increase with its strength.

• The average duration of dominance for a stimulus is independent of its strength.

• The speed with which dominance switches between stimuli increases as the strength of one stimulus increases.

• The speed with which dominance switches between stimuli increases as the strength of both stimuli increases. Increasing the contrast of one stimulus, rather than increasing the time of dominance of that eye, reduces the time of suppression of the eye receiving enhanced contrast (Blake, 1977; Fox and Rasche, 1969; Levelt, 1965).

**OUR MODEL**

A software package (NeuroSolutions V.3.022, The Neural Network Simulation Package) was chosen to build the neural net. The model was loosely based on Dayan's, but included a much more extensive input layer and a far more sophisticated recognition layer.

Two "eyes" for input were constructed with a visual pathway comprising four layers eventually combining to form a binocular network (figure 18.1).

The first layer models the LGN via an $81 \times 81$ matrix of inputs whose excitation varied over an 8-bit range (256 gray levels). The "receptive fields" of these units had no orientation tuning, somewhat like the pixels of a video camera sensor (i.e., without surround). Layer 2 modeled the striate cortex and was represented by a $27 \times 27 \times 4$ cell matrix, the last dimension representing possible orientations of $0°$, $45°$, $90°$, and $135°$. The third layer modeled early extrastriate cortex with an oriented $9 \times 9 \times 4$ matrix of cells (again limited to four orientations), combining inputs from the striate cortical units. The outputs from the separate pathways were merged as they entered the fourth layer, using a Kohonen "winner-take-all" neural network classifier that assigned its inputs just one of a group of classifications (which we will refer to as categorical cells—much like the idea of "grandmother cells").

We chose to implement ten such categorical cells. It should be clear that the receptive field properties of these categorical cells are not usually available from such a Kohonen network, and this feature provided a challenging limitation to rectify. Kohonen maps are artificial neural network components that assign each of the inputs to one of a group of classifications based on the features the network itself extracts from the input data. In addition, a Kohonen map classifies inputs topographically, with the algorithm forcing nearby classifier cells to respond to images that have similar features. In this sense, the Kohonen classifiers demonstrate features similar to neurons in primate inferotemporal cortex that possess

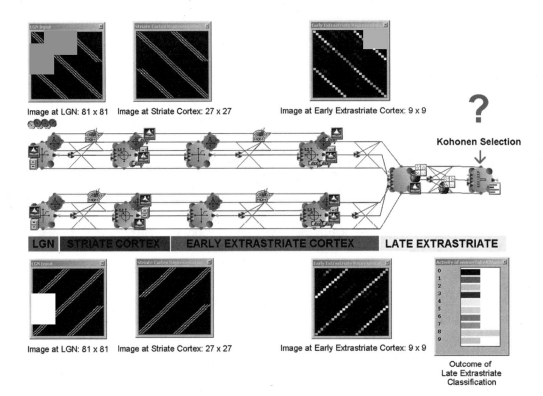

**Figure 18.1** Breadboard layout of the neural network. The layers and their connections are shown as two independent processing networks that undergo modification at levels labeled LGN (lateral geniculate nucleus), Striate Cortex, Early Extrastriate Cortex, and Late Extrastriate Cortex. It is between these last two axons that binocular interaction first occurs. Graphs above and below the eye inputs represent the simple 81 × 81 array at the LGN level, a 27 × 27 array at the Striate Cortex, and an image at the 9 × 9 level of Early Extrastriate. The final level is a winner-take-all Kohonen classifier that selects which of ten categorical cells is perceived.

highly complex receptive fields organized in columns with much greater similarity in receptive field within columns than between columns (Tanaka, 1993, 2003; Wang, Fujita, and Murayama, 2000).

**TRAINING**

Because we were not concerned with the process of creating orientation specificity for the cells of level 2 (V1), a developmentally plausible training algorithm was not required. Thus, backpropagation, the most efficient training algorithm, was used. The input data consisted of binary matrices,

D. P. Crewther and colleagues

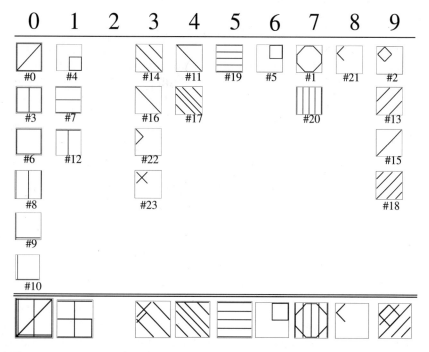

**Figure 18.2** An array of 24 input stimuli organized into columns according to the categorical cell with which they associated after training. The set of images at the bottom of the figure represents "collations" used as a means of representing each categorical cell.

used to train and to test the network (see top section of figure 18.2). During training, the network used a data set of 24 images (of $81 \times 81$ pixels), with eyes viewing a pair of matching inputs at contrasts 1, 0.9, 0.7, and 0.5 (i.e., bioptically). These input images were transformed by synaptic weights as they passed up to the striate layer. The output of this transformation was then compared with a previously prepared orientation-selective representation of the input image.

The process was repeated for all images and constituted one training run or epoch. Since NeuroSolutions provided graphical output probes to monitor the progress of the network, training was ceased when no visually recognizable improvement in the 8-bit gray scale representation could be seen (i.e., the output of the orientation-selective striate and extrastriate cells matched the input pattern). During the training phase for orientation specificity, the Kohonen map was not active.

After training for orientation specificity, the Kohonen network used these paired matching inputs to classify each representation into one of ten different classes (the categorical cells). The Kohonen network is often used in recognition software and is characterized by a "winner-take-all" response, with a single solution from the network being provided by the cell that gains maximum activation. Since the network did not allow recurrent connections as an inbuilt option of NeuroSolutions, a separately programmed module implemented as a dynamic link library (DLL) was coded. This served two functions. During training, the DLL calculated the average of the left- and right-eye firing strengths for each cell. This representation was added to any existing representation of the same categorical cell output. This creates a "collation," a superimposed image comprising all representations for each of the ten categorical cell outputs (see bottom section of figure 18.2). The training set needed to be executed only once to create such a collation.

## HYPOTHESIS FOR PREDICTING RIVALRY

Given the 24 input states (stimuli) and the ten categorical cells in the model, it is clear that more than one input state will associate with the same categorical cell (see figure 18.2). Indeed, for the input set of stimuli used, six input stimuli associated with categorical cell 1 but no input stimuli formed an association with categorical cell 2. Rivalry in this model is seen as a competition at the level of the categorical cells between inputs trying to claim association. Thus, our expectation was that input stimuli which associate with the same categorical cell should not rival, while stimuli that associate with different categorical cells during training will rival.

## Testing

When the training was completed and testing began, pairs of images were presented to the eyes (with $24^2 = 576$ possibilities). Each pair was shown to the "eyes" for 100 presentations, corresponding to 100 units of time. The Kohonen map was forced to make a classification based on the mismatching data. The second function of the DLL was to determine which of the images was "seen" by the Kohonen map and to modify the strengths of the neural connections being fed back to the late extrastriate layer based on this perception. The DLL compared each cell of the left eye and the right eye against the collated image of the current Kohonen selection. Calculating the absolute value of the difference between these two numbers for each cell and accumulating a total difference value finds a measure of similarity between the current Kohonen selection and the left- and right-eye representations. The eye with greater similarity to the Kohonen selection was chosen as the winner or dominant eye.

Two variables, termed left modifier and right modifier, altered the strength of the inputs at the early extrastriate layer. Initially, both these modifiers were set to 1. The dominant-eye modifier decreased the strength of the winning representation at the early extrastriate layer by 0.1, and the suppressed-eye modifier increased the representation by 0.1 for each iteration. The suppressed eye came into dominance when the total difference value indicated that the suppressed eye was now more similar to the current Kohonen output than the previously dominant eye. When this occurred, both the left and the right modifier were multiplied by a value derived from the ratio between the total difference of the left eye and that of the right eye. Thus the strength for the newly dominant eye was raised by this value and that for the suppressed eye was decreased by the same amount. Though artificial, these factors were intended to represent the processes loosely termed "habituation" and "selective attention/ suppression."

## RESULTS

The output files generated by the network were saved in spreadsheet form for later analysis. Overall averages for mean left-eye and right-eye dominance length, mean left and right dominance percentage, switching frequency, total percentage of stimuli that rivaled, and consistency between expected and actual behaviors were investigated.

### Summary of Cases

Given the 24 input states, the whole set of cases of potential rivalry or its lack could not be reasonably presented. However, several interesting cases have been included as an appendix in which the predictions of rivalry or lack of rivalry are described in detail. These cases are presented diagrammatically in figure 18.3.

It is clear that the model incorporates a nonrealistic regular fluctuation, as might be expected from the gradual fatigue built into the model. The figures show the strength modifiers for each eye's input, the similarity measure between each input and the current Kohonen "winning" classifier, and the Kohonen selection (that which is closest to percept). Thus rivalry is regular, nonexistent, slow, rapid, or irregular, depending on interactions between the network weightings associated with stimulus input.

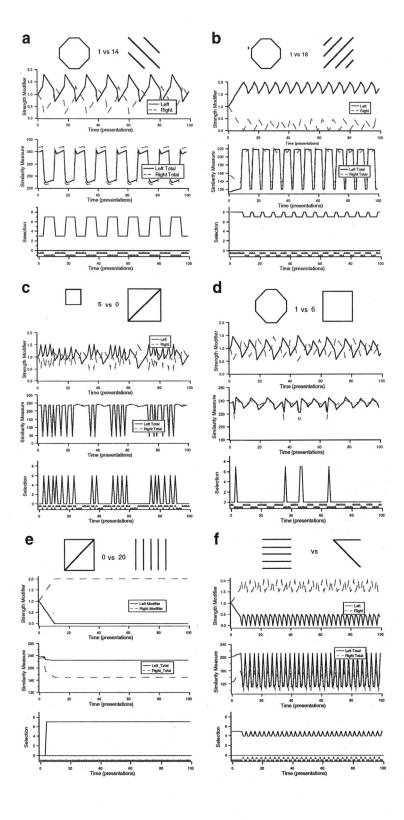

## Rivalry Prediction Performance

Given the relatively large set of input stimuli (24), the total number of possible pair combinations ($24^2 = 576$ cases) was sufficiently large to test statistical relations. All 576 cases were tested. The summary statistics for rivalry were as follows:

Nonrivalry (cases where the two input stimuli were associated during training with the same categorical cell) was correctly predicted in 97.2% of 85 cases.

Rivalry occurred in 81.4% of the 491 cases in which it was predicted (cases where the two input stimuli were associated during training with different categorical cells).

## Rivalry Parameters as a Function of Contrast

As indicated earlier, the network was trained under two conditions of varying contrast. The first variation involved altering the contrast presented to the right eye (0.5, 0.7, 0.9, 1.0), while the contrast of the left eye was fixed (1.0). This condition was termed "the interocular contrast difference condition."

The second variation involved presenting stimuli with the same contrast to the two eyes but altering the contrast across blocks of trials (0.5, 0.7, 0.9, 1.0)—this was termed "equal-eye contrast variation."

Under conditions of interocular contrast variation, a distinct behavior was observed in mean dominance periods as a function of contrast. Where unequal contrast was presented to the two eyes, rather than the mean dominance of the stronger eye stimulus becoming greater, the mean dominance period of the weaker eye was reduced (see figure 18.4).

◄ **Figure 18.3** Six cases of heterogeneous input to the two eyes and the variety of outcomes that ensue. The input stimuli are shown at the top of each figure, and three graphs are presented for each rivalry case. The top graph shows the behavior of the left and right modifiers over 100 iterations or presentations. The middle graph shows the behavior of the similarity measures for left and right stimuli. The bottom graph shows the behavior of the Kohonen classifier (solid line) as well as the "winner" (triangular markers) across the 100 presentations. (*a*) Stim 1 vs. stim 14—rivalry expected (regular rivalry occurred). (*b*) Stim 1 vs. stim 18—rivalry expected (rival alternation between nonexpected categorical cells occurred). (*c*) Stim 5 vs. stim 0—rivalry expected (rapid, irregular rivalry observed). (*d*) Stim 1 vs. stim 6—rivalry expected (very irregular switching observed). (*e*) Stim 0 vs. stim 20—rivalry expected (after initial switch, no rivalry observed). (*f*) Stim 19 vs. stim 11—rivalry expected (very rapid alternation observed).

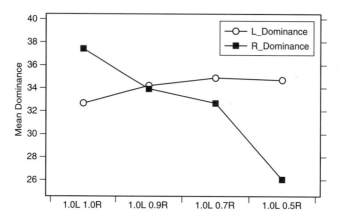

**Figure 18.4** Mean dominance period for the left- and right-eye stimuli under varied interocular contrast. The contrast for the left eye was maintained at 1.0, while that for the right eye was varied from 1.0 to 0.5. All cases where rivalry was expected have been included. While left-eye dominance remained approximately constant, a distinct trend to shorter mean dominance is observed as the contrast of the weaker stimulus is reduced.

Analysis of variance (ANOVA) was used to assess the results of contrast variation, using a $2 \times 4$ factorial design. In addition, a one-way ($1 \times 4$) design was used to investigate the dynamics of switching as a function of contrast. While for the interocular contrast difference condition a systematic drop in the mean percentage of left-eye dominance with increasing right-eye contrast was observed, the main effect of interocular contrast on total percent dominance was not significant ($F_{3,191} = 0.1$, $p > 0.05$). The interaction between interocular contrast and left- and right-eye percent total dominance was also not significant ($F_{3,191} = 0.47$, $p > 0.05$).

The frequency of dominance switching between eyes showed an interesting trend, with an increase in mean switching frequency as the right-eye contrast was increased from 0.5 to 1.0. However, significance was again lacking ($F_{3,95} = 0.96$, $p > 0.05$).

When both eyes were presented with the same contrast, the frequency of switching increased with contrast in a significant fashion: $F_{3,95} = 3.52$, $p < 0.05$ (figure 18.5).

### DISCUSSION

The model of binocular rivalry, as created, clearly provides a theoretical arena in which to investigate the properties of perception and suppression. The model was large enough in terms of input complexity and

D. P. Crewther and colleagues

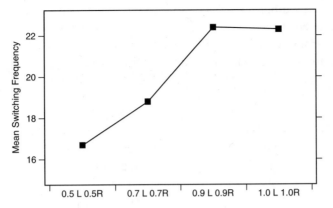

**Figure 18.5** Mean switching frequency (number of switches per 100 presentations) shown as a function of stimulus contrast for equal-contrast stimuli presented to the two eyes across the cases where rivalry was expected. A significant increase in switching frequency was observed.

output sophistication to investigate properties of rivalry across a range of stimuli presented to the two eyes, such that the relations between low- and high-order processing of the stimuli could be related to the dynamics of their rivalry.

The first aim, that the model would exhibit rivalry (i.e., dominant and suppressive phases when presented with dissimilar stimuli) was clearly supported by the results. Indeed, under normal, high-contrast conditions, the prediction of rivalry was confirmed at a rate of over 80%, and the prediction of nonrivalry was confirmed on a case-by-case basis at a rate of 97%. It is also apparent, from the series of cases demonstrated in figure 18.3, that the dynamics of rivalry was not fixed, with varying rates of alternation and irregular switching of dominant and suppressive phases. This was a requirement for biological plausibility (Levelt, 1966). However, it is also obvious that the distribution of alternations for any particular pair of our rival stimuli is far more regular than the gamma distribution experimentally observed (Fox and Herrmann, 1967; Levelt, 1966).

This regularity is largely due to the deterministic manner in which strength modifiers increase and decrease in value. It is plausible that if there were a noise contribution to the strength modifier, then a more natural distribution would result.

It is important to acknowledge the degree to which the network reflects the theoretical assumptions hardwired into its design. We expected to achieve rivalry in the gross sense because of two input features. First, the

A Neural Network Model of Top-Down Rivalry

use of a winner-take-all network to provide an answer to the question of what percept the network is "seeing" means that a solution is assured for all iterations in terms of one of ten categorical cells. The second input feature is that of habituation. While this factor may not have been necessary to achieve rivalry in some cases, its presence can be argued as logical on the basis of single-cell electrophysiological studies where habituation is a common observation of recordings from cortex.

The issue of bottom-up or top-down theories of rivalry has not been directly addressed by this neural network attempt. An inspection of figure 18.1 shows that there is segregation of the visual information through the first couple of stages and that interaction between the two eyes really occurs only at the penultimate stage, just before the Kohonen classifier. In the current model it is the activity in the early extrastriate cortex that causes rivalry for dominance at the late extrastriate level. The result of the late extrastriate decision on the winner is fed back to the activity levels at the early extrastriate layer. Thus the current model embraces aspects of both theories. Also, the model does not really mimic the human visual system, where binocular interaction occurs at the level of striate cortex and where pipelining of information to "categorical cortex" in the inferotemporal regions occurs via several more synaptic steps utilizing predominantly binocular neurons.

The model does not give a prediction regarding cortical localization or hemispheric switching (Miller et al., 2000), largely because there is only one higher cortical region in the model. However, it is clear from the way in which attention was (somewhat artificially) implemented that the model would respond to neural firing changes accompanying such a hemispheric stimulation. Also, it is clear that rivalry does not require the presence of two hemispheres to compete, because the properties of the categorical cells are sufficient.

The one feature of this model that was not an input was not engineered, and yet gave plausibility to the top-down approach was the emergence of a principle of prediction of rivalry which was validated with high reliability. Consider the system from the bottom up and from the top down. A priori there is nothing from the bottom-up direction that allows a prediction of rivalry in particular choices of stimuli presented to the two eyes. While one might guess that stimuli with like contours are less likely to rival, it is only when the system has actually learned and categorized the set of stimulus images into one of ten categorical cells that one can predict with almost complete certainty which pairs of stimuli will not rival. The human visual system also shows a preference for images that it has learned. Yu and Blake (1992) showed that in rivalry, a face stimulus predominated more than a pattern stimulus equated for spatial frequency, luminance, and contrast.

The Kohonen classifier is interesting in that neighboring classifiers are closer in terms of similarity than are more distant ones. This was seen in some of the rivalry cases where the expected categorical cells did not participate, but a neighboring categorical cell was involved. Also, rivalry comparison at high and low contrast showed, for example, that a stimulus may have been classified as GC#3 at low contrast but GC#4 at high contrast.

In principle, the model could be extended to provide an account of other bistable phenomena, where the low-level part of the network receives invariant input. Practically, this could be achieved through the training of images with binocular disparity (e.g., the two alternate 3D views of the Necker cube) and then testing with 2D (zero disparity) stimuli presented to the two eyes.

In conclusion, the results of this and other computational studies of binocular rivalry indicate that both bottom-up and top-down approaches yield rivalry behaviors that mimic well parts of the experimental literature. Thus it is likely that composite models, where rivalry may emerge from interactions at several levels of neural processing, need to be investigated.

## REFERENCES

Alais, D., and Blake, R. (1999). Grouping visual features during binocular rivalry. *Vision Research*, 39, 4341–4353.

Andrews, T. J., and Blakemore, C. (1999). Form and motion have independent access to consciousness. *Nature Neuroscience*, 2, 405–406.

Blake, R. (1977). Threshold conditions for binocular rivalry. *Journal of Experimental Psychology: Human Perception and Performance*, 3, 251–257.

Blake, R. (1989). A neural theory of binocular rivalry. *Psychological Review*, 96, 145–167.

Bullier, J. (2001). Integrated model of visual processing. *Brain Research Review*, 36, 96–107.

Dayan, P. (1998). A hierarchical model of binocular rivalry. *Neural Computation*, 10, 1119–1135.

Epstein, R., and Kanwisher, N. (1998). A cortical representation of the local visual environment. *Nature*, 392, 598–601.

Fox, R., and Herrmann, J. (1967). Stochastic properties of binocular rivalry alternations. *Perception and Psychophysics*, 2, 432–436.

Fox, R., and Rasche, F. (1969). Binocular rivalry and reciprocal inhibition. *Perception and Psychophysics*, 5, 215–217.

Hupé, J. M., James, A. C., Girard, P., Lomber, S. G., Payne, B. R., and Bullier, J. (2001). Feedback connections act on the early part of the responses in monkey visual cortex. *Journal of Neurophysiology*, 85, 134–145.

Kanwisher, N., McDermott, J., and Chun, M. M. (1997). The fusiform face area: A module in human extrastriate cortex specialized for face perception. *Journal of Neuroscience*, 17, 4302–4311.

Kovács, I., Papathomas, T. V., Yang, M., and Fehér, A. (1996). When the brain changes its mind: Interocular grouping during binocular rivalry. *Proceedings of the National Academy of Sciences of the United States of America*, 93, 15508–15511.

Lamme, V. A., Super, H., Landman, R., Roelfsema, P. R., and Spekreijse, H. (2000). The role of primary visual cortex (V1) in visual awareness. *Vision Research*, 40, 1507–1521.

Lamme, V. A., Van Dijk, B. W., and Spekreijse, H. (1992). Texture segregation is processed by primary visual cortex in man and monkey. Evidence from VEP experiments. *Vision Research*, 32, 797–807.

Lee, S. H., and Blake, R. (2002). V1 activity is reduced during binocular rivalry. *Journal of Vision*, 2, 618–626.

Lehky, S. R. (1988). An astable multivibrator model of binocular rivalry. *Perception*, 17, 215–228.

Leopold, D. A., and Logothetis, N. K. (1996). Activity changes in early visual cortex reflect monkeys' percepts during binocular rivalry. *Nature*, 379, 549–553.

Levelt, W. J. M. (1965). *On Binocular Rivalry*. Soesterberg, The Netherlands: Institute for Perception RVO-TNO.

Levelt, W. J. M. (1966). The alternation process in binocular rivalry. *British Journal of Psychology*, 57, 225–238.

Liu, L., Tyler, C. W., and Schor, C. M. (1992). Failure of rivalry at low contrast: Evidence of a suprathreshold binocular summation process. *Vision Research*, 32, 1471–1479.

Logothetis, N. K. (1998a). Object vision and visual awareness. *Current Opinion in Neurobiology*, 8, 536–544.

Logothetis, N. K. (1998b). Single units and conscious vision. *Philosophical Transactions of the Royal Society of London*, B353, 1801–1818.

Logothetis, N. K., Leopold, D. A., and Sheinberg, D. L. (1996). What is rivalling during binocular rivalry? *Nature*, 380, 621–624.

Logothetis, N. K., and Schall, J. D. (1989). Neuronal correlates of subjective visual perception. *Science*, 245, 761–763.

Lumer, E. D. (1998). A neural model of binocular integration and rivalry based on the coordination of action-potential timing in primary visual cortex. *Cerebral Cortex*, 8, 553–561.

Miller, S. M., Liu, G. B., Ngo, T. T., Hooper, G., Riek, S., Carson, R. G., and Pettigrew, J. D. (2000). Interhemispheric switching mediates perceptual rivalry. *Current Biology*, 10, 383–392.

Mueller, T. J. (1990). A physiological model of binocular rivalry. *Vision Neuroscience*, 4, 63–73.

Mueller, T. J., and Blake, R. (1989). A fresh look at the temporal dynamics of binocular rivalry. *Biological Cybernetics*, 61, 223–232.

Polonsky, A., Blake, R., Braun, J., and Heeger, D. J. (2000). Neuronal activity in human primary visual cortex correlates with perception during binocular rivalry. *Nature Neuroscience*, 3, 1153–1159.

Puce, A., Allison, T., Gore, J. C., and McCarthy, G. (1995). Face-sensitive regions in human extrastriate cortex studied by functional MRI. *Journal of Neurophysiology*, 74, 1192–1199.

Seghier, M., Dojat, M., Delon-Martin, C., Rubin, C., Warnking, J., Segebarth, C., and Bullier, J. (2000). Moving illusory contours activate primary visual cortex: An fMRI study. *Cerebral Cortex*, 10, 663–670.

Sugie, N. (1982). Neural models of brightness perception and retinal rivalry in binocular vision. *Biological Cybernetics*, 43, 13–21.

Super, H., Spekreijse, H., and Lamme, V. A. (2001). Two distinct modes of sensory processing observed in monkey primary visual cortex (V1). *Nature Neuroscience*, 4, 304–310.

Tanaka, K. (1993). Neuronal mechanisms of object recognition. *Science*, 262, 685–688.

Tanaka, K. (2003). Columns for complex visual object features in the inferotemporal cortex: Clustering of cells with similar but slightly different stimulus selectivities. *Cerebral Cortex*, 13, 90–99.

Tong, F., and Engel, S. A. (2001). Interocular rivalry revealed in the human cortical blind-spot representation. *Nature*, 411, 195–199.

Tong, F., Nakayama, K., Vaughan, J. T., and Kanwisher, N. (1998). Binocular rivalry and visual awareness in human extrastriate cortex. *Neuron*, 21, 753–759.

Tononi, G., Srinivasan, R., Russell, D. P., and Edelman, G. M. (1998). Investigating neural correlates of conscious perception by frequency-tagged neuromagnetic responses. *Proceedings of the National Academy of Sciences of the United States of America*, 95, 3198–3203.

Wang, Y., Fujita, I., and Murayama, Y. (2000). Neuronal mechanisms of selectivity for object features revealed by blocking inhibition in inferotemporal cortex. *Nature Neuroscience*, 3, 807–813.

Wolfe, J. M. (1983). Influence of spatial frequency, luminance, and duration on binocular rivalry and abnormal fusion of briefly presented dichoptic stimuli. *Perception*, 12, 447–456.

Yu, K., and Blake, R. (1992). Do recognizable figures enjoy an advantage in binocular rivalry? *Journal of Experimental Psychology: Human Perception and Performance*, 18, 1158–1173.

## APPENDIX: SAMPLE CASES OF RIVALRY AND NONRIVALRY

Given the overall hypothesis of the study concerning the chance of rivalry—that stimuli which attract the same categorical cell to respond should not rival, while stimuli which associate with different categorical cells during training will rival—several cases exhibit the success (and variations of success) of the hypothesis.

### Expect Rivalry—Get Regular Rivalry

Stim 1 versus stim 14. In this situation, with stim 1 presented to one eye and stim 14 presented to the other, rivalry was expected because stim 1 associated with categorical cell 7, while stim 14 associated with categorical cell 3 (see figure 18.3a). The figure shows a graphical representation of the rivaling stimuli as well as a representation across the 100 iterations (Time) of the left and right strength modifiers. Notice the regular alternation between the modifiers, with reciprocal weakening and strengthening (0.1 per iteration) until the point at which the "winner" (bottom graph, triangle symbols) changes identity. At this point the strength of the winning eye is enhanced by a factor (perhaps analogous to attention), with a corresponding drop in strength for the suppressed stimulus.

The overall strength of this factor was arbitrary, but was fixed throughout all of the network calculations. The similarity measure for the left and right eyes is shown in the second trace. It also shows regularity in alternation that is highly correlated with the switch in Kohonen choice (categorical selection) (lower trace). The "winner" is shown as a series of triangular markers taking on one of two states (upper = right, lower = left). In this case the change in "winner" occurs at precisely the same time as the change in Kohonen choice.

### Expect Rivalry—Get Rivalry with Erroneous Percept

Stim 1 versus stim 18. Given the two stimuli, rivalry was expected between categorical cell 7 (stim 1) and categorical cell 9 (stim 18). However, as figure 18.3b shows, though rivalry was observed, it was between categorical cells 7 and 8 (bottom graph—selection), rather than GC7 and GC9. Note that the strength modifiers for the left and right eyes are again mirror

D. P. Crewther and colleagues

images around the value 1. Again the rivalry is quite regular, after an initial longer settling period—this appears to be associated with the relatively large change in similarity measure for each eye between the one percept and the other, what one might call "strong rivalry." It is interesting that while "false" percept was generated, the incorrect categorical cell (GC8 rather then GC9) is a neighboring Kohonen classifier of the expected one, with the implication of some similarity relation between the neighbors. Such erroneous percept (disagreeing with either monocular input) is possible experimentally (Kovács et al., 1996).

**Expect Rivalry—Get Irregular Rapid Rivalry**   Stim 5 (GC6) versus stim 0 (GC0). The lowest graph of figure 18.3c shows a rapid alternation between GC6 and GC0. While the rivalry is between the expected categorical cell representations, the frequency of alternation is irregular. This irregularity possibly arises because of the close similarity measures for the two eyes.

**Expect Rivalry—Get Irregular, Infrequent Rivalry**   Stim 1 (GC7) versus stim 6 (GC0). While the strength modifiers overlap in a fashion very similar to that exhibited in figure 18.3a, the rivalry results are dramatically different. The similarity measures for the two eyes are not at all similar in shape, and the "winner" graph at the extreme bottom of figure 18.3d shows an irregularity in switching. This irregularity is further teased out by the Kohonen selection graph (lowest solid curve, figure 18.3d). The switching between categorical cells is not well predicted by the switching in winner. This possibly is due to the relatively small difference in similarity measure between dominance and suppression states for the two eyes (roughly of amplitude 30, compared with over 100 for figure 18.3a). This might be termed "weak rivalry."

**Failed Rivalry—When Expected**

Stim 0 (GC0) versus stim 20 (GC7). One switch in percept near the start of the iteration was observed. After this time, the percept remained stuck at categorical cell 7 (see figure 18.3e). This failure of rivalry (when expected from the difference in categorical cell preference for the two stimuli) can be identified as due to the fact that the similarity measures never approached a crossing point.

## Expect Regular Rivalry—Get Rapid Rivalry

Stim 19 (GC5) versus stim 11 (GC4). The alternation between GC5 and GC4 occurred as expected. However, the frequency of alternation was considerably higher than would be expected from the 10% per iteration change in strength modifier, for which (e.g., figure 18.3a) occupancy of each dominant state of about seven iterations is observed. This "standard" rivalry corresponds to a frequency of 15 alternations per 100 iterations. However, for the rapid rivalry observed in this case (figure 18.3f), more than 60 alternations per 100 iterations were observed.

# Contributors

David Alais
Department of Physiology and
Institute for Biomedical Research
School of Medical Science
University of Sydney
Sydney, Australia

Timothy J. Andrews
University Laboratory of
Physiology
University of Oxford
Oxford, United Kingdom

Department of Psychology
University of Durham
Durham, United Kingdom

Randolph Blake
Department of Psychology
Vanderbilt University
Nashville, Tennessee

Colin Blakemore
University Laboratory of
Physiology
University of Oxford
Oxford, United Kingdom

Thomas Carlson
Department of Psychology
University of Minnesota
Minneapolis, Minnesota

O. L. Carter
Vision Touch and Hearing
Research Centre
School of Biomedical Sciences
University of Queensland
Brisbane, Australia

Miguel Castelo-Branco
Faculty of Medicine
Instituto Biomédico de
Investacão de Luz e Imagem
Coimbra, Portugal

Xiangchuan Chen
University of Science and
Technology of China
Department of Neurobiology and
Biophysics
Hefei, Anhui, People's Republic of
China

Tiffany Conway
Laboratory of Vision Research
Rutgers University
Piscataway, New Jersey

Paul M. Corballis
Center for Cognitive Neuroscience
Dartmouth College
Hanover, New Hampshire

D. P. Crewther
Brain Sciences Institute
Swinburne University of
Technology
Melbourne, Australia

S. Crewther
School of Psychological Science
La Trobe University
Melbourne, Australia

Michal Eisenberg
Department of Psychology and
Laboratory of Vision
Research/Center for Cognitive
Science
Rutgers University
Piscataway, New Jersey

Andreas K. Engel
Institute of Neurophysiology
and Pathophysiology
University Hospital Hamburg-
Eppendorf
Hamburg, Germany

Robert Fox
Department of Psychology and
Department of Biomedical
Engineering
Kennedy Center Scientist
Vanderbilt University
Nashville, Tennessee

Alan W. Freeman
School of Biomedical Sciences
University of Sydney
Lidcombe, Australia

Itzhak Fried
Division of Neurosurgery and
Department of Psychiatry and
Biobehavioral Sciences
David Geffen School of Medicine
University of California
Los Angeles, California

Functional Neurosurgery Unit
Tel Aviv Medical Center and
Sackler School of Medicine
Tel Aviv University
Tel Aviv, Israel

Pascal Fries
F.C. Donders Centre for Cognitive
Neuroimaging
Nijmegen, The Netherlands

Department of Biophysics
University of Nijmegen
The Netherlands

Sheng He
Department of Psychology
University of Minnesota
Minneapolis, Minnesota

Zijiang J. He
Department of Psychological and
Brain Sciences
University of Louisville
Louisville, Kentucky

Ian P. Howard
Centre for Vision Research
York University
Toronto, Ontario, Canada

Jean-Michel Hupé
Center for Neural Science
New York University
New York, New York

R. Jones
School of Psychological Science
La Trobe University
Melbourne, Australia

Christof Koch
Computation and Neural Systems
Program
California Institute of Technology
Pasadena, California

Ilona Kovács
Department of Psychology and
Laboratory of Vision
Research/Center for Cognitive
Science
Rutgers University
Piscataway, New Jersey

Gabriel Kreiman
Division of Neurosurgery and
Department of Psychiatry and
Biobehavioral Sciences
David Geffen School of Medicine
University of California
Los Angeles, California

Computational and Neural
Systems Program
California Institute of Technology
Pasadena, California

David A. Leopold
Department of Physiology of
Cognitive Processes
Max Planck Institute for Biologic
Cybernetics
Tübingen, Germany

Unit on Cognitive
Neurophysiology and Imaging
National Institutes of Health
Bethesda, Maryland 20892

Nikos K. Logothetis
Department of Physiology of
Cognitive Processes
Max Planck Institute for Biologic
Cybernetics
Tübingen, Germany

Alexander Maier
Department of Physiology of
Cognitive Processes
Max Planck Institute for Biologic
Cybernetics
Tübingen, Germany

J. Munro
School of Psychological Science
La Trobe University
Melbourne, Australia

Vincent A. Nguyen
School of Biomedical Sciences
University of Sydney
Lidcombe, Australia

Teng Leng Ooi
Department of Basic Sciences
Pennsylvania College of
Optometry
Elkins Park, Pennsylvania

Robert P. O'Shea
Department of Psychology
University of Otago
Dunedin, New Zealand

Thomas V. Papathomas
Department of Biomedical
Engineering and Laboratory of
Vision Research
Rutgers University
New Brunswick, New Jersey

J. D. Pettigrew
Vision Touch and Hearing
Research Centre
School of Biomedical Sciences
University of Queensland
Brisbane, Australia

T. Price
School of Psychological Science
La Trobe University
Melbourne, Australia

S. Pulis
School of Psychological Science
La Trobe University
Melbourne, Australia

Nava Rubin
Center for Neural Science
New York University
New York, New York

Frank Sengpiel
University Laboratory of
Physiology
University of Oxford
Oxford, United Kingdom

School of Biosciences
Cardiff University
Cardiff, United Kingdom

Wolf Singer
Max Planck Institut für
Hirnforschung
Frankfurt, Germany

Frank Tong
Department of Psychology
Princeton University
Princeton, New Jersey

Nicholas J. Wade
Department of Psychology
University of Dundee
Dundee, Scotland

Melanie Wilke
Department of Physiology of
Cognitive Processes
Max Planck Institute for Biologic
Cybernetics
Tübingen, Germany

Hugh R. Wilson
Centre for Vision Research
York University
Toronto, Ontario, Canada

# Name Index

Adams, P. A., 11
Adelson, E. H., 137, 140, 152, 197, 199, 269
Aguilonius, F., 35
Ahlstrom, U., 89
Akasu, T., 294
Alais, D., xi, 7, 17, 22, 47, 84, 89, 128, 132, 152, 155, 164, 166, 197, 248, 250, 269, 272, 307, 308, 309, 310, 313, 339
Albright, T. D., 199, 233, 269
Alexander, L. T., 83
Alhazen, 34, 252
Allman, J., 19, 215, 227
Alonso, J. M., 260
Amira, L., 90
Andersen, R. A., 59, 233, 235
Anderson, B. L., 172, 174
Anderson, J. D., 85
Andrews, T. J., xiii, 21, 77, 89, 165, 187, 198, 199, 200, 201, 203, 205, 249, 296, 339
Angelucci, A., 242
Asher, H., 1
Ashida, H., 87
Atkinson, J., 11, 102
Avoli, M., 319, 320, 321
Azouz, R., 260

Bagby, J. W., 11
Baitch, L. W., 90
Bakin, J. S., 132, 242, 247
Barlow, H. B., 188, 246, 312
Barnard, N., 102
Barrett, R. K., 294
Bauer, J., 103, 113

Baumgartner, G., 132
Baylis, G. C., 203
Bechtoldt, H. P., 85
Beck, D. M., 65
Becklen, R., 165
Behnke, E., 227
Benzer, S., 293
Bettinger, L. A., 19, 261
Bilotta, J., 248
Blackburn, S., 174, 176
Blake, R., vii, 1, 3, 4, 6, 7, 10, 13, 14, 15, 17, 19, 20, 21, 49, 51, 56, 63, 69, 71, 75, 76, 77, 81, 83, 84, 85, 86, 87, 89, 90, 92, 93, 106, 120, 128, 132, 143, 149, 150, 153, 155, 164, 165, 166, 182, 187, 188, 191, 193, 194, 196, 197, 199, 200, 206, 215, 234, 242, 245, 248, 250, 260, 269, 283, 284, 292, 295, 302, 305, 308, 309, 310, 312, 313, 317, 318, 320, 323, 325, 326, 327, 333, 337, 338, 339, 340, 341, 351
Blakemore, C., xiii, 55, 89, 133, 187, 189, 190, 191, 192, 194, 195, 199, 200, 235, 236, 246, 266, 312, 339
Bloor, D. C., 15, 155
Blundo, C., 226
Boer, G. J., 292
Bogen, J. E., 301
Bokander, I., 11
Bonneh, Y., 233, 249, 286, 287, 293, 294
Born, R. T., 233
Borsellino, A., 283, 322, 332
Borsting, E., 118, 245
Bossink, C. J., 83, 84, 143, 153

Bower, T. G. R., 85
Boynton, G. M., 68
Braddick, O. J., 102, 138, 152, 191
Bradley, D. C., 233, 235
Bravo, M., 15
Breese, B. B., xviii, 7, 8, 9, 10, 11, 12, 15, 20, 76, 92, 292
Brewster, D., 32, 35, 36, 37, 38, 39, 40, 41, 42, 43
Britten, K. H., 204
Broadbent, D., x
Brown, R. J., 64, 103, 113
Bruner, J., 12
Bullier, J., 76, 338
Burke, D., 84, 152
Burkhalter, A., 246
Burns, D. E., 294
Burton, H. E., 169

Calvert, G. A., 203
Camisa, J., 49, 194, 245, 248
Campbell, F. W., 11, 233, 249
Campbell, T., 296
Candy, T. R., 103, 113
Carkeet, A., 102
Carlson, T. A., xiii, 81, 88, 90, 91
Carney, T., 89, 199
Carpenter, W. B., 39, 41
Carter, O. L., x, 283, 284, 286, 287, 288, 292, 294
Castelo-Branco, M., 259, 271, 273, 274, 277, 278
Cavanagh, P., 59, 113, 247
Cave, C., 22
Chang, G. C., 233, 235
Charles, E. R., 82, 85, 86
Check, R., 13, 193, 234, 245
Chen, X., xiii, 81, 93
Cheng, K., 69, 84, 226
Chow, C. C., 149, 150, 317, 322, 323, 330
Chun, M. M., 201, 337
Ciner, E. B., 102
Cobb, W. A., 64
Cogan, R., 305
Connor, C. E., 246
Connors, B. W., 320
Conte, M. M., 272

Conway, T. E., xiii, 155
Cooperman, A., 233, 249, 286
Corballis, P. M., xi, 92, 301, 303, 304, 305, 306, 307, 308, 309, 310
Cowey, A., 203
Crassini, B., 85, 234
Creed, R. S., 155, 199
Crewther, D. P., xi, 102, 337
Crewther, S., xi, 102, 337
Crick, F., 1, 77, 78, 215, 227
Crovitz, H. F., 92
Culham, J., 87
Cumming, B. G., 246, 247
Curtin, K. D., 294

Dacey, D. M., 82
Dakin, S. C., 58
Das, A., 311, 325
Dayan, P., 339, 340, 341
DeAngelis, G. C., 246, 277
De la Iglesia, H. O., 285, 291
DeLange, H., 85
De Marco, A., 19
Dember, W. N., 12
Derrington, A. M., 82, 83, 84, 85
Desaguliers, J. T., 33, 34
Desimone, R., 60
De Weert, C. M. M., 83, 84, 143, 153, 160, 164
DeYoe, E. A., 82
Diaz-Caneja, E., 22, 155, 250, 307, 308, 311, 313
Dodd, J. V., 233, 235
Dohle, C., 110
Dolan, R. J., 113, 204
Dörrenhaus, W., 17
Douglas, R. J., 194
Downing, P. E., 204
Dowse, H. B., 294
Dubé, S., 137, 153
Dubner, R., 200
Duensing, G., 129
Duke, P. A., 178, 179, 181
Dunbabin, K. M. D., 31
Du Tour, E.-F., 188

Ehrenstein, W. H., 102
Eichenbaum, H., 218, 226

Eisenberg, M., xi, 7, 101
Ekman, P., 218
Emerson, E., 40, 41, 43
Engel, A., xiii, 259
Engel, S., 14, 51, 56, 69, 70, 72, 73, 75, 133, 200, 226, 235, 317, 338
Enoksson, P., 260
Epstein, R., 201, 337
Erdelyi, M. H., 12
Erlanger, J., 294
Ettlinger, G., 64
Eysel, U. T., 194

Fahle, M., 92, 292
Favreau, O. E., 59
Fechner, G. T., 18, 43
Fehér, A., 164, 166
Felleman, D. J., 204, 213, 218, 246
Fennema, C. L., 269
Feynman, R. P., 284, 294, 295
Fox, R., xviii, 7, 11, 12, 13, 14, 15, 19, 20, 21, 77, 81, 83, 89, 117, 193, 199, 234, 245, 248, 261, 305, 322, 323, 341, 349
Freeman, A. W., x, xi, 47, 56, 77
Freeman, T. C. B., 191, 192, 206
Fried, I., xiii, 213, 214, 215, 218, 219, 222, 223, 226, 227, 237
Friedman, H. S., 132, 233, 242, 247
Fries, P., xiii, 259, 261, 268
Frisby, J. P., 182
Friston, K. J., 65, 93, 133, 226, 302, 305, 308, 313
Fujita, I., 242
Fukuda, H., 248
Funk, A. P., 293

Gauthier, I., 204
Gazzaniga, M. S., 301, 303, 308, 313
Gelade, G., 131
Giaschi, D., 102
Gibson, B. S., 248
Gibson, J. J., 1
Gilbert, C. D., 110, 132, 194, 242, 247, 311, 325
Gill, A. T., 36
Gillam, B., 118, 174, 175, 176, 245
Gobbini, M. I., 203
Goebel, R., 78

Goldstein, A. G., 85
Golin, E. S., 110
Goodale, M. A., 110, 111
Gopnik, A., 110
Gordon, M. M., 43
Gorea, A., 160
Govan, D. G., 7, 84, 312
Grabowecky, M., 155, 164, 251
Gray, C. M., 260
Graziano, M. S. A., 59
Green, D., 223
Greenwald, M. J., 193, 260
Gregory, R., 85, 231, 233
Grindley, G. C., 10, 129
Grossberg, S., 14, 118
Grossman, E., 13
Grunewald, A., 233, 235
Grzywacz, N. M., 152
Gutnick, M. J., 320
Gwiazda, J., 103, 113
Gyoba, J., 165

Habak, C., 56
Haffenden, A. M., 111
Haley, L. J., 85
Halgren, E., 66
Hall, J. C., 294
Hall, S., 110
Haller, A. von, 31
Halpern, D. L., 75
Hanisch, C., 110
Hansell, N., 293
Harrad, R., 55, 90, 190, 206, 235, 236
Hasselmo, M. E., 203
Hasson, U., 204
Hasuo, H., 294
Haxby, J. V., 201, 203
He, S., xiii, 81, 88, 90, 91
He, Z. J., x, xii, 117, 121, 124, 125, 129, 131, 132, 133, 164, 165
Hebb, W., x
Heider, B., 233, 242, 247
Hekel, A. P., 294
Held, R., 103, 113
Helfrich-Förster, C., 293
Helmholtz, H. von, 7, 42, 43, 117, 128, 252
Hering, K. E., 7, 85, 312

Herrmann, J., 305, 322, 349
Herzberg, C., 102
Hickey, T. L., 326
Hinkle, D. A., 246
Hoffman, E. A., 203
Hollants-Gilhuijs, M. A., 102
Hollins, M., 6
Holopigian, K., 193
Horowitz, F. D., 102
Horton J., 69, 325
Howard, I. P., xii, 33, 169, 171, 178, 179, 181,
    182, 183, 184, 185, 243, 245, 252
Howell, E. R., 11, 233, 249
Howie, D., 12
Hoyt, W. F., 325
Huang, Z. J., 294
Hubel, D. H., 17, 82, 84, 85, 86, 89, 196, 200,
    260, 261, 295, 331
Hupé, J-M., xii, 21, 137, 140, 141, 146, 147,
    148, 151, 153, 242, 284, 287, 338

Jackendoff, R., 227
James, W., 4, 8
Janssen, P., 246
Jessell, T., 218
Joseph, J., 131
Julesz, B., x, 246, 252

Kakizaki, S., 11
Kanizsa, G., 164
Kanwisher, N., 201, 204, 337
Karrer, R., 90
Kaufman, L., 85
Kerkhof, G. A., 287
Kim, C. Y., 13
Kim, J., 149, 152
Kisvárday, Z. F., 194
Kleinschmidt, A., 203
Koch, C., xiii, 1, 77, 78, 213, 215, 217, 218,
    219, 222, 223, 226, 227, 237
Koffka, K., 231, 233
Kohler, W., ix
Konczak, J., 110
Konopka, R. J., 293, 294
Kontsevich, L. L., 90
Kovács, I., xi, xiii, 3, 7, 17, 76, 101, 102,
    108, 110, 111, 113, 126, 128, 155, 156,

160, 161, 164, 165, 234, 250, 317, 338,
    339, 355
Krauskopf, J., 85, 199, 269
Kreiman, G., xiii, 78, 213, 214, 215, 217, 218,
    219, 220, 222, 223, 226, 227, 237
Krupa, B., 320, 331, 332
Kulikowski, J. J., 82, 86, 164, 250
Kuskowski, M., 113
Kyriacou, C. P., 294

Lacan, E., 39
Lack, L., xviii, 7, 11, 117
Laing, C. R., 149, 150, 317, 322, 323, 330
Lamme, V. A., 78, 233, 242, 338
Lansing, R. W., 64
Lee, B. B., 82
Lee, D. K., 60
Lee, S. H., 3, 6, 14, 21, 56, 69, 77, 81, 120, 166,
    200, 234, 250, 269, 283, 318, 320, 325, 326,
    327, 338
Lee, T. S., 233
Legge, G. E., 82
Lehky, S. R., 19, 63, 142, 143, 144, 145, 149,
    150, 188, 189, 226, 235, 283, 317, 322,
    323, 339
Lehman, M. N., 292
Lehmkuhle, S. W., 15, 89, 199, 234, 248
Lejeune, A., 188
Lema, S. A., 191
Lennie, P., 82, 83, 84, 85
Leopold, D. A., x, 3, 14, 21, 48, 56, 59, 60,
    63, 65, 69, 74, 76, 77, 81, 93, 132, 145, 153,
    155, 200, 217, 226, 231, 233, 234, 235, 237,
    240, 250, 260, 289, 290, 291, 317, 318, 327,
    329, 331, 333, 337, 340
Leung, E. H. L., 86
Levelt, W. J. M., xviii, xix, 11, 17, 18, 19, 20,
    21, 54, 63, 71, 83, 92, 122, 142, 145, 149,
    150, 151, 152, 153, 233, 248, 283, 292, 317,
    323, 324, 326, 340, 341, 349
Levi, D. M., 90, 102
Lewy, A. J., 285
Liden, L., 152
Lillakas, L., 245
Liu, L., 84, 152, 174, 175, 340
Livingstone, M. S., 82, 84, 86, 89

Logothetis, N. K., 14, 15, 17, 48, 56, 59, 60,
  63, 65, 67, 68, 69, 74, 76, 77, 81, 86, 88, 106,
  132, 133, 145, 153, 155, 165, 187, 200, 215,
  217, 218, 226, 227, 231, 233, 234, 235, 237,
  238, 239, 240, 242, 248, 259, 260, 261, 284,
  295, 317, 318, 331, 333, 337, 339, 340
Loop, M. S., 86, 312
Lovegrove, W., 17
Lumer, E. D., 133, 302, 305, 308, 312, 313, 339
Lund, J. S., 194

MacDonald, K. A., 215
Mackeben, M., 131, 132
Magnussen, S., 249
Maier, A., 231
Makous, W., 49
Malach, R., 201, 325
Manny, R. E., 102
Mapperson, B., 17
Marr, D., 117, 125
Marroquin, J. L., 331, 332
Martin, K. A. C., 194
Mather, G., 251
Matsumiya, K., 185
Maunsell, J. H. R., 83, 189, 226, 235, 246
Mayhew, J. E. W., 182
McCormick, D. A., 320, 321, 332, 333
McDermott, D., 284, 295
McDermott, J., 201, 317
McGinnies, E., 12
McIntyre, C., 7, 19, 305, 323
McNamara, T., 22
Meenes, M., 6
Meijer, J. H., 291
Miezin, F., 19, 215
Menaker, M., 285
Meng, M., 65
Meskenaite, V., 233, 242, 247
Metelli, F., 126, 127
Miller, B., 129
Miller, J. E., 90
Miller, J. G., 311
Miller, S. M., 93, 286, 289, 302, 311, 313, 350
Milner, A. D., 110, 111
Minors, D. S., 289
Mittag, M., 289
Mooney, C. M., 110, 111, 113

Moore, C., 113
Morre, D. J., 295
Morre, D. M., 295
Morton, H. B., 64
Movshon, J. A., 137, 140, 142, 152, 197, 199,
  200, 269, 271, 273
Mueller, T. J., 6, 20, 51, 81, 83, 92, 106, 143,
  153, 196, 196, 250, 283, 292, 302, 312, 325,
  333, 339
Murayama, Y., 342
Myerson, J., 19, 215

Nagai, Y., 325
Nakayama, K., 118, 125, 126, 129, 131, 132,
  155, 169, 171, 172, 174, 176, 242, 245,
  246, 247
Necker, L. A., 30, 32, 43, 187, 233
Neisser, U., 165
Nelson, C. A., 101
Neuenschwander, S., 274
Newsome, W. T., 246, 277
Ngo, T. T., 128, 302
Nguyen, V., xi, 47, 56, 77
Nicoll, A., 194
Nishida, S., 87
Norcia, A. M., 64, 103, 113
Norman, H. F., 248
Norman, J. F., 248

O'Connell, D. N., 233
O'Craven, K. M., 204
Ogle, K. N., 11
Ojemann, G. A., 215
Ono, H., 245
Ooi, T. L., x, xii, 117, 132, 133, 164, 165, 312
Optican, L., 131
Orban, G. A., 246
O'Shea, R. P., xi, 1,6, 7, 21, 51, 84, 85, 86, 87,
  90, 92, 106, 182, 196, 197, 234, 250, 301,
  302, 303, 304, 305, 306, 307, 308, 309, 310,
  312, 325, 333
Overton, R., 13, 14, 51, 81, 93, 132, 234

Pack, C. C., 233
Panum, P. L., 34, 35, 244, 245, 250, 252
Papathomas, T. V., xiii, 128, 155, 160,
  164, 165

Paradiso, M. A., 233
Parker, A. J., 247
Pascual-Leone, A., 78
Patterson, R., 75
Peckham, R. H., 7
Perrett, D. I., 203
Perry, V. H., 83
Perry, R. J., 292
Peterhans, E., 132, 233, 242, 247
Peterson, M. A., 248
Petrig, B., 102
Pettigrew, J. D., x, 21, 246, 283, 284, 285, 286,
    287, 288, 289, 292, 293, 294, 302, 308, 311,
    312, 313
Phillips, G. C., 49
Platz, A., 311
Pocock, S., 15, 155
Poggio, G., 117, 246, 331
Pollen, D. A., 78
Polonsky, A., 56, 68, 69, 73, 74, 75, 165, 200,
    226, 235, 317, 338
Pöppel, E., 283, 284
Porta, J. della, 33, 35, 37, 39, 42, 317
Posner, M. I., 128, 129
Postman, L., 12
Powell, D. J., 14
Pritchard, R. M., 233, 249
Puce, A., 337
Purves, D., 21, 77, 165, 187, 200, 231, 249, 296

Raaijmakers, J. G. W., 160
Ramachandran, V. S., 86, 126, 199, 271,
    292, 305
Rasche, F., 7, 20, 83, 341
Rauschecker, J. P., J., 11
Reade, J., 40, 43
Rees, G., 65, 78, 93, 133, 226, 227, 302, 305,
    308, 313
Refinetti, R., 285
Regal, D., 102
Regan, D., 102
Rehman, J., 289
Reid, R. C., 260
Reisenhuber, M., 331
Reuter-Lorenz, P. A., 301
Reynolds, J. H., 268
Ricci, C., 226

Richards, W., 323
Riess, B. F., 11
Rieth, C., 102
Rietveld, W. J., 291
Rifkin, R., 225, 227
Ringo, J. M., 294
Rittenhouse, C. D., 233
Rittenhouse, D., 31
Rock, I., 110, 233
Rockland, K. S., 194
Rodriguez- Rodriguez, V., 233
Rodriguez, E., 113
Roelfsema, P. R., 78, 242
Roenneberg, T., 289
Rogers, B. J., 171, 243, 245, 252
Rogers, R. L., 17
Rogers, S. W., 17
Rolls, E., 203, 226
Rosbash, M., 294
Rossi, A. F., 233
Rubin, E., 32, 187, 206, 233, 248
Rubin, N., xii, 21, 137, 140, 141, 146, 147,
    148, 151, 153, 284, 287
Ruby, N. F., 204
Ruijter, J. M., 102
Ruttiger, K. F., 311

Sagi, D., 233, 249, 286
Saleem, K. S., 218, 226
Salin, P. A., 76
Salinas, E., 260
Sanders, R. K., 49
Sasaki, H., 165
Sato, T., 87
Schall, J. D., 56, 60, 65, 132, 155, 200, 226,
    233, 235, 261, 340
Schanel-Klitsch, E., 102
Schiller, P. H., 82, 85, 86, 88
Schiller, P. V., 233
Schoepfle, G. M., 294
Schor, C. M., 6, 84, 152, 174, 175, 185, 340
Schrauf, M., 102
Schröder, J. H., 261, 268
Schwartz, J., 218
Seedorff, H. H., 311
Seghier, M., 339
Sejnowski, T. J., 260

Sengpiel, F., xiii, 55, 77, 133, 187, 188, 189, 190, 191, 192, 193, 194, 195, 196, 200, 235, 236, 266
Seymour, S. E., 301
Shadbolt, G., 39
Shadlen, M., 89, 199
Shapley, R., 83, 137
Sheinberg, D. L., 14, 21, 48, 56, 60, 65, 67, 74, 76, 77, 81, 133, 145, 153, 155, 200, 215, 218, 226, 227, 234, 235, 236, 237, 238, 239, 242, 259, 265, 317, 318, 327, 329, 333, 337, 340
Sherrington, C. S., 4
Shimojo, S., 102, 103, 113, 118, 125, 126, 132, 155, 169, 171, 172, 245, 246
Sims, A. J. H., 7, 84, 312
Singer, W., xiii, 259, 274
Sireteanu, R., 102
Skottun, B. C., 272
Smith, A. M., 31
Smith, E. L., 86, 234, 248
Smith, R., 31
Snowden, R. J., 59
Sobel, K. V., 17, 20, 128, 283, 292
Somers, D. C., 235
Sommer, M. A., 323
Somogyi, P., 194
Spekreijse, H., 102, 233, 338
Spelke, E., 101
Sperry, R. W., 301
Squire, L. R., 218, 226
Stadler, M., 19
Stalmeier, P. F., 83, 84, 143, 153
Sternfels, S., 113
Stettler, D. D., 242
Stevenson, S. B., 174, 175
Stirling, W., 155
Stoner, G. R., 199, 233, 269, 275, 276
Strong, D. S., 169, 171
Strüber, D., 19
Sugie, N., 14, 339
Sugita, Y., 132, 233
Super, H., 338
Suzuki, S., 155, 164, 251
Suzuki, W. A., 218, 226
Swets, J., 223
Switkes, E., 89, 199

Taira, M., 246
Tait, P. G., 40, 41
Takahashi, J. S., 294
Takeya, M., 294
Tanaka, K., 69, 218, 226, 342
Tarr, M. J., 204
Teller, D. Y., 102
Testaferrata, E., 35
Thiele, A., 275, 276
Thomas, O. M., 247, 255
Thompson, W. B., 269
Todd, S., 19, 261
Tolhurst, D. J., 82
Tong, F., xiii, 3, 14, 51, 56, 63, 65, 66, 67, 69, 73, 74, 75, 78, 133, 200, 203, 226, 235, 317, 330, 337, 338
Tononi, G., 64, 266, 339
Tootle, J. S., 17
Townsend, V., 10, 129
Treisman, A. M., 11, 14, 90, 131, 164
Troxler, D., 233, 249
Ts'o, D. Y., 194
Tsai, J. J., 182
Tyler, C. W., 84, 90, 152, 185, 340
Tzourio, N., 292

Uhr, L., 311
Uka T., 246
Usrey, W. M., 260

Van de Grind, W. A., 88
Van der Zwan, R., 15, 89, 128
Van Dijk, B. W., 338
Van Essen, D. C., 82, 204, 213, 218, 246
Van Esseveldt, K. E., 292
Van Lier, R. J., 164
Vapnik, V., 224, 225
Victor, J. D., 182, 272
Vogels, R., 246
Von der Heydt, R., 132, 233, 242, 247
Von Grunau, M., 137, 153
Von Noorden, G. K., 260

Wade, N. J., xii, 4, 14, 15, 33, 35, 37, 38, 77, 85, 86, 206, 245, 317
Waggoner, R. A., 69
Wakefield, J. M., 11

Wales, R., 13, 17, 193, 234, 248
Walker, P., 14, 165, 283
Wallach, H. , 11, 137, 140, 142, 196, 233
Wallin, J. E. W., 33
Walsh, V., 78, 164
Wang, Y., 342
Wang, Y-Z., 58
Waterhouse, J. M., 289
Weintraub, D. J., 110
Weisstein, N., 248
Weitzman, B. A., 248
Welch, L., 272
Wenderoth, P. M., 15, 56, 84, 89, 128, 152
Wertheimer, M., 251
Westendorf, D. H., 13, 14, 19, 51, 81, 93, 132,
   155, 234
Westheimer, G., 242
Wheatstone, C., 4, 6, 7, 8, 32, 33, 34, 35, 37,
   38, 39, 42, 43,169, 187, 188, 206
White, K. D., 15,
Whitteridge, D., 194
Whittle, P., 11, 15, 16, 17, 21, 22, 83, 155
Wiesel, T. N., 17, 194, 196, 200, 260, 261,
   295, 331
Wiesenfelder, H., 15, 89, 199
Wilke, M., 217, 231
Wilkinson, F., 56, 320, 331, 332
Williams, D. R., 86
Williamson, A., 320, 321, 332, 333
Wilson, C., 215
Wilson, H. R., xi, 3, 6, 14, 49, 56, 90, 120, 147,
   149, 152, 250, 283, 317, 318, 320, 321, 322,
   323, 325, 326, 327, 328, 329, 330, 331, 332
Wirz-Justice, A., 289
Wist, E. R., 102
Wolfe, J. M., 1, 51, 85, 90, 92, 155, 189, 217,
   218, 235, 236, 265, 318, 322, 329, 338
Wong, E., 248
Wuerger, S., 137

Yang, Y., 7, 90
Yantis, S., 129, 131
Yonas, A., 113
Yu, K., 10, 13, 155, 248, 351
Yuille, A. L., 152

Zanker, J., 102
Zeki, S., 200
Zhou, H., 132, 233, 242, 247
Zimba, L. D., 22
Zola-Morgan, S., 218, 226

# Subject Index

Aftereffects, ix, 15, 89, 234, 248, 251
Alhazen, 34, 252
Anaglyph, 3, 103, 104
Apparent motion, 89, 129–130, 199
Attention, vii, viii, x, xii, xv, 3, 7, 11, 33, 60, 63, 65, 128–132, 165, 204, 217, 268, 275, 277–279, 312, 345, 350, 354
Awareness, vii, viii, xiii, xiv, xv, 1, 3, 12, 13, 63–67, 71, 75, 77–78, 91, 187, 197, 201, 204, 232, 283, 297

Brightness, 18–19, 296
Broadbent, x
Brown, Alexander Crum, 36–37, 39, 42
Binding, 268–269, 273, 279
Binocular beats, 88, 90
Binocular corresponding boundaries, 118–121, 124, 125
Binocular luster, 183–185
Binocular rivalry. *See* Eye rivalry
Binocular vision, vii, x, xii, 10, 33, 34, 38, 43, 103, 117, 194, 199, 244–248, 251
Biological cycles and oscillators
circadian, 283–285, 287, 289–296
nasal, 287, 294, 295
ultradian, 283–284, 285, 287, 290, 294–296
Bistability and fMRI activity, 201, 276–279
Bistability and perceptual ambiguity, xii-xiv, xviii, 3, 19, 21, 29, 31–33, 78, 93, 106, 108, 110, 137–152, 187, 188, 200–204, 224, 234, 235, 269, 276, 277, 279, 283, 284, 296, 351
Bistable alternations, 31, 43, 137–152, 233, 235, 248–249, 251, 279, 283, 286, 290–291, 292, 322

Bistability in plaid motion
component motion, 196–198, 200, 269, 271–273, 274, 276–278
pattern motion (coherent motion), xii, 137, 138, 140, 142, 144–149, 151, 153, 196–200, 269, 272–273, 274, 276–277
transparent motion, xii, 137, 138, 140, 142, 144–149, 151, 153, 269, 271, 272–273, 274–276
Blind spot, 51, 69–71, 244, 317
Bottom-up processes, 155, 156, 165, 338, 350, 351
Breese, B. B., xviii, 8–11, 12, 15
Brewster, David, 32, 35–43

Camouflage, 171–174, 177, 179, 181, 182
Categorical cells, 340–344, 347, 350, 351, 354–355
Cattell, James McKeen, 8
Cheshire cat illusion, 14, 129
Chimenti da Empoli, Jacopo, 35
Chimenti pictures, 35–37, 39–43
Computational modeling, xi, 317–333, 330, 339, 337–351
Contour collinearity, 16–17, 271, 274, 275, 276 309–310, 325–327
Contrast, 14, 19, 20, 49–56, 58–59, 68, 70–71, 75, 77–78, 82–86, 92, 121–123, 126, 132, 138, 142–143, 149, 151–152, 184–185, 192–193, 199, 201, 203, 232, 248–249, 265, 268, 269, 274, 286, 292, 312, 323, 325–326, 340–341, 347–349, 351
Contrast-response function, 55, 82, 193
Contrast sensitivity, 49–50, 52–56, 77, 83–85

Corpus callosum, xi, 301, 308–311, 313
  callosotomy, xi, 303, 311
Cortex, primate
  amygdala, 215, 218–220
  anterior commissure, 308, 311, 313
  entorhinal cortex, 215, 218
  frontal lobe, 64–65, 226–227
  frontoparietal, 65, 302, 312, 313
  FFA, 66–67, 75, 201–205, 337
  hippocampus, 214, 215, 218
  human medial temporal lobe, 218, 222,
    226, 227
  IT, 226, 227, 238–239, 242, 259, 260
  LGN, 82, 85, 188–189, 226, 235, 341, 342
  lateral occipital complex, 201–204
  lunate sulcus, 237
  MST, 59, 89
  occipital lobe, 64–65, 111, 201–204
  PPA, 66–67, 75, 201–203, 215, 218, 337
  parietal lobe, 111, 113
  primary visual cortex (V1) , xiii, 51, 56, 58,
    63, 65, 68–78, 82, 101, 102, 111, 132, 165,
    188, 189, 191, 193–196, 200, 226, 231, 235,
    237–242, 243, 246–247, 252, 260, 261, 263,
    272, 302, 312, 313, 317, 325–327, 331,
    337–339, 340, 341–343
  superior temporal sulcus, 201–203
  suprachiasmatic nucleus, 285, 291
  temporal lobe, 188, 204
  TEO, 260
  V2, 69, 165, 235, 237–242, 247, 260
  V3/V3A, 69, 165, 277, 278
  V4/V4V, 60, 65, 66, 69, 73, 165, 226,
    237–241, 260, 331
  V5/MT/ hMT+, 60, 65, 89, 200, 226, 272,
    276–279, 331
Cortex, cat
  area 18, 271, 273, 274, 276
  PMLS, 271, 273, 274–275
Cortical electrophysiology,
  single-unit, 64, 65, 73, 74–75, 76, 77, 101,
    165, 189, 193, 214, 223, 226, 236, 237, 331,
    338, 350
  multiple-unit, xviii, 214, 237, 240, 241
Cortical magnification, 196, 250, 252, 325
Crussaire, Pierre, 30–32, 206
Cyclopean vision, 245, 252

Depth electrodes, 213, 215
Development of rivalry, xi, 7, 101–114
Dichoptic stimulation, 4, 261, 263
Dichoptic plaid, 84–85, 196–200
Dichoptic motion/flicker, 88, 90, 91, 188
Distributed cortical processing in rivalry,
  xiii, 20, 69, 81, 101, 102, 103, 113, 117,
  132–133, 188, 203, 231, 242, 284, 318,
  329–330, 331
Dominance duration, 8, 19, 20, 71, 94, 106,
  140–143, 145, 149–151, 153, 292, 318, 323,
  328, 330, 332–333, 340
Dominance waves, 6, 324–327
Dominant eye, 93, 189, 191–192, 261,
  263–266, 268, 345

Ebbinghaus illusion, 110, 111
Eccentricity. *See* Retinal eccentricity
Emerson, Edwin, 40–41, 43
Epilepsy, 213, 215, 218, 301
Equiluminant color, 86, 156, 160
Euclid, 169
Exclusive dominance, 7, 15–17, 71, 75, 86,
  88, 106, 157–163, 183, 185, 198, 247, 249,
  305, 311
Exclusive interocular grouping, 17, 156,
  161–163, 308
Eye dominance, xiii, 35, 106, 164, 234, 249,
  261, 265, 268, 348
Eye of origin, xiii, 95, 119, 132, 155–157, 160,
  163, 164, 188, 245–246
Eye movements, 7, 8, 18–19, 250, 261, 269
Eye rivalry, 48, 49–51, 54, 73, 77, 81, 155,
  163, 165–166, 235, 246, 295, 317–318,
  327–328, 330, 331, 338, 339, 350–351
  vs. stimulus rivalry, 53–54, 76–77, 81, 295,
  317–318, 327–330, 331, 338–339,
  350–351
Eye swapping paradigm, 155, 318,
  327–330

False fusion, 51, 338
Fechner's paradox, 18
Figural grouping (perceptual grouping),
  xiii, 15, 17, 22, 31, 76, 125–126, 128,
  155–156, 157, 164, 231, 251, 269, 292,
  308–311

Flash suppression, xiii, xviii, 4, 14, 19, 189, 213–224, 235–241, 265

Flicker, 21, 64, 69–70, 83, 85, 88, 90, 101–102, 113, 269, 318, 327, 329

Flicker and swap paradigm, 318, 327–330, 333

Fox, Robert, xviii, 11–15

Fusion, vii, xii, xiv, 11, 35, 84, 85, 86, 87, 89, 152, 189, 191, 194, 244–245, 250, 252, 312, 338

Galen, 34–35

Gamma distribution/function, 18–19, 106, 107, 109, 145, 166, 305, 307, 322–323, 330, 332, 340, 349

Gamma-frequency synchronization, 113, 259, 264–268

Gestalt, 31, 111, 250, 251, 269

Global context, 7, 110, 165, 187, 232–233, 248, 292–293

Global motion, 17, 137, 276–277

Hallucinogenics, 287–288

Hebb, D. O., x

Helmholtz, H. von, 7, 42–43, 128

Hemispheres (cerebral), xi, 10, 66, 95, 293, 301–311, 313

Hemispheric oscillator, 285

Hemispheric switching, 93, 292, 302, 313, 350

Horopter, 35, 252

Illusory contours, 122, 123, 332

Image segmentation, 76, 102, 138, 146, 149, 151–152, 269, 273, 276, 279

Individual differences, ix, x–xi, 75, 289, 332

Interhemispheric switching, 285, 291–292, 302, 350

Interocular competition (suppression; mutual inhibition)

reciprocal inhibition, xi, xii, xv, 4, 8, 13–14, 53, 54, 55–56, 63, 64, 69, 73–74, 76–77, 117–118, 124, 149–152, 155, 156, 164, 187–188, 189–194, 194–196, 200, 240, 259–260, 266, 268, 283–284, 318–323, 325–327, 329–333, 339

Interocular grouping, 17, 76, 155, 164, 250, 307, 313, 338

with motion stimuli, 156–160, 163–165

Interocular rivalry, 76, 259–260, 333. *See also* Eye rivalry

Interocular transfer, 87, 234, 251

James, William, 4, 8

Joint predominance, 15, 309–310

Julesz, Bela, x, 118, 246

Kohonen classifier, 341–345, 347, 350–351, 354–355

Kohler, Wolfgang, ix

Levelt, Willem J. M., xviii, xix, 17–21, 149–152, 153, 292, 323–324, 326

Levelt's second proposition, xix, 19, 20, 149–152, 153, 248, 292, 323–324, 326, 340

Lobed circles, 56–58

Local ambiguity, 231, 232

Log-normal dominance distribution, 145

Long-range intrinsic connections, 194, 195, 242, 311, 325

Magnocellular pathway, xiii, 81–86, 88–91, 95

Monocular occlusion, xii, 169, 171–177, 180, 185

Monocular rivalry , 10–11, 76, 294

Monocular transparency, 171, 177–182, 185

Mooney images, 110, 111, 113

Motion aftereffect, 15, 86, 89, 199, 251

Motion-induced blindness, 286–287

Multistable perception, xvii, 31, 106, 233, 235, 248, 249, 284

Mutual exclusivity, 139, 152

Necker, L. A., 32, 43

Necker cube, 29–32, 43, 139, 187, 233, 290, 332, 351

Neural correlates, 59–60, 63–67, 193, 200, 213, 215, 226, 235, 261, 338

Neuronal synchronization, xiv, 15, 113, 224, 259–261, 263–269, 271–276, 279, 339

Nondominant eye, 189, 191–193, 261, 263–266, 288.

Nonius lines, 121, 122, 174, 175

Nonlinear dynamics, xviii, 318–319, 323, 327, 330
Nonselectivity of suppression, xii, 13–14, 48, 49, 194, 195

Occlusion, xii, 33, 155, 172, 173, 232, 245
Occlusion constraint, 117–121, 124–125, 245
Occlusion zone, 169, 170–172, 182, 185
Ocular dominance (cortical), 14, 17, 69, 194–195, 326, 331
Orientation, 13, 14, 49, 50, 77, 102, 108, 110, 159, 163–165, 189–200, 232, 239, 246, 261, 272, 339, 341

Panum's fusional area, 244, 245, 250, 252
Parvocellular pathway, xiii, 81–82, 83–89, 90, 91, 101
Perceptual organization, 111, 156, 164–165, 231, 234, 235, 245, 247–250, 251, 259
Perceptual switches, 65, 150, 203, 277, 278, 279, 283, 338
Periphery. See Retinal eccentricity
Permanent suppression, 312
Piecemeal rivalry (mixed dominance), viii, ix, x, 6, 7, 51, 75, 76, 103, 106, 108, 113, 152, 158, 164, 196, 197, 200, 224, 249–250
Plaid transparency, 137, 140, 142, 144–149, 151, 153, 269, 271, 273–276
Pop-out, 131–132
Porta, Giambattista della, 33, 35, 37, 39, 42, 317
Predominance, 6–10, 15, 17–21, 126, 127, 157, 160–163, 292, 309–310
Preferential looking, 102–103, 113
Probe technique, ix, xi-xii, xiii, 11–15, 57, 248
Pseudoscopic, 40–42
Pseudo disparity, 179–182
Pseudorivalry, 303–305, 310, 312. *See also* Stimulus alternation
Ptolemy, 31, 33, 34, 206

Recurrent excitation, 78, 320, 330, 340
Recurrent inhibition, 78, 322, 329, 333, 340
Retinal eccentricity, 6, 33, 75, 84, 92, 196, 250, 312, 325
Reversible figures, viii, 3, 26

Rival depth, 182
Rivalry alternations, ix, xii, xiii, 1, 6, 7, 8, 9, 10, 15, 18–21, 29, 31, 32, 43, 63, 65–66, 67–68, 71, 72, 74–77, 93, 95, 101–108, 110, 113, 118, 121, 123, 124, 128, 149, 151, 160, 200, 203, 204, 215, 217, 233–234, 249, 260, 276–277, 283–284, 286, 287, 290–291, 292, 303–304, 305, 311–312, 321–322, 325, 328–333, 337–338, 341, 347, 348, 349, 354–356
  rate of , 3, 7, 9, 15, 20, 83, 92, 103, 106–108, 110, 140–143, 153, 291, 293–294, 311, 328, 340, 345, 348, 349, 354–356
Rivalry and EEG activity, 63, 64–65, 73
Rivalry and fMRI activity, xiii, 51, 65–73, 74–76, 77, 78, 165, 201, 302, 312–313, 317, 330, 338, 339
Rivalry and perceptual history, 93, 290
Rivalry and visual field asymmetries, 6, 75, 92–93, 196, 250, 312, 325
Rivalry dominance, ix, x, xii-xv, 1, 3, 6–10, 13–21, 29, 35, 47–50, 54, 57–59, 63, 71, 75, 86, 92–94, 106, 117, 120, 121–124, 126, 127, 129, 131–132, 143, 149, 150–152, 157, 159–160, 161–165, 183, 185, 188, 194, 195, 198, 226, 234–236, 239–240, 247–251, 260–261, 265, 266, 268, 283, 288, 292, 305, 307, 309, 310, 312, 318, 322–333, 340, 341, 345, 347, 348, 350, 355
Rivalry suppression, vii-ix, xi-xv, 10, 11–15, 18–21, 35, 47–60, 64, 69, 76, 77, 83, 84, 86, 89, 90, 92, 95, 118, 124, 129, 130, 132, 165, 187, 188–196, 200, 215–224, 234–241, 243, 245, 247–249, 251, 261, 264, 265–267, 268, 283, 287, 292, 297, 312–313, 338–339, 340, 341, 345, 348, 355
Rivalry with motion stimuli, viii, xiii, 10, 13, 15, 17, 58–59, 65, 86–89, 128, 129–130, 188, 196–200, 233, 269–271, 287, 339
Roman mosaics, 30–31

Self-adaptation, 319, 321, 329
Sieve effect, 182–185
Spatial frequency, 6, 13, 82, 83, 84–85, 156, 159, 161, 164, 189, 191–192, 193, 250, 292, 312, 351
Split-brain observers, 92, 301–303, 305–306, 308, 310–311, 313

Stereogram, 118, 172, 174–177, 180–182, 185, 303

Stereopsis, vii, xii, 4, 11, 15, 175, 194, 246, 247, 312

   da Vinci stereopsis, 169–171

   from rival stimuli, 89–91

Stereoscope, 4–5, 8, 30, 32–40, 42, 179, 237, 303, 304

Stereoscopic depth, 33, 34, 47, 246

Stereoscopic vision, 4, 37, 42, 102, 174, 245, 246

Stimulus (physical) alternations, 64–69, 71–75, 104, 241, 303–305, 310, 312

Stimulus/figural organization, xiii, 16, 155–156, 157, 163, 165, 250, 307

Stimulus rivalry, 48, 49–51, 76, 77, 81, 155, 234, 295, 317–318, 328–329, 330, 331, 338–339, 350–351

Stimulus strength, xii, 8, 18, 19–20, 54, 84, 92, 130, 138, 142–143, 149–151, 153, 212, 292–293, 324, 340–341

Strabismus, xiv, 191, 193, 248, 250, 260–261, 265, 266, 268

Suppression depth, 11–15, 47–50, 54, 56–60, 58, 77, 86, 193, 248

Suppression theory, 1, 35

Surface occlusion, 118, 119, 124

Synchronous rivalry, 16

Temporal frequency, 82–83, 85, 88, 90, 197, 318

Threshold, vii-x, xii, xv, 50, 54, 55, 57–60, 84, 85, 91, 190, 193, 248, 272, 319, 321, 339

Tilt aftereffect, 15

Top-down processes, 11, 73, 113, 165, 337–351

Transcranical magnetic stimulation, 293, 302

Transients, xiii, 14, 20, 54, 65, 74, 82, 85, 91, 129, 132, 219, 239, 318, 321, 322, 329, 333

Troxler's fading, 21, 130

Unpaired boundary, 121, 124, 125

Unpaired zones, 71, 118, 171–172, 243–245

Utrocular discrimination, 246, 252

Vase/face illusion (Rubin's illusion), 3, 32, 110, 187, 201, 203, 205, 206, 248–249

Vinci, Leonardo da, 169, 171, 185, 245

Visual development, 101–103

Wallach, Hans, ix, 137

Wheatstone, Charles, 4–8, 32–35, 37–39, 42–43, 169, 206

Whittle, Paul, 15–17, 21, 22

*Zeitgebers*, 284–286, 289, 291, 292